STRESS
AND DIGESTIVE MOTILITY

Scientific committee :

Lionel Buéno (Toulouse)
Steve Collins (Hamilton)
Jacques Frexinos (Toulouse)
Jean-Louis Junien (Paris)
Juan Malagelada (Barcelone)
David Wingate (Londres)

Proceedings of the International Workshop
on Stress and Digestive Motility
"Stress and Digestive Motor Disturbances : New Insights"
organized by Jouveinal Laboratoires
Mont Gabriel, Canada March 29 - 31 1989

STRESS
AND DIGESTIVE MOTILITY

Mont Gabriel, Canada March 29 - 31 1989

Editors :

Lionel Buéno
Steve Collins
Jean-Louis Junien

John Libbey
EUROTEXT
LONDON · PARIS

British Library Cataloguing in Publication Data
International Workshop on Stress and Digestive Motility
(1989 : Mont Gabriel, Canada)
Stress and digestive motility,
1. Man. Gastrointestinal tract. Diseases. Role of stress
I. Title. II. Buéno, Lionel. III. Collins, Steve . IV. Junien, Jean-Louis
616.3'3071

ISBN 0-86196-212-5

Editions John Libbey Eurotext
6, rue Blanche, 92120 Montrouge, France.
Tél. : (1) 47.35.85.52

John Libbey Company Ltd
13, Smith Yard, Summerley Street, London SW18 4HR, England
Tél. : (01) 947.27.77

FOREWORD

Many workshops or meetings have been devoted to the effects of stress since the 30's when Selye first spoke about "the general adaptation syndrome" to stress. Most of these meetings have dealt with the well known consequences of stress on the central nervous system and behaviour, the cardiovascular system, the immune system or the occurrence of ulcers, which are certainly the most dramatic, acute and chronic consequence of stress. It is however accepted that virtually all organs are to varying extents affected by stress, depending on the stressors, the individuals or the species. It is obvious that "a general adaptation syndrome" is a rather simple view and that stress includes both a non specific response and also an "adaptative response" in relation to the type of stress.

It is widely recognized, at least in acute conditions, that stress induces disturbances in G.I. motility. For several years now, an increasing number of papers have been published on stress induced changes in G.I. function but no special meeting, to our knowledge, has so far been organized to address this issue.

For this meeting, the organisers gathered together researchers working in this field in order to consider what is known on the mechanisms of stress and its neuroendocrinological alterations, to discuss the relevance and the predictivity of models in man and animals, the importance of the type of stressor, consequences of acute VS chronic stress, the possible pharmacological interactions and, most importantly to consider the pathological consequences. We are sure this meeting will increase knowledge and understanding about stress and will give suggestions for future research.

The Editors.

List of participants
Liste des participants

Akkermans, Division of Surgery, Academic Hospital Utrecht Catharijnesingel 101, 3500 Utrecht, Netherlands.

Barrowman, 300 Pric Philio Dr., St John's Newfoundland A1B 3V6, Canada.

Bass P., Center for Health Sciences, School of Pharmacy, 425 North Carter Street, Madison, Wisconsin 53706, U.S.A.

Bassoti G., Instituto di Clinica, Medica Generale E Terapia Medica, Policlinico Monteluce, 06100 Perugia, Italy.

Bastien Y., Jouveinal Inc. 1950 32e Avenue, Lachiné, Québec, H8T 3J7 Canada

Beck, 166 Brock St. Kingston, Ontario, K7L 5G2, Canada.

Berard H., Jouveinal Laboratoires, 1, rue des Moissons, B.P. 100, 94265 Fresnes Cedex, France.

Boivin, 1058 St. Denis, Montréal, Québec, H2X 3J4 Canada.

Brunin C., Jouveinal Laboratoires, 1, rue des Moissons, B.P. 100, 94265 Fresnes Cedex, France.

Buéno L., Département de Pharmacologie, INRA, 180, chemin de Tournefeuille, 31300 Toulouse, France.

Burks T.F., Department of Pharmacology, University of Arizona, Health Science Center, Tucson, Az. 85724, U.S.A.

Caulin C., A.D.M.2., Service Médecine A, Hôpital Lariboisière, 75475 Paris Cedex 10, France.

Chaussade, Service Hépato-Gastro-Entérologie, Hôpital Cochin, 27, rue du fg. Saint-Jacques, 75674 Paris Cedex 14, France.

Collins S., Institute of Disease Research, Mc Master University, Room 355 C, 1200 Main Street West, Hamilton, Ontario, L8N 3Z5 Canada.

Cook I.J.S., Division of Gastroenterology, Department of Medicine, Adelaide Hospital, North Terrace, Adelaide 5000, Australia.

Corazziari, Cattedra di gastroenterologia 1, Viale des Policlinico, 00161 Rome, Italy.

Couturier D., Service Hépato-Gastro-Entérologie, Hôpital Cochin, 27, rue du fg. Saint-Jacques, 75674 Paris Cedex 14, France.

Creed F., Department of Psychiatry, Manchester Royal Infirmary, Manchester, United Kingdom.

Dantzer R., Labo de Neurobiologie des comportements, Université Bordeaux 11, 146, rue Léo Saignat, 33076 Bordeaux, France.

Davison J., University of Calgary, Calgary, Alberta, T2N 4N1, Canada.

Devroede G., Département de Chirurgie, Centre Hospitalier Sherbrooke, Sherbrooke, Québec, J1H 5N4, Canada.

Diamant N.E., Division of Gastroenterology, Toronto Western Hospital, 399 Bathurst St. Ste 504, Toronto, Ontario M5T 2S8, Canada.

Diop L., Jouveinal Laboratoires, 1, rue des Moissons, B.P. 100, 94265 Fresnes Cedex, France.

Dubois, Uniformed Services University of the Health Sciences, F. Edouard Herbert School of Medicine, 4301 Jones Bridge Road, Bethesda, Maryland, U.S.A.

Dunn A.J. Department of Pharmacology and Therapeutics, School of Medicine, in Shreveport, 1501 King's Height Way, P.O.B. 33932, Shreveport, La., 71130-3332, U.S.A.

Ehrlein, Universität Hohenheim, Institut für Zoophysiologie, 7000 Stuttgart 70, Hehenheim, F.R.G.

Enck P., Universität Düsseldorf, Medizinische Klinik und Poliklinik, Moorenstrasse 5, 4000 Düsseldorf, F.R.G.

Erckenbrecht J.F., Department of Internal Medicine, University Hospital, 4000 Düsselforf, F.R.G.

Fielding J.F., Department of Medicine, Beaumont Hospital, P.O. Box 1297, Beaumont Rd., Dublin 9, Ireland.

Fioramonti J., Laboratoire de Pharmacologie, INRA, 180, chemin de Tournefeuille, 31300 Toulouse, France.

Fraitag B., Jouveinal Laboratoires, 1, rue des Moissons, B.P. 100, 94265 Fresnes, France.

Garrick T., Wadsworth and Brentwood Divisions, Wilshire and Sawelle Boulevards, Los Angeles, Ca. 90073, U.S.A.

Geyer S., Department of Medical Sociology, University of Marburg, Marburg, F.R.G.

Groll, Queen's University, Kingston, Ontario, K7L 3J7 Canada.

Gué M., Département de Pharmacologie, INRA, 180, chemin de Tournefeuille, 31300 Toulouse, France.

Harding, Radiation Biology Department, Defense Res. Establishment, Ottawa, Ontario K1AOZ4, Canada.

Henke P.G., Department of Psychology, St. Francis Xavier University, Antigonish, Nova Scotia, B2G 1VO, Canada.

Holtman G., Department of Medicine, University of Essen, Hufefandstr. 4300 Essen, F.R.G.

Henry J.F., Jouveinal Laboratoires, 1, rue des Moissons, B.P. 100, 94265 Fresnes Cedex, France.

Hostein, Centre Hospitalier de Grenoble, Centre de Gastro-Entéro-Hepatologie, B.P. 217 X, 38043 Grenoble Cedex, France.

Jenkins R., Jouveinal Inc, 1950, 32e ave E., Lachiné, Québec, H8T 3J7 Canada.

Junien J.L., Jouveinal Laboratoires, 1, rue des Moissons, B.P. 100, 94265 Fresnes Cedex, France.

Koch K.L., Gastroenterology Division, The Milton S Hershey Medical Center, Hershey, Pa. 17033, U.S.A.

Kumar D., Gastro Intestinal Science Research Unit, 26 Ashfield St, E1 2AJ London, United Kingdom.

Leonard B., Department of Pharmacology, University College Galway, Galway, Ireland.

Lichter, Jewish General Hospital, 3755 ch de la Cote Ste Catherine, Montréal, Québec, H3T 1E2 Canada.

Malagelada J., Department of Gastroenterology, Hospital General Vall d'Hebron, Passai Vall d'Hebron, 08035 Barcelona, Spain.

Marzio L., Instituto di Patalogia Medica, O.R. S.S. Annunziata 66100 Chieti, Italy.

Meunier P., Laboratoire d'Exploration Fonctionnelle, Hôpital Debrousse, 69322 Lyon Cedex 05, France.

Pascaud X., Jouveinal Laboratoires, 1, rue des Moissons, B.P. 100, 94265 Fresnes Cedex, France.

Peeters T., Division of Gastroenterology, University of Leuven, 3000 Leuven, Belgium.

Poitras P., Hôpital Saint-Luc, Centre de Recherche Clinique, 1058 rue St Denis, Montréal, Québec H2X 3J4 Canada.

Raybould H.E., Center for Ulcer Research and Education, V.A. Wadsworth Medical Center, Building 115, Room 115, Los Angeles, Ca. 90073, U.S.A.

Read N.W., Clinical Research Unit, Royal Hallanshire Hospital, Sheffield S10 2TN, United Kingdom.

Riou D., Jouveinal Laboratoires, 1, rue des Moissons, B.P. 100, 94265 Fresnes Cedex, France.

Rivier C., Clayton Foundation Laboratories, Salk Institute, La Jolla, Ca. 92037, U.S.A.

Rozé C. INSERM U 239, Faculté de Médecine, Hôpital Bichat, 75018 Paris, France.

Sarna S.K., Medical College of Wisconsin, Milwaukee, Wisconsin 53295, U.S.A.

Snape W., JR Harbor, UCLA Medical Center, 1000 West Carson Street, Torrance, Ca. 90509, U.S.A.

Stanghellini V., Institute of Clinical Medecine, University of Bologna, Via Massarenti 9, 40138 Bologna, Italy.

Staumont G., INRA, Laboratoire de Pharmacologie, 180, chemin de Tournefeuille, 31300 Toulouse, France.

Taché Y., Center for Ulcer Research VA Wadworth Medical Center, Building 115, Room 203, Los Angeles, Ca. 90074, U.S.A.

Thompson D.G., Department of Medicine, Eccles Old Road, Salford M6 8HD, United Kingdom.

Tougas, Mc Master University, Intestinal disease research unit, Room HSC-3N5C, 1200 Main Street West, Hamilton, Ontario L8N 3Z5, Canada.

Uvnäs Moberg K., Division of Pharmacology, Karolinska Institutet, Box 60400, 10401 Stockholm, Sweden.

Vantrappen G., Department of Medicine and Medical Research, University of Leuven, 3000 Leuven, Belgium.

Vermillion D., Mc Master University, Intestinal Disease Research Unit, Room HSC 3N5C, 1200 Main Street West, Hamilton, Ontario L8N 3Z5, Canada.

Wechsler, GI Laboratory, De Soto at O'Hara Streets, Pittsburg, Pennsylvania 15213-2582, U.S.A.

Wingate D.L., Gastrointestinal Science Research Unit, 26 Ashfield Street, London E1 2AJ, United Kingdom.

CONTENTS

. Foreword ... V
. List of participants ... VII

I Neuroendocrinal and behavioral components

- Stress : Definition and neuroendocrine evaluation. **C. Rivier** ... 3
- CRF as mediator of stress responses. Neurochemical and behavioral aspects. **A.J. Dunn**.. 13
- Behavioral responses to stressors. **R. Dantzer** ... 23
- Assessing life events in stress-related disease. **S. Geyer, J. Siegrist** ... 31
- Clinical identification of stress related disorders of the gastrointestinal tract in adults. **J. Fielding** ... 41
- Hormone levels and personality in individuals with functional disorders of the gastrointestinal tract. **K. Uvnäs-Moberg** ... 45
- Constipation, anxiety and personality : what comes first ? **G. Devroede, M. Bouchoucha, G. Girard**.. ... 55

II Experimental approach in humans

- Disturbances of gastric myoelectrical and neuroendocrine activity and the stress of motion sickness. **K.L. Koch, R.M. Stern, T.S. Harrison, J.F. Seton, L.M. Demers** ... 63
- The influence of psychological stress on esophageal motility. **I.J.S. Cook** ... 71
- Gastric emptying and intestinal transit in pain stress. **D.G. Thompson** ... 75
- The influence of psychological stress on intestinal motility. **D.L. Wingate, R.M. Valori, D. Kumar** . 85
- Noise and intestinal motor alterations. **J.F. Erckenbrecht** ... 93

- Correlations of cardiovascular and gastroduodenal motility responses to acute mental stress. **G. Holtmann, R. Kriebel, M.V. Singer** 97
- Effect of cold pressure test on gallbladder contraction induced by a standardized meal in normal human subjects. **L. Marzio, F. DiFelice, V. Celiberti, M. Grazia Laico** 105
- Influence of cold water stress on colonic myoelectrical spiking activity in irritable bowel syndrome patients. **J. Frexinos, G. Staumont, M. Delvaux, J. Fioramonti, L. Buéno** 109

Animals models and mechanisms

III

- Restraint stress and intestinal transit in rats. **T.F. Burks, J.M. Peterson, C.L. Williams, T.H. Kramer** 115
- Stress-induced alterations of gastric emptying. **Y. Taché** 123
- Influence of different stressors on gastric emptying in mice and rats. **M. Gué, J. Fioramonti, L. Buéno** 133
- Role of corticotropin-releasing factor in genesis of gastrointestinal motor disturbances induced by stress : an overview. **L. Buéno** 141
- The effects of repeated acoustic or hypothermic stress on smooth muscle and enteric nerve function *in vitro* in the rat; a model for studying hyperresponsiveness in irritable bowel syndrome. **S. Collins, D. Vermillion, P. Blennerhassett, B. Randall** 151
- Postprandial hormonal status and gastric emptying in stress dogs. **T. Peeters, M. Gué, I. Depoortere, L. Buéno, G. Vantrappen** 157
- A novel stress model to investigate stress effects on gastrointestinal transit in the rat. **P. Enck** 165
- TRH and CRF injected into the brain have opposite effects on gastric contractility in the rat. **T. Garrick, R. Stephens, H. Yang, H. Weiner, Y. Taché** 169
- Inhibition of gastric motor function by circulating corticotropin-releasing factor in rats. **H.E. Raybould, Y. Taché** 171
- Cold restraint and tail shock stimulate gastric contractility in the rat. **T. Garrick, H. Weiner, P. Bass** 175

Pharmacological and clinical observations

IV

- Involvement of opiate and adrenergic pathways on stress-induced gastrointestinal motor disturbances. **V. Stanghellini, R. Corinaldesi, L. Barbara** 181
- Central and peripheral opioid inhibitory pathways on stress-induced gastric motor alteration in fasted dogs : a pharmacological approach. **J.L. Junien, M. Gué, X. Pascaud, L. Buéno** 187
- The effects of dopamine antagonists on stress-induced alterations of intestinal motor activity. **D. Kumar, R.M. Valori, D.L. Wingate** 197
- Environmental stress, psychiatric disorder and functional abdominal pain. **F. Creed, T. Craig** 205
- Simultaneous measurement of intraluminal pressure and transit; a newly developed technique for the study of colonic function under different conditions. **W.J. Snape, S. Narasimha Reddy, G. Bazzocchi, J. Villanueva-Meyer, I. Mena, E. Moreno-Osset** 215
- Evaluation of the effect of stress on the gut, clinical implications. **N.W. Read** 225
- Influence of sudden awakening on colonic contractile activity in man. **G. Bassotti, C. Betti, A. Morelli** 243
- N-methyl-D-aspartate receptors and stress : gastric ulcers, hippocampal long-term potentiation, and coping. **P.G. Henke** 247
- Is MMC sick in intestinal disease ? **S.K. Sarna** 251

CONCLUDING REMARKS. J. Malagelada 257

1st SESSION :

Neuroendocrinal and behavioral components

Moderators : *Y. Tache, D. Wingate*

Stress : definition and neuroendocrine evaluation

Catherine Rivier

The Clayton Foundation Laboratories for Peptide Biology, The Salk Institute, 10010 North Torrey Pines Road, La Jolla, CA 92037, U.S.A.

In the 19th century, the French physiologist Claude Bernard proposed the concept that in order to have a free and independent existence, the body must maintain the consistency of its "milieu interieur", which means that the organism must make appropriate hormonal, autonomic and/or behavioral changes so as to retain homeostasis. In this context, stress can be defined as the demand placed upon an organism when it is subjected to a real or perceived threat or challenge -be it physical or psychological.

This chapter will be devoted to the studies, carried out in our laboratory, to elucidate some of the mechanisms which lead to changes in pituitary activity in an organism exposed to stress. Two particular types of stresses will be considered: exposure to mild electroshocks and exposure to an immunologic challenge.

A. STRESS: ELECTROSHOCKS

While many stimuli are recognized as stressful by rats, it is often difficult to quantitate their intensity (for example, in the case of immobilization) or precisely control their duration (for example, in the case of surgical trauma). For this reason, we have chosen mild electroshocks, delivered to the paws of the rats, as representing well defined stimuli of controllable intensity. In this paradigm, shock intensity is defined as the product of the intensity (in milliamperes) and the duration (in seconds) of each shock, and is expressed as a coulometric relation (Fanselow, 1984). Scrambled inescapable shocks are delivered by Coulbourn shockers to the grid floors of plexiglass chambers. A program run by an Apple 2E computer is used to enter the length of the shock session, the duration of each shock, and the minimal interval allowed between each shock (Rivier & Vale, 1987). The shocks are randomly distributed over time.

1. ACTH SECRETION DURING ELECTROSHOCKS:

We have shown that using this model, we could generate voltage-dependent increases in the plasma levels of ACTH, β-endorphin and corticosterone (Rivier & Vale, 1987) (Fig. 1). Interestingly, such a response can only be elicited in rats 3 weeks or older (Walker et al., 1986a), a phenomenon which we attributed to a significantly higher pituitary sensitivity to glucocorticoid feedback during the first weeks of life in the rat (Walker et al., 1986b).

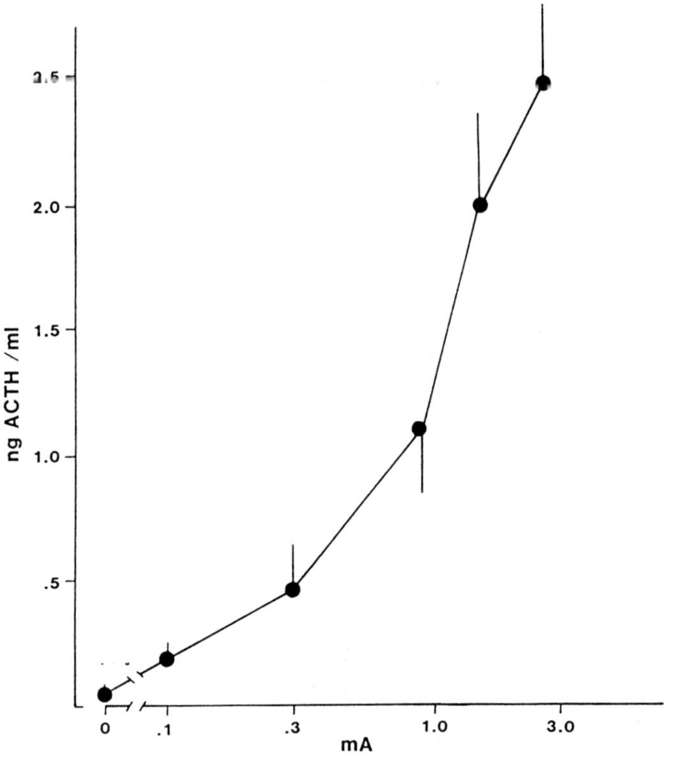

Fig. 1. Increasing shock intensity (expressed as milliamperes, mA) caused dose-related increases in plasma ACTH levels. Blood samples were obtained after one 10 min shock session. The shocks were delivered for 1 sec, at an average frequency of 2 shocks/min. Each point represents the mean ± SEM of 5 rats.

Because corticotropin-releasing factor (CRF) is released during stress (Plotsky & Vale, 1984), we evaluated the possible modulating role of endogenous CRF in mediating the increased ACTH release in rats exposed to electroshocks, by injecting either a CRF antiserum (Rivier & Vale, 1985) or a CRF antagonist (Rivier et al., 1984) immediately prior to the stress. We have demonstrated that immunoneutralization of CRF, or blockade of CRF receptors, significantly reduced the effect of stress (Rivier et al., 1982; Rivier & Vale, 1983b). However, the persistence of measurable elevations of plasma ACTH levels over baseline values in stressed rats treated with the CRF antiserum or antagonist, suggested the additional presence of a modulating factor other than CRF. Therefore, because vasopressin has also been documented as a secretagogue capable of modulating ACTH secretion, we tested the ability of a vasopressin antagonist to interfere with stress-induced ACTH release. Indeed, while the antagonist given alone slightly lowered plasma ACTH levels in shocked rats, the combination of the vasopressin antagonist and the CRF antiserum completely abolished the ability of the stress to stimulate pituitary function (Rivier & Vale, 1983b). These results suggested that while endogenous CRF represents the main physiological modulator of ACTH released by shocked rats, vasopressin also plays a role. This hypothesis agrees with previous reports showing that CRF and vasopressin interact to modulate ACTH secretion both in *in vitro* (Vale et al., 1983) and *in vivo* (Rivier & Vale, 1983a) models.

2. *LH SECRETION DURING ELECTROSHOCKS:*

Exposure to stress has long been known to interfere with reproductive functions. Is there a possible connection between the effects of stress on the hypothalamic-pituitary-adrenal axis, and those on gonadotropin and sex steroid secretion?

Because, as mentioned above, CRF is released during stress (Plotsky & Vale, 1984), we first evaluated the ability of CRF to alter LH secretion. While the peripheral injection of this peptide was without effect, we measured a dose-dependent inhibition of LH release following the injection of CRF into the lateral ventricle of the brain of castrated rats (Rivier & Vale, 1984). We then observed that while exposure of rats to electroshocks markedly decreased their plasma LH levels, the administration of a CRF antagonist into the brain reversed the effect of stress (Rivier et al., 1986). We concluded from these experiments that endogenous CRF mediates some deleterious effects of noxious stimuli on reproduction.

Because endogenous opioid peptides are also activated during stress (Millan et al., 1981; Rossier et al., 1977), and decrease LH levels when injected centrally (Blank et al., 1979; Bruni et al., 1977; Cicero et al., 1979), we then explored the role of these peptides in the stress-induced inhibition of LH release. The presence of three opioid peptide systems in the hypothalamus [i.e., endorphin, enkephalin and dynorphin (Roth et al., 1983; Swanson et al., 1983)], led us to evaluate the effect of μ, Δ and κ receptor blockers. Immunoneutralization of β-endorphin and pharmacological blockade of κ receptors, completely reversed electroshock-induced decreases in LH concentration (Petraglia et al., 1986). The injection of β-funaltrexamine, an irreversible μ1-opiate receptor antagonist, only partially blocked the inhibitory action of stress. Finally, neither passive immunization with anti-enkephalin antiserum, nor pretreatment with a Δ-opiate antagonist, modified the effect of stress (Petraglia et al., 1986). These results strongly suggested that the activation of central β-endorphin pathways played an important role in mediating stress-induced inhibition of reproductive functions. Furthermore, our observation that an antiserum or antagonist to β-endorphin also blocked the inhibitory action of CRF on LH secretion (Petraglia et al., 1986), indicated a possible functional interaction between CRF and opiate peptides in modulating stress-induced decreases in LH secretion.

B. STRESS: IMMUNOLOGIC CHALLENGE

1. *ACTH SECRETION DURING IMMUNOLOGIC CHALLENGE:*

An organism exposed to a bacterial invasion or some other immunologic challenge responds with an array of metabolic, behavioral and/or endocrine changes which are collectively referred to as the "acute-phase response" (Kushner, 1982). Interestingly, the comparison between the effects of an immunologic challenge on pituitary activity, and those of stress, indicate striking similarities. For example, both the immunologic challenge, often provided experimentally by the administration of a lipopolysaccharide (LPS), a bacterial endotoxin, and exposure to stress, markedly elevate plasma ACTH levels (Fig. 2). As in the case of the effect of stress (Rivier & Plotsky, 1986), the stimulatory action of LPS can be altered by adrenal steroids (Fig.3). Even more interestingly, the ACTH-stimulating activity of LPS appears to depend upon endogenous CRF, as illustrated by the ability of a CRF antiserum to markedly abolish this effect (Fig. 4).

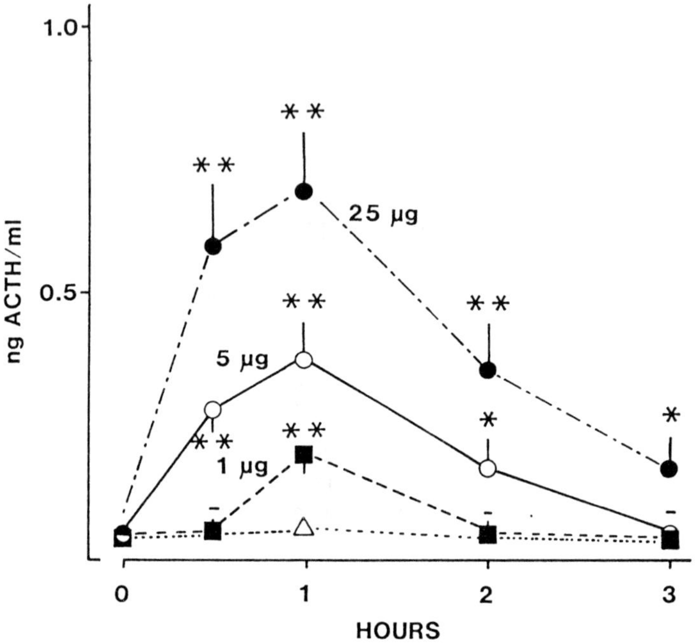

Fig. 2. The iv injection of a bacterial endotoxin lipopolysaccharide causes dose-related increases in plasma ACTH levels measured 45 min later. Each point represents the mean ± SEM of 5 rats. -, $P > 0.05$; *, $P \leq 0.05$; **, $P \leq 0.01$.

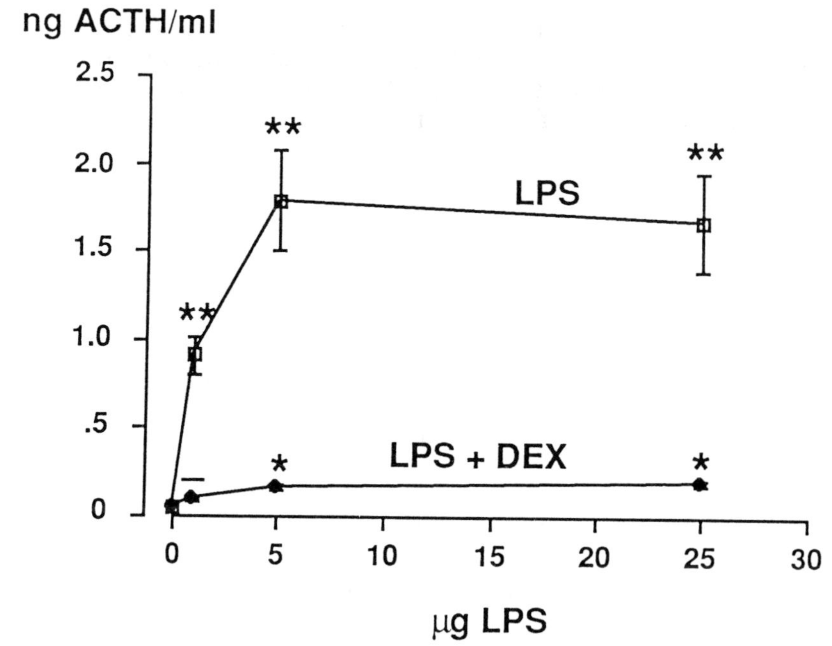

Fig. 3. The synthetic corticosteroid dexamethasone [(DEX); (100 µg/kg sc, -18h)] interferes with the stimulatory action of a bacterial lipopolysaccharide (LPS) on ACTH secretion. Blood samples were obtained 45 min after administration of LPS. Each point represents the mean ± SEM of 5 rats. -, P > 0.05; *, P ≤ 0.05; **, P ≤ 0.01.

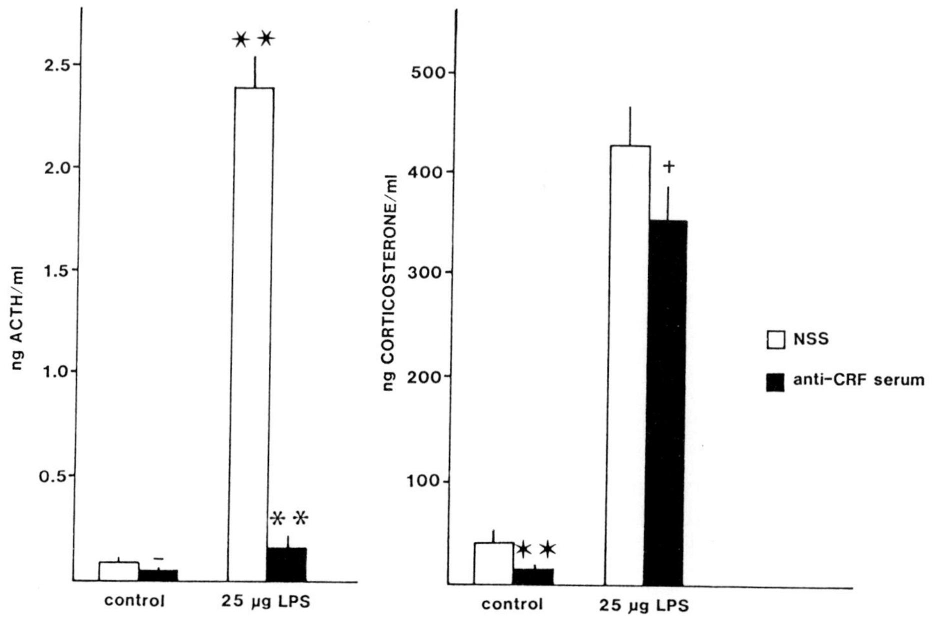

Fig. 4. Effect of a CRF antiserum on the ability of a bacterial lipopolysaccharide to stimulate ACTH secretion. Each point represents the mean ± SEM of 5 rats. -, P > 0.05; *, P ≤ 0.05; **, P ≤ 0.01.

Perhaps the most fundamental event in the initiation of the "acute-phase response" mentioned above, is the production of interleukin-1 (Il-1) (Kushner, 1982). Il-1 belongs to a group of proteins called cytokines (Dinarello & Mier, 1986; Dinarello & Mier, 1987), which mediate important regulatory functions between leukocytes in the immune system. In particular, Il-1 is produced by macrophages shortly after immunological activation, then can enter the circulation and act as an endocrine signal .

A growing number of studies have led to the hypothesis that Il-1 represents an essential mediator of the bidirectional communication existing between the immune and the neuroendocrine systems. Consequently, the growing belief that the immune system can, in particular, activate the adrenocortical axis, has led a number of investigators to study the effect of Il-1 on ACTH and CRF secretion. While a direct pituitary effect of Il-1 has been reported (Beach et al., 1989; Bernton et al., 1987; Weigent & Blalock, 1987), our laboratory has consistently observed that in short-term *in vitro* experiments, this lymphokine does not measurably alter the secretion of any of the pituitary hormones measured (Sapolsky et al., 1987). In contrast, both the peripheral (Sapolsky et al., 1987; Uehara et al., 1987b) and the central (Fig. 5) administration of Il-1 has been shown to significantly increase the circulating plasma levels of ACTH and β-endorphin, a phenomenon presently believed to involve the release of endogenous CRF (Sapolsky et al., 1987; Uehara et al., 1987a).

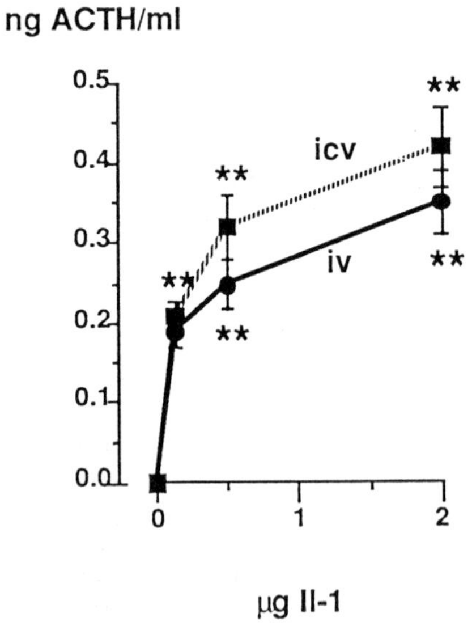

Fig. 5. Comparison between the intravenous (iv) and the intracerebroventricular (icv) injection of interleukin-1α (Il-1) on ACTH secretion by intact adult male rats. Each point represents the mean ± SEM of 5 animals. **, $P \leq 0.01$.

It therefore appears that cells of the immune system synthesize hormones which act on the hypothalamic-pituitary-adrenal axis, thus providing the basis for the postulated interaction between the immune and the neuroendocrine systems.

2. *GONADOTROPIN AND SEX STEROID SECRETION DURING IMMUNOLOGICAL CHALLENGE:*

Infection and inflammation are sometimes accompanied by an inhibition of reproductive parameters. The observation that Il-1 released endogenous CRF (Sapolsky et al., 1987), coupled with our earlier report that CRF acted within the brain to inhibit LH secretion (Rivier & Vale, 1984), led to the hypothesis that Il-1 might alter gonadotropin release. Indeed, we noticed that while the injection of even large doses of Il-1 α into the jugular vein did not measurably modify plasma LH levels, administration of 0.1 to 3 μg Il-1α significantly decreased LH values (Rivier & Vale, 1989). In addition, Il-1 acts peripherally to lower both basal and gonadotropin-induced sex steroid secretion (Rivier & Vale, 1989). Because this effect can be observed in hypophysectomized rats, it does appear to take place directly at the level of the gonads (Rivier & Vale, 1989). These results may provide the basis for one of the mechanisms through which stimulation of the immune system can interfere with reproductive functions.

ACKNOWLEDGEMENTS

Research supported by NIH grants AA06420 and AM26741. Research conducted in part by the Clayton Foundation for Research, California Division. CR is a Clayton Foundation investigator. The author thanks David Hutchinson, Rosalia Chavarin, and Leah Gandara for expert technical help and Bethany Coyne for secretarial assistance.

REFERENCES

Beach, J.E., Smallridge, R.C., Kinzer, C.A., Bernton, E.W., Holaday, J.W. & Fein, H.G. (1989): Rapid release of multiple hormones from rat pituitaries perifused with recombinant interleukin-1. Life Sci 44, 1-7.

Bernton, E.W., Beach, J.E., Holaday, J.W., Smallridge, R.C. & Fein, H.G. (1987): Release of multiple hormones by a direct action of interleukin-1 on pituitary cells. Science 238, 519-521.

Blank, M.S., Panerai, A.E. & Friesen, H.G. (1979): Opioid peptides modulate luteinizing hormone secretion. Science 203, 1129-1131.

Bruni, J.F., VanVugt, D., Marshall, S. & Meites, J. (1977): Effects of naloxone, morphine and methionine enkephalin on serum prolactin, luteinizing hormone, follicle stimulating hormone, thyroid stimulating hormone and growth hormone. Life Sci 21, 461-466.

Cicero, T.J., Schainker, B.A. & Mayer, E.R. (1979): Endogenous opioids participate in the regulation of the hypothalamus pituitary-luteinizing hormone axis and testosterone negative feed-back control of luteinizing hormone. Endocrinology 104, 1286-1291.

Dinarello, C.A. & Mier, J.W. (1986): Interleukins. Ann Rev Med 37, 173-178.

Dinarello, C.A. & Mier, J.W. (1987): Lymphokines. New Eng J Med 317, 940-945.

Fanselow, M.S. (1984): Shock-induced analgesia on the formalin test: effects of shock severity, naloxone, hypophysectomy and associative variables. Behav Neurosci 98, 79-98.

Kushner, I. (1982): The phenomenon of the acute phase response. Ann NY Acad Sci 389, 39-48.

Millan, M.J., Tsang, Y.F., Przewlocki, R., Hollt, V. & Herz, A. (1981): The influence of foot-shock stress upon brain, pituitary and spinal cord pools of immunoreactive dynorphin in rats. Neurosci Lett 24, 75-79.

Petraglia, F., Vale, W. & Rivier, C. (1986): Opioids act centrally to modulate stress-induced decrease in luteinizing hormone in the rat. Endocrinology 119, 2445-2450.

Plotsky, P.M. & Vale, W. (1984): Hemorrhage-induced secretion of corticotropin-releasing factor-like immunoreactivity into the rat hypophysial portal circulation and its inhibition by glucocorticoids. Endocrinology 114, 164-169.

Rivier, C.L. & Plotsky, P.M. (1986): Mediation by corticotropin-releasing factor (CRF) of adenohypophysial hormone secretion. In *Annual Review of Physiology"* , pp. 475-494.

Rivier, C., Rivier, J. & Vale, W. (1982): Inhibition of adrenocorticotropic hormone secretion in the rat by immunoneutralization of corticotropin-releasing factor (CRF). Science 218, 377-379.

Rivier, C., Rivier, J. & Vale, W. (1986): Stress-induced inhibition of reproductive functions: Role of endogenous corticotropin-releasing factor. Science 231, 607-609.

Rivier, C. & Vale, W. (1983a): Interaction of corticotropin-releasing factor (CRF) and arginine vasopressin (AVP) on ACTH secretion *in vivo*. Endocrinology 113, 939-942.

Rivier, C. & Vale, W. (1983b): Modulation of stress-induced ACTH release by corticotropin-releasing factor, catecholamines and vasopressin. Nature 305, 325-327.

Rivier, C. & Vale, W. (1984): Influence of corticotropin-releasing factor (CRF) on reproductive functions in the rat. Endocrinology 114, 914-919.

Rivier, C. & Vale, W. (1985): Effects of CRF, Neurohypophysial Peptides and Catecholamines on Pituitary Function. Fed Proc 44, 189-195.

Rivier, C. & Vale, W. (1987): Diminished responsiveness of the hypothalamic-pituitary-adrenal axis of the rat during exposure to prolonged stress: A pituitary-mediated mechanism. Endocrinology 121, 1320-1328.

Rivier, C. & Vale, W. (1989): In the rat, interleukin-1α acts at the level of the brain and the gonads to interfere with gonadotropin and sex steroid secretion. Endocrinology in press.

Rivier, J., Rivier, C. & Vale, W. (1984): Synthetic competitive antagonists of corticotropin releasing factor: Effect on ACTH secretion in the rat. Science 224, 889-891.

Rossier, J., French, E.D., Rivier, C., Ling, N., Guillemin, R. & Bloom, F.E. (1977): Foot-shock induced stress increases β-endorphin levels in brain. Nature 270, 618-620.

Roth, K.A., Weber, E. & Barchas, J.D. (1983): Immunoreactive dynorphin- (1-8) and corticotropin-releasing factor in subpopulation of hypothalamic neurons. Science 219, 189-191.

Sapolsky, R.M., Rivier, C., Yamamoto, G., Plotsky, P. & Vale, W. (1987): Interleukin-1 stimulates the secretion of hypothalamic corticotropin-releasing factor. Science 238, 522-524.

Swanson, L.W., Sawchenko, P.E., Rivier, J. & Vale, W. (1983): Organization of ovine corticotropin releasing factor immunoreactive cells and fibers in the rat brain: an immunocytochemical study. Neuroendocrinology 36, 165-186.

Uehara, A., Gottschall, P.E., Dahl, R.R. & Arimura, A. (1987a): Interleukin-1 stimulates ACTH releae by an indirect action which requires endogenous corticotropin releasing factor. Endocrinology 121, 1580-1582.

Uehara, A., Gottschall, P.E., Dahl, R.R. & Arimura, A. (1987b): Stimulation of ACTH release by human interleukin-1β, but not by interleukin-1α, in conscious, freely-moving rats. Biochem Biophys Res Commun 146, 1286-1290.

Vale, W., Vaughan, J., Smith, M., Yamamoto, G., Rivier, J. & Rivier, C. (1983): Effects of synthetic ovine CRF, glucocorticoids, catecholamines, neurohypophysial peptides and other substances on cultured corticotropic cells. Endocrinology 113, 1121-1131.

Walker, C.D., Perrin, M., Vale, W. & Rivier, C. (1986a): Ontogeny of the stress response in the rat: Role of the pituitary and the hypothalamus. Endocrinology 118, 1445-1451.

Walker, C.D., Sapolsky, R.M., Meaney, M.J., Vale, W.W. & Rivier, C.L. (1986b): Increased pituitary sensitivity to glucocorticoid feedback during the stress nonresponsive period in the neonatal rat. Endocrinology 119, 1816-1821.

Weigent, D.A. & Blalock, J.E. (1987): Interactions between the neuroendocrine and immune systems: Common hormones and receptors. Immunol Rev 100, 79-108.

CRF as mediator of stress responses
Neurochemical and behavioral aspects

Adrian J. Dunn

Department of Pharmacology and Therapeutics, Louisiana State University Medical Center, P.O. Box 33932, Shreveport, LA 71130-3932, U.S.A.

Selye (1950) defined stress as the nonspecific response of an organism to perturbations of its environment. Response was included in the definition because a treatment (i.e. a stressor) that was stressful to one organism might not be stressful to another, and what was stressful to one organism at one time might not be stressful to the same organism at another time. He characterized the response as nonspecific because he considered that certain physiological responses in stress were not specific for a particular stressor, but were observed generally in all stressful situations. This was not to deny that responses specific to the stressor could occur, but that certain responses appeared consistently during stress. Selye believed there were two responses characteristic of stress: the activation of the sympathetic nervous system and adrenal medulla (originally discovered by Cannon); and the activation of the adrenal cortex to secrete glucocorticoids, discovered by himself. Mason (1968) performed a very careful analysis of a number of hormones whose secretion was known to be influenced by stress, including the catecholamines, glucocorticoids, aldosterone, growth hormone, insulin, thyroxin, and various gonadal steroids, including testosterone and estradiol. He concluded that during stress there was a complex set of hormonal changes, and that the particular pattern did indeed vary with the stress. Nevertheless, he found that psychological stress was invariably associated with an activation of the pituitary-adrenal system, and that catecholamine systems (the sympathetic nervous system and the adrenal medulla) were almost always involved. Various subsequent commentators have cited Mason's research and scholarly reviews (e.g., Mason, 1971) as refuting Selye's nonspecific response hypothesis. The dispute appears to be more semantic than real, because few, if any, disagree that the catecholamine and pituitary-adrenal systems are activated in stress, and none has proposed a definition of stress superior to that involving pituitary-adrenal activation.

Twenty years later we can add to the list of physiological responses in stress. We now know that the activation of the pituitary-adrenal system occurs largely following secretion of corticotropin-releasing factor (CRF) from hypothalamic cells, located primarily in the paraventricular nucleus (PVN). The CRF is released from terminals in the median eminence region of the hypothalamus into the portal blood which carries it in relatively high concentrations to the anterior pituitary where it stimulates the secretion of adrenocorticotropin (ACTH) from pituitary corticotrophs. Circulating ACTH subsequently initiates the synthesis and secretion of glucocorticoid from the adrenal cortex - corticosterone in rats and mice, and cortisol in most other species. Thus the pituitary-adrenal system has become the hypothalamic pituitary-adrenal (HPA) axis, and the critical event in stress is the stimulation of hypothalamic CRF secretion. While a number of other factors (such as vasopressin and β-endorphin) may participate in the activation of this axis, and there are complex regulatory mechanisms, the importance of these three hormones is unchallenged.

An important addition of the last decade or so is the involvement of cerebral systems in stress. A large number of investigators has noted changes of brain catecholamine metabolism during stress. While the initial focus was on noradrenergic systems, perhaps as a CNS counterpart to the sympathetic nervous system, it is now clear that dopaminergic and adrenergic systems are commonly involved, as well as serotonin (see reviews by Stone, 1975; Anisman, 1978; Dunn & Kramarcy, 1984; Glavin, 1985). In the past few years some attention has been focussed on a role for CRF within the brain. This has occurred because there is evidence for a neurotransmitter-like role for CRF, aside from its primary role in initiating the HPA activation, and because studies involving CRF administered into the brain have shown it to be an extraordinary potent activator of a number of endocrine, physiological, neurochemical, and behavioral responses.

In this paper I shall summarize our own data and that of others on the neurochemical changes observed in stress and the neurochemical and behavioral responses to intracerebral CRF administration. I will review the data that indicate that CRF can produce a number of physiological, neurochemical, and behavioral responses characteristic of stress, which have led others to propose that CRF can coordinate a whole body response in stress (Gold & Chrousos, 1985; Koob & Bloom, 1985). I shall also examine the hypothesis that secretion of cerebral CRF may be both necessary and sufficient to initiate a stress response. Our temporary conclusion will be that intracerebral administration of CRF can simulate a wide range of responses regarded as characteristic of stress, and that there is already substantial evidence that intracerebral CRF may indeed be the mediator of many of these responses during stress.

METHODS

Male CD-1 mice (25-35 g) were obtained from Charles River (Wilmington, MA) and were maintained on a 12-12 light-dark cycle (lights on 07:00). Human/rat CRF and α-helical-CRF_{9-41} (ahCRF) were generous gifts from Jean Rivier (Salk Institute). Mice requiring ICV injections were implanted with polyethylene cannulae as described by Guild and Dunn (1982). ICV injections were given to unanesthetized mice and consisted of a total volume of 4 μl divided equally between the two cannulae and given over a 30-45 sec period. Footshock and restraint were administered as previously described (Dunn, 1988b,c).

The multicompartment testing chamber (MCC) was based on that designed by Arnsten and Segal (1979). For mice this chamber (38 x 38 x 23 cm) consisted of nine interconnecting compartments within each of which a wire mesh stimulus (3.0 cm sphere) was recessed in a 2.5 cm hole below the floor. The animal was placed in this chamber and observed for a 25-30 min period. The MCC was brightly lit, and background sounds were masked using a white noise generator. Testing was conducted between the hours of 09:00 and 15:30. During the observation period the duration and frequency of a number of behaviors were recorded using an event recorder. Behaviors recorded include: Measures of contact with the stimuli: total number of contacts; total duration of contacts; mean time per contact (total duration of contacts/total number of contacts); Measures of locomotor activity: total number of compartment entries; total number of rears, time spent grooming.

After decapitation trunk blood was collected into heparinized 1.5 ml Eppendorf tubes for assay of plasma corticosterone, and the brain was rapidly removed from the skull. Brain regions were dissected as previously described (Dunn, 1988b) and tissue samples weighed frozen on dry ice and homogenized by brief ultrasonication in 0.1 M $HClO_4$ containing 0.1 mM EDTA. The samples were thawed and centrifuged briefly immediately prior to HPLC analysis with electrochemical detection as described previously (Dunn, 1988b).

RESULTS

Stress-induced changes in cerebral catecholamine metabolism

Following a brief period (15-30 min) of footshock to mice, we observed increases in the cerebral concentrations of the catabolites of norepinephrine (NE) (i.e. 3-methoxy,4-hydroxyphenylglycol, MHPG), dopamine (DA) (i.e. 3,4-dihydroxyphenylacetic acid, DOPAC and homovanillic acid, HVA), and serotonin (5-HT) (i.e. 5-hydroxyindoleacetic acid) (Dunn, 1988a,b; Figure 1). This suggests that there is not only an activation of cerebral noradrenergic systems, but also of dopaminergic and serotonergic systems. Free tryptophan concentrations were also increased in all regions (Dunn, 1988a). The activation of dopaminergic systems occurred in all brain regions studied although the magnitude of the response was the greatest in prefrontal cortex. A similar pattern of responses was observed following conditioned footshock (replacement in the apparatus in which they received footshock on the previous day), restraint (Dunn, 1988c), or during the training or testing of mice in passive avoidance behavior (Dunn et al., 1986).

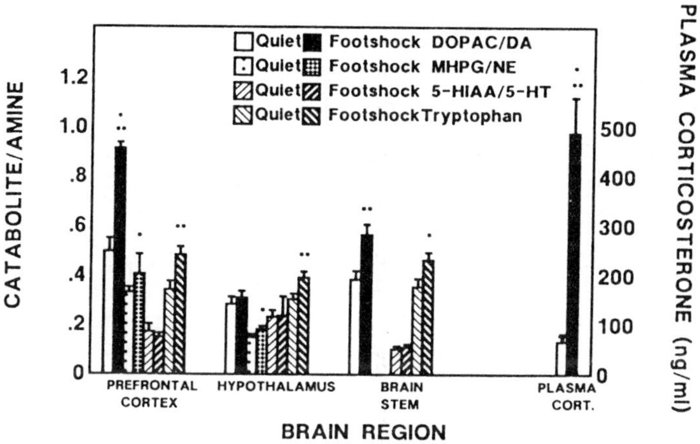

Figure 1. The effect of footshock treatment of mice (20 shocks 0.3 mA in 15 min) on the DOPAC:DA, MHPG:NE, and 5-HIAA:5-HT ratios, and the tryptophan content of prefrontal cortex, hypothalamus, and brain stem. Data for plasma corticosterone are also included. *Significantly different from quiet mice (Student's *t*-test $P < 0.05$. **$P < 0.01$, ***$P < 0.001$: $n = 6$).

The role of glucocorticoids and CRF

Prior adrenalectomy of the mice did not substantially alter any of these responses, nor did we detect any activation of cerebral catecholaminergic systems by administration of corticosterone (Dunn, 1988b). However, when we administered CRF there were substantial changes. ICV or SC injections of CRF caused changes in brain catecholamine metabolites that closely resembled those we observed following footshock or restraint. DOPAC:DA ratios were significantly increased in prefrontal cortex, septum, hypothalamus, and brain stem, and MHPG:NE ratios were increased in prefrontal cortex, hypothalamus, and brain stem (Dunn & Berridge, 1987). Free tryptophan, however, was not altered in any brain region. The increased MHPG is consistent with the observations of Valentino et al. (1983) who found that ICV CRF increased the firing rate of neurons in the locus coeruleus. Recently, these results have essentially been confirmed by Butler et al. (1988) who observed an increase in cerebral 3,4-dihydroxyphenylethyleneglycol (DHPG) following ICV or direct local application of CRF in the rat. These results offer the possibility that intracerebral CRF may mediate changes in catecholamine metabolism during stress.

Behavioral Effects of CRF administration

CRF-like immunoreactivity and bioactive CRF have been identified in many extrahypothalamic regions of the brain (Merchenthaler, 1984; Sawchenko & Swanson, 1985; Nakane et al., 1986). The highest concentration of extrahypothalamic immunoreactive CRF is found in neocortex, areas of the limbic system, and regions involved in the regulation of the autonomic nervous system. High-affinity binding sites for CRF have been observed with a similar regional distribution, using both quantitative autoradiographic and biochemical techniques (Wynn et al., 1984; De Souza et al., 1985). Moreover, CRF-like immunoreactivity has been shown to be released from samples of fresh brain tissue by K^+ in a Ca^{2+}-dependent manner (Smith et al., 1986). Finally, responses to iontophoretically applied CRF have been recorded. In the thalamus and lateral septum inhibition occurred, whereas there was excitation in the cerebral cortex and hypothalamus (Eberly et al., 1983). These observations suggest that cerebral CRF has a neurotransmitter function in brain, separate from its ability to activate the HPA axis. Regionally specific changes in the cerebral concentrations of CRF have been reported following both acute and chronic stressful treatments (Chappell et al., 1986).

ICV administration of CRF has been reported to elicit a number of behaviors characteristic of stress (see also below), therefore we investigated its effect on exploratory behavior. Arnsten et al. (1985) had previously shown that the time rats spent investigating novel objects in holes in the floor of a multicompartment chamber (MCC) was decreased by prior stressful treatments (restraint, noise, or tail pinch). Using mice, we first showed that 30 minutes of restraint had a similar effect on the mean time they made contact with similar "stimuli" in a scaled down version of the same apparatus (Berridge & Dunn, 1986). We then showed that ICV CRF resulted in effects closely resembling those of restraint (Berridge & Dunn, 1986). Doses as low as 5 ng significantly reduced the mean contact times (Berridge & Dunn, 1989). Notably, CRF at these low doses did not alter other behavioral measures such as locomotor activity, rears, or grooming. The effect of CRF on exploratory behavior was independent of pituitary-adrenal activation because it was observed in hypophysectomized mice just as was the effect of restraint (Berridge & Dunn, submitted). The effect of CRF on exploratory behavior, like that of restraint, was prevented by prior treatment with naloxone. We have also observed similar effects of ICV CRF in rats (unpublished observations).

A stress-like effect of CRF was not confined to this task. In the social interaction test, a test designed to be sensitive to agents that affect the anxiety state of the animals, ICV doses of 100 or 300 ng CRF significantly decreased interactions (Dunn & File, 1987). This effect is characteristic of anxiogenic agents, and opposite to that observed with anxiolytic drugs, such as the benzodiazepines. Consistent with this, chlordiazepoxide reversed the effect of CRF.

A CRF antagonist reverses the stress-related changes in behavior

To test whether or not the effect of stress on exploratory behavior in the MCC was mediated by CRF, we employed the CRF-antagonist, α-helical $CRF_{9\text{-}41}$ (ahCRF). This peptide has been shown to inhibit the CRF-induced activation of ACTH release from the isolated anterior pituitaries (Rivier et al., 1984). Unfortunately, its affinity for CRF-receptors is markedly less than that of CRF itself, and an IV dose of 3 mg/kg was necessary to inhibit stress-related ACTH and corticosterone secretion in intact rats. We injected 10, 20, 50 or 100 μg of ahCRF ICV into mice immediately prior to 40 minutes restraint. The peptide had no statistically significant effect on mean stimulus-contact times in unrestrained mice, but in restrained animals there was a dose-dependent effect of the ahCRF, such that doses of 10, 20, and 50 μg significantly reversed the restraint-induced decrease in contact times (Berridge & Dunn, 1987a; Figure 2). These results provides good evidence that endogenous CRF in the brain mediates this restraint-induced behavioral change.

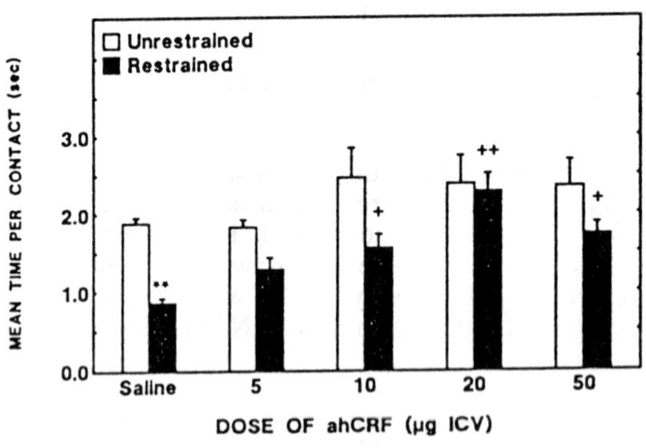

Figure 2. Effect of ahCRF on the restraint-induced decrease in the mean time per contact. Open bars represent unrestrained, and solid bars represent restrained mice. **P < 0.01 compared to saline-unrestrained. +P < 0.05, ++P < 0.01 compared to saline-restrained.

Cerebral NE mediates stress-related exploratory behavior
Idazoxan (1 mg/kg SC), an α_2-antagonist known to increase LC firing, decreased stimulus-contact times, and clonidine (25 µg/kg SC), an α_2-agonist known to decrease LC firing, increased stimulus-contact times (Berridge & Dunn, 1987b). These results are thus consistent with noradrenergic mediation of the behavioral response to restraint. Treatment with the NE-specific neurotoxin, DSP-4 (50 mg/kg IP, 3 days) and clonidine (25 µg/kg SC, 5 minutes before restraint for 40 minutes) reversed the effect of restraint on exploratory behavior (Berridge & Dunn, 1989). Also, the α_1-selective agonist, phenylephrine (50 or 100 ng ICV 10 minutes before testing) had a restraint-like effect on behavior in the MCC, and the α_1-antagonist, prazosin (200 µg/kg SC 45 minutes before testing), completely prevented the effect of restraint in the MCC.

Interactions between NE and CRF
Our results thus support the hypotheses that both CRF and noradrenergic systems in the brain are involved in the restraint-induced decrease in exploratory behavior. Above we described our results indicating that CRF can activate noradrenergic systems. An extensive literature supports the idea that noradrenergic systems in the brain regulate the release of CRF. Although older studies supported an inhibitory role for NE, more recent studies suggest that the effect of NE in the PVN is to stimulate CRF-containing neurons (Plotsky, 1987; Szafarczyk et al., 1987; Al-Damluji, 1988). The question that remains is whether the effects of CRF and NE are independent or related, and if they are related whether CRF modulates the activation of NE neurons or *vice versa.*

We first showed that the effects of CRF on exploratory behavior in the MCC were unaffected by DSP-4 or prazosin pretreatment. Then we determined that ahCRF at a dose of 20 mg ICV completely reversed the effects of ICV phenylephrine (50 or 100 ng). These results appear to exclude an activation of noradrenergic systems by CRF as responsible for the behavioral effects of restraint, and strongly suggest that the restraint-induced activation of noradrenergic neurons stimulates the release of CRF via an α_1-receptor. The CRF released into the ventricles or certain brain sites then affects the behavior.

SUMMARY AND DISCUSSION

CRF can elicit endocrine, behavioral, electrophysiological, and neurochemical effects resembling those observed in stress. The effects can be summarized as follows:

Neuroendocrine responses to CRF
As initially demonstrated by Vale et al. (1981), CRF activates the HPA axis. It also inhibits the secretion of growth hormone (Ono et al., 1984; Rivier & Vale, 1984) and luteinizing hormone (Ono et al., 1984), but not thyroid-stimulating hormone (Ono et al., 1984) or prolactin (Ono et al., 1985).

Physiologic responses to CRF
CRF activates sympathetic and adrenomedullary output, increasing the circulating concentrations of NE, epinephrine, glucagon, and glucose, as well as increasing mean arterial pressure, heart rate, and oxygen consumption in both rats and dogs (Brown & Fisher, 1985). ICV CRF also increases the electrophysiological activity in the splanchnic nerve (Kurosawa et al., 1986). The effect appears to be central because peripheral administration of antibody to CRF which prevents the elevation of plasma ACTH by ICV CRF, does not prevent the effects on plasma NE and epinephrine (Brown & Fisher, 1985).

CRF also has profound effects on the gastrointestinal system. ICV CRF decreases gastric acid secretion in rats and dogs (Tache et al., 1983; Lenz et al., 1985; Bueno & Fioramonti, 1986). Vagotomy blocked this effect of CRF in rats (Tache et al., 1983), but not in dogs (Lenz et al., 1987), in which the effects were blocked by chlorisondamine. In rats, ICV CRF also decreased gastric emptying and decreased small intestinal transit, while increasing large intestine transit and fecal excretion (Williams et al., 1987; Lenz et al., 1988). Each of these gastrointestinal responses changes observed during stress.

Electrophysiological responses to CRF
ICV CRF produced a dose-dependent activation of the electroencephalogram with signs of both EEG and behavioral arousal predominating at low doses, and epileptiform activity and seizures observed at

higher doses (Ehlers et al., 1983). ICV CRF also increases firing of locus coeruleus (LC) neurons in anesthetized and awake rats (Valentino et al., 1983). Similar effects are observed following local injection of CRF on to LC neurons (Valentino & Foote, 1988). In the latter study, CRF was found to increase the basal firing rate, without affecting that due to noxious stimuli.

Neurochemical responses to CRF
As reported above, CRF activates cerebral NE and DA systems as indicated by the increased production of DHPG, MHPG and DOPAC in various brain regions (Dunn & Berridge, 1987; Butler et al., 1988).

Behavioral responses to CRF
CRF increased grooming in mice and rats (Britton et al., 1982; Dunn et al., 1987; Morley & Levine, 1982; Sutton et al., 1982; Veldhuis & de Wied, 1984), and decreased feeding but not drinking in rats (Morley & Levine, 1982; Krahn et al., 1986). Sexual behavior was reduced in both male and female rats (Sirinathsinghji, 1985, 1987). Kalin (1985) reported depression-like effects of ICV CRF in monkeys.

Intracerebral administration of CRF to rats produced a dose-dependent activation of locomotor behavior in a familiar environment (Sutton et al., 1982), whereas in a novel open field it decreased locomotion and rears and increased freezing, results that were interpreted to reflect an increase in the aversive nature of the novel environment (Sutton et al., 1982). CRF decreased approaches to food in a novel open-field (Britton et al., 1982). This effect was opposite to that seen following administration of benzodiazepines, suggesting that CRF enhances the anxiogenic nature of the novel environment. In a conflict test, CRF decreased punished responding, whereas benzodiazepines increased this response (Britton et al., 1985). CRF also exacerbated the acoustic startle response (Swerdlow et al., 1986)and shock-induced freezing (Sherman & Kalin, 1988). CRF has complex effects on avoidance behavior (Sahgal et al., 1983; Veldhuis & de Wied, 1984). As reported above, we showed that ICV CRF reduced a measure of exploratory behavior in both rats and mice (Berridge & Dunn, 1986), and decreased social interaction in rats (Dunn & File, 1987).

The involvement of the HPA axis in the effects of CRF
In every case where it has been tested, these behavioral effects appear to be independent of the the pituitary-adrenal axis. Hypophysectomized animals administered CRF showed a grooming response (Morley & Levine, 1982), increased locomotor activity (Eaves et al., 1985), and decreased exploratory behavior (Berridge & Dunn, submitted). Moreover, the sympathetic nervous system activation caused by ICV CRF was present in hypophysectomized and adrenalectomized rats (Fisher et al., 1983). The decreased gastric acid secretion and inhibited gastric emptying responses to ICV CRF were likewise not affected by hypophysectomy (Tache et al., 1983; Lenz et al., 1985). The locomotor activating effects of ICV CRF were not prevented by dexamethasone treatment, which suppresses CRF-induced ACTH release from the pituitary (Britton et al., 1986a,b). Dexamethasone did not alter the CRF-induced decreases in responding in the conflict test (Britton et al., 1986a), nor did it alter the ICV CRF-induced increases in grooming (Dunn et al., 1987; Britton et al., 1986a), or decreases in feeding (Britton et al., 1986a). Moreover, the actions of CRF appear to be directly on the brain; they are not elicited by peripheral injections at similar doses.

The effects of CRF-antagonists on stress-related responses
These stress-like effects of CRF suggest, but do not prove that CRF may be an endogenous mediator of stress responses. The CRF administration could merely be stressful, activating the endogenous stress systems. However, a number of stress-related phenomena have now been shown to be attenuated or reversed by the intracerebral administration of antisera to CRF or the CRF-antagonist, ahCRF. Rivier et al. (1982, 1984) initially demonstrated the ability of immunoneutralization or ahCRF to reverse the ether stress-induced secretion of ACTH. Subsequently, the same group showed that ICV ahCRF could reverse the electric shock-induced decreases in growth hormone (Rivier & Vale, 1985) and LH secretion in male rats (Rivier et al., 1986). Brown et al. (1985) found that ICV ahCRF could reverse the ether-induced increase in plasma epinephrine (but curiously not NE). Williams et al. (1987) showed that ICV ahCRF prevented the restraint-related increases of large intestinal transit time and fecal secretion, and Stephens et al. (1988) showed that intracisternal ahCRF reversed the surgery-related inhibition of gastric acid secretion. There appear also to be peripheral effects of CRF on the gastrointestinal system, because an antiserum to CRF administered reversed the effects of acoustic or cold stress in mice (Bueno & Gue,

1988). So far as the behavioral effects are concerned, Krahn et al. (1986) demonstrated that ICV ahCRF attenuated the shock-induced decrease in feeding. As reported above, we found that ICV ahCRF reversed the effect of restraint on exploratory behavior in mice (Berridge & Dunn, 1987a). Tazi et al. (1987a) found that ahCRF blocked footshock-induced fighting in rats, and, more recently, Kalin et al. (1988) found that ahCRF prevented footshock-induced freezing behavior in rats.

These results provide compelling evidence that endogenous CRF mediates at least some of the behavioral and physiological changes that occur in stress. Nevertheless, we do not know the sites of action for any of these effects. In all cases reported, the responses to CRF are elicited with intracerebroventricular injections. While this suggests a periventricular site of action for the peptide, this is not necessarily the case. Brown (1986) could find no particular active site for the sympathetic activating effects of ICV CRF, and Tazi et al. (1987b) reported a forebrain site for the locomotor activation effects. We have preliminary evidence that the effect of ICV CRF on exploratory behavior is exerted via a third ventricle rather than a fourth ventricle site (Berridge, Spadaro, Baldwin & Dunn, unpublished). But our experiments would not reveal the final site of action of the CRF which could be in the cortex. Likewise, we do not know the location of the NE-CRF interaction involved in the behavioral changes in the MCC (if it occurs directly). Whereas it is possible that it is in the PVN, such that collaterals of CRF neurons projecting to the median eminence are responsible for the behavioral effects, it could just as easily be in the cortex, or anywhere else in the brain that both NE terminals and CRF-containing neurons appear.

The studies reviewed above suggest that CRF administration can reproduce many of the well characterized endocrine, physiological, neurochemical, and behavioral responses in stress. Experiments with CRF antagonists administered to stressed animals indicate that several of the stress-related changes can be attenuated or reversed, suggesting that endogenous CRF may indeed mediate certain stress responses. Thus we can extend the hypothesis of Gold and Chrousos (1985) and Koob and Bloom (1985) to suggest that release of endogenous CRF from brain sites may be both necessary and sufficient to initiate a stress response. I propose that we consider using the secretion of CRF as a definition of stress, and that we should seek similar physiological definitions for related states such as arousal, anxiety, fear, or panic. Accordingly, experimental manipulations that do not result in CRF secretion should not be regarded as stressful.

REFERENCES

Al-Damluji, S. (1988): Adrenergic mechanisms in the control of corticotrophin secretion. *J. Endocrinol.* 119, 5-14.

Anisman, H. (1978): Neurochemical changes elicited by stress. In *Psychopharmacology of Aversively Motivated Behavior*, ed. H. Anisman & G. Bignami, pp. 119-172. New York: Plenum Press.

Arnsten, A.F.T. & Segal, D.S. (1979): Naloxone alters locomotion and interaction with environmental stimuli. *Life Sci.* 25, 1035-1042.

Arnsten, A.F.T., Berridge, C.W. & Segal, D.S. (1985): Stress produces opioid-like effects on investigatory behavior. *Pharmacol. Biochem. Behav.* 22, 803-809.

Berridge, C.W. & Dunn, A.J. (1986): Corticotropin-releasing factor elicits naloxone-sensitive stress-like alterations in exploratory behavior in mice. *Regulat. Peptides* 16, 83-93.

Berridge, C.W. & Dunn, A.J. (1987a): A corticotropin-releasing factor antagonist reverses the stress-induced changes of exploratory behavior in mice. *Horm. Behav.* 21, 393-401.

Berridge, C.W. & Dunn, A.J. (1987b): α_2-noradrenergic agonists and antagonists alter exploratory behavior in mice. *Neurosci. Res. Commun.* 1, 97-103.

Berridge, C.W. & Dunn, A.J. (1989): Norepinephrine-stimulated CRF release mediates stress-induced changes in exploratory behavior. In *Molecular Biology of Stress, UCLA Symposia on Molecular and Cellular Biology, New Series*, ed. S. Breznitz & O. Zinder, pp. 57-66. New York: Alan R. Liss.

Berridge, C.W. & Dunn, A.J.: CRF and restraint stress decrease exploratory behavior in hypophysectomized mice. Submitted for publication.

Britton, D.R., Koob, G.F., Rivier, J. & Vale, W. (1982): Intraventricular corticotropin-releasing factor enhances behavioral effects of novelty. *Life Sci.* 31, 363-367.

Britton, D.R., Varela, M., Garcia, A. & Rosenthal, M. (1986a): Dexamethasone suppresses pituitary-adrenal but not behavioral effects of centrally administered CRF. *Life Sci.* 38, 211-216.
Britton, K.T., Morgan, J., Rivier, J., Vale, W. & Koob, G.F. (1985): Chlordiazepoxide attenuates response suppression induced by corticotropin-releasing factor in the conflict test. *Psychopharmacol.* 86, 170-174.
Britton, K.T., Lee, G., Vale, W., Rivier, J. & Koob, G.F. (1986b): Corticotropin releasing factor (CRF) receptor antagonist blocks activating and 'anxiogenic' actions of CRF in the rat. *Brain Res.* 369, 303-306.
Brown, M. R. (1986): Corticotropin-releasing factor: central nervous system sites of action. *Brain Res. 399, 10-14.*
Brown, M.R. & Fisher, L.A. (1985): Corticotropin-releasing factor: effects on the autonomic nervous system and visceral systems. *Fed. Proc.* 44, 243-248.
Brown, M.R., Fisher, L.A., Webb, V., Vale, W.W. & Rivier, J.E. (1985): Corticotropin-releasing factor: a physiologic regulator of adrenal epinephrine secretion. *Brain Res.* 328, 355-357.
Bueno, L. & Fioramonti, J. (1986): Effects of corticotropin-releasing factor, corticotropin and cortisol on gastrointestinal motility in dogs. *Peptides* 7, 73-77.
Bueno, L. & Gue, M. (1988): Evidence for the involvement of corticotropin-releasing factor in the gastrointestinal disturbances induced by acoustic and cold stress in mice. *Brain Res.* 441, 1-4.
Butler, P.D., Weiss, J.M., Stout, J.C., Kilts, C.D., Cook, L.L. & Nemeroff, C.B (1988): Corticotropin-releasing factor produces anxiogenic and behavioral activating effects following microinfusion into the locus coeruleus. *Soc. Neurosci. Abstr.* 114.14.
Chappell, P.B., Smith, M.A., Kilts, C.D., Bissette, G., Ritchie, J., Anderson, C. & Nemeroff, C.B. (1986): Alterations in corticotropin-releasing factor-like immunoreactivity in discrete rat brain regions after acute and chronic stress. *J. Neurosci.* 6, 2908-2914.
De Souza, E.B., Insel, T., Perrin, M., Rivier, J., Vale, W. & Kuhar, M. (1985): Corticotropin-releasing factor receptors are widely distributed within the rat central nervous system: an autoradiographic study. *J. Neurosci.* 5, 3189-3203.
Dunn, A.J. (1988a): Changes in plasma and brain tryptophan and brain serotonin and 5-hydroxyindoleacetic acid after footshock stress. *Life Sci.* 42, 1847-1853.
Dunn, A.J. (1988b): Stress-related changes in cerebral catecholamine and indoleamine metabolism: lack of effect of adrenalectomy and corticosterone. *J. Neurochem.* 51, 406-412.
Dunn, A.J. (1988c): Stress-related activation of cerebral dopaminergic systems. *Ann. N.Y. Acad. Sci.* 537, 188-205.
Dunn, A.J. & Berridge, C.W. (1987): Corticotropin-releasing factor administration elicits a stress-like activation of cerebral catecholaminergic systems. *Pharmacol. Biochem. Behav.* 27, 685-691.
Dunn, A.J. & File, S.E. (1987): Corticotropin-releasing factor has an anxiogenic action in the social interaction test. *Horm. Behav.* 21, 193-202.
Dunn, A. J. & Kramarcy, N. R. (1984): Neurochemical responses in stress: relationships between the hypothalamic-pituitary-adrenal and catecholamine systems. In *Handbook of Psychopharmacology*, Vol. 18, eds. L. L. Iversen, S. D. Iversen & S. H. Snyder, pp. 455-515. New York: Plenum Press.
Dunn, A.J., Elfvin, K.L. & Berridge, C.W. (1986): Changes in plasma corticosterone and cerebral biogenic amines and their catabolites during training and testing of mice in passive avoidance behavior. *Behav. Neural Biol.* 46, 410-423.
Dunn, A.J., Berridge, C.W., Lai, Y.I. & Yachabach, T.L. (1987): CRF-induced excessive grooming behavior in rats and mice. *Peptides* 8, 841-844.
Eaves, M., Thatcher-Britton, K., Rivier, J., Vale, W. & Koob, G.F. (1985): Effects of corticotropin releasing factor on locomotor activity in hypophysectomized rats. *Peptides* 6, 923-926.
Eberly, L.B., Dudley, C.A. & Moss, R.L. (1983): Iontophoretic mapping of corticotropin-releasing factor (CRF) sensitive neurons in the rat forebrain. *Peptides* 4, 837-841.
Ehlers, C.L., Henriksen, S.J., Wang, M., Rivier, J., Vale, W. & Bloom, F.E. (1983): Corticotropin-releasing factor produces increases in brain excitability and convulsive seizures in rats. *Brain Res.* 278, 332-336.
Fisher, L.A., Jessen, G. & Brown, M.R. (1983): Corticotropin-releasing factor (CRF): mechanism to elevate mean arterial pressure and heart rate. *Reg. Peptides* 5, 153-161.
Glavin, G.B. (1985): Stress and brain noradrenaline: A review. *Neurosci. Biobehav. Rev.* 9, 233-243.

Gold, P.W. & Chrousos, G. (1985): Clinical studies with corticotropin-releasing factor: implications for the diagnosis and pathophysiology of depression, Cushing's disease, and adrenal insufficiency. *Psychoneuroendocrinol.* 10, 401-419.
Guild, A.L. & Dunn, A.J. (1982): Dopamine involvement in ACTH-induced grooming behavior. *Pharmacol. Biochem. Behav.* 17, 31-36.
Kalin, N.H., (1985): Behavioral effects of ovine corticotropin-releasing factor administered to rhesus monkeys. *Fed. Proc.* 44, 249-254.
Kalin, N.H., Sherman, J.E. & Takahashi, L.K. (1988): Antagonism of endogenous CRH systems attenuates stress-induced freezing behavior in rats. *Brain Res.* 457, 130-135.
Koob, G.F. & Bloom, F.E. (1985): Corticotropin-releasing factor and behavior. *Fed. Proc.* 44, 259-263.
Krahn, D.D., Gosnell, B.A., Grace, M. & Levine, A.S. (1986): CRF antagonist partially reverses CRF- and stress-induced effects on feeding. *Brain Res. Bull.* 17, 285-289.
Kurosawa, M., Sato, A., Swenson, R.S. & Takahashi, Y. (1986): Sympatho-adrenal medullary functions in response to intracerebroventricularly injected corticotropin-releasing factor in anesthetized rats. *Brain Res.* 367, 250-257.
Lenz, H.J., Hester, S.E. & Brown, M.R. (1985): Corticotropin-releasing factor. Mechanisms to inhibit gastric acid secretion in conscious dogs. *J. Clin. Invest.* 75, 889-895.
Lenz, H.J., Raedler, A. Greten, H. & Brown, M. (1987): CRF initiates biological actions within the brain that are observed in response to stress. *Am. J. Physiol.* 252, R34-39.
Lenz, H.J., Burlage, M., Raedler, A. & Greten, H. (1988): Central nervous system effects of corticotropin-releasing factor on gastrointestinal transit in the rat. *Gastroenterol.* 94, 598-602.
Mason, J.W. (1968): A review of psychoendocrine research on the pituitary-adrenocortical system. *Psychosomat. Med.* 30, 576-607.
Mason, J.W. (1971): A re-evaluation of the concept of 'non-specificity' in stress theory. *J. Psychiat. Res.* 8, 323-333.
Merchenthaler, I. (1984): Corticotropin releasing factor (CRF)-like immunoreactivity in the rat central nervous system. Extrahypothalamic distribution. *Peptides* 5 (Suppl. 1), 53-69.
Morley, J.E. & Levine, A.S. (1982): Corticotrophin releasing factor, grooming and ingestive behavior. *Life Sci.* 31, 1459-1464.
Nakane, T., Audhya, T., Hollander, C.S., Schlesinger, D.H., Kardos, P., Brown, C. & Passarelli, J. (1986): Corticotrophin-releasing factor in extra-hypothalamic brain of the mouse: demonstration by immunoassay and immunoneutralization of bioassayable activity. *J. Endocrinol.* 111, 143-149.
Ono, N., Lumpkin, M.D., Samson, W.K., McDonald, J.K. & McCann, S.M. (1984): Intrahypothalamic action of corticotrophin-releasing factor (CRF) to inhibit growth hormone and LH release in the rat. *Life Sci.* 35, 1117-1123.
Ono, N., Samson, W.K., McDonald, J.K., Lumpkin, M.D., Bedran de Castro, J.C. & McCann, S.M. (1985): Effects of intravenous and intraventricular injections of antisera directed against corticotropin-releasing factor on the secretion of anterior pituitary hormones. *Proc. Natl. Acad. Sci. USA.* 82, 7787-7790.
Plotsky, P. M. (1987): Facilitation of immunoreactive corticotropin-releasing factor secretion into the hypophysial-portal circulation after activation of catecholaminergic pathways or central norepinephrine injection. *Endocrinology* 121, 924-930.
Rivier, C & Vale, W. (1984): Corticotropin-releasing factor (CRF) acts centrally to inhibit growth hormone secretion in the rat. *Endocrinol.* 114, 2409-2411.
Rivier, C. & Vale, W. (1985): Involvement of corticotropin-releasing factor and somatostatin in stress-induced inhibition of growth hormone secretion in the rat. *Endocrinol.* 117, 2478-2482.
Rivier, C., Rivier, J. & Vale, W. (1982): Inhibition of adrenocorticotropic hormone secretion in the rat by immunoneutralization of corticotropin-releasing factor. *Science* 218, 377-379.
Rivier, J., Rivier, C. & Vale, W. (1984): Synthetic competitive antagonists of corticotropin-releasing factor: effects on ACTH secretion in the rat. Science 224, 889-891.
Rivier, C., Rivier, J. & Vale, W. (1986): Stress-induced inhibition of reproductive functions: role of endogenous corticotropin-releasing factor. *Science* 231, 607-609.
Sahgal, A., Wright, C., Edwardson, J.A. & Keith, A.B. (1983): Corticotropin releasing factor is more potent than some corticotropin-related peptides in affecting passive avoidance behavior in rats. *Neurosci. Letts* 36, 81-86.
Sawchenko, P.E. & Swanson, L.W. (1985): Localization, colocalization, and plasticity of corticotropin-releasing factor immunoreactivity in rat brain. *Fed. Proc.* 44, 221-227.

Selye, H. (1950): The Physiology and Pathology of Exposure to Stress. Montreal: *Acta Med. Publ.*
Sherman, J.E. & Kalin, N.H. (1988): ICV-CRH alters stress-induced freezing behavior without affecting pain sensitivity. *Pharmacol. Biochem. Behav.* 30, 801-807.
Sirinathsinghji, D.J.S. (1985): Modulation of lordosis behavior in the female rat by corticotropin releasing factor, β-endorphin and gonadotropin releasing hormone in the mesencephalic central gray. *Brain Res.* 336, 45-55.
Sirinathsinghji, D.J.S. (1987): Inhibitory influence of corticotropin releasing factor on components of sexual behavior in the male rat. *Brain Res.* 407, 185-190.
Smith, M.A., Slotkin, T.A., Knight, D.L. & Nemeroff, C.B. (1986): Release of corticotropin-releasing factor from rat brain regions in vitro. *Endocrinology* 118, 1997-2001.
Stephens, R.L., Yang, H., Rivier, J. & Tache, Y. (1988): Intracisternal injection of CRF antagonist blocks surgical stress-induced inhibition of gastric secretion in the rat. *Peptides* 9, 1067-1070.
Stone, E.A. (1975): Stress and catecholamines. In *Catecholamines and Behavior. Vol. 2 Neuropsychopharmacology*, ed. A.J. Friedhoff, pp. 31-72. New York: Plenum Press.
Sutton, R.E., Koob, G.F., Le Moal, M., Rivier, J. & Vale, W. (1982): Corticotropin releasing factor produces behavioral activation in rats. *Nature* 297, 331-333.
Swerdlow, N.R., Geyer, M.A., Vale, W.W. & Koob, G.F. (1986): Corticotropin-releasing factor potentiates acoustic startle in rats: blockade by chlordiazepoxide. *Psychopharmacol.* 88, 147-152.
Szafarczyk, A., Malaval, F., Laurent, A., Gibaud, R. & Assenmacher, I. (1987): Further evidence for a central stimulatory action of catecholamines on adrenocorticotropin release in the rat. *Endocrinology* 121, 883-892.
Tache, Y., Goto, Y., Gunion, M., Vale, W. Rivier, J. & Brown, M. (1983): Inhibition of gastric acid secretion in rats by intracerebral injection of corticotropin-releasing factor. *Science* 222, 935-937.
Tazi, A., Dantzer, R., Le Moal, M., Rivier, J., Vale, W. & Koob, G. F. (1987a): Corticotropin-releasing factor antagonist blocks stress-induced fighting in rats. *Regulat. Peptides* 18, 37-42.
Tazi, A., Swerdlow, N. R., Le Moal, M., Rivier, J., Vale, W. & Koob, G. F. (1987b): Behavioral activation by CRF: evidence for the involvement of the ventral forebrain. *Life Sci.* 41, 41-49.
Vale, W., Spiess, J., Rivier, C. & Rivier, J. (1981): Characterization of a 41-residue ovine hypothalamic peptide that stimulates secretion of corticotropin and β-endorphin. *Science* 213, 1394-1397.
Valentino, R.J. & Foote, S.L. (1988): Corticotropin-releasing hormone increases tonic but not sensory-evoked activity of noradrenergic locus coeruleus neurons in unanesthetized rats. *J. Neurosci.* 8, 1016-1025.
Valentino, R.J., Foote, S.L. & Aston-Jones, G. (1983): Corticotropin-releasing factor activates noradrenergic neurons of the locus coeruleus. *Brain Res.* 270, 363-367.
Veldhuis, H.D. & de Wied, D. (1984): Differential behavioral actions of corticotropin-releasing factor (CRF). *Pharmacol. Biochem. Behav.* 21, 707-713.
Williams, C.L., Peterson, J.M., Villar, R.G. & Burks, T.F. (1987): Corticotropin-releasing factor directly mediates colonic responses to stress. *Amer. J. Physiol.* 253, G582-G586.
Wynn, P.C., Hauger, R.L., Holmes, M.C., Millan, M.A., Catt, K.J. & Aguilera, G. (1984): Brain and pituitary receptors for corticotropin releasing factor: localization and differential regulation after adrenalectomy. *Peptides* 5, 1077-1084.

ACKNOWLEDGEMENTS

The research reported in this review was supported by grants from the National Institutes of Health (MH25486 and NS27283).

Behavioral responses to stressors

Robert Dantzer

INRA-INSERM U. 259, Psychobiologie des Comportements Adaptatifs, rue Camille Saint-Saëns, 33077 Bordeaux Cedex, France

Traditional descriptions of the responses of animals to stressors are either stimulus-oriented or response-oriented, depending on which side of the stimulus-response chain they emphasize. Regardless of the orientation, the emphasis is mainly on responses to standardized external stressors such as electric shock (escape-avoidance behavior) and to aggressive conspecifics (attack and defense). Stress is usually viewed as a nonspecific reaction to many different stimuli that threaten homeostasis.

Current views on stress reactions depart from this unitary concept. Animals are equipped with different defense systems, each of which has specific triggering stimuli and organizes specific patterns of behavior. Within each system, there are different response patterns or different strategies that are possible depending on the way the organism is able to cope with the stressful situation. Each strategy consists of a set of closely inter-related behavioral, neuro-endocrine and autonomic responses. By discussing the main features of the most important defense systems and the way they integrate behavioral and visceral components, the aim of this review paper is to illustrate the usefulness of a multiunitary concept of stress.

I. THE SKIN DEFENSE SYSTEM

The skin defense system is aroused by external dangers that threaten the psychological and physical integrity of the individual. Its output consists of a set of species-specific defense reactions which are hierarchically organized depending on the nature and intensity of the stressor and the organism's ability to predict and control it.

Because of the easiness with which it can be studied and the traditional interest of experimental psychologists for punishment and avoidance, the skin defense system has been extensively studied. Electric shock has been the negative reinforcement most commonly used in these experiments. Controversies have raged for decades about the best way to account for suppressing effects of punishment on positively reinforced behavior and on maintenance of avoidance behavior (what is reinforcing avoidance responding since, by definition, there is no more shock when the subject is successfully avoiding?). The aridity of this literature has reduced the interest of the rest of the scientific community in this field and is responsible for a purely technologically oriented use of the tools of instrumental conditioning by other scientists. In addition, because of the emphasis on learning and conditioning other more natural behaviors such as aggressive behavior have been relatively neglected.

This situation has changed during recent years. Thus, the ethological dimension of the behavior under study has been considered instead of attending only to response curves. One of the pioneers in this area was Robert Bolles from the University of Washington at Seattle (Bolles, 1970). He showed that the different rates at which different avoidance responses are learned can be accounted for by the importance of response topography within the context of evolution. In contradiction to prevailing Skinnerian theories, he pointed out that animals come into the experimental avoidance situation with a set of species-specific defense reactions (SSDR) that have been selected by evolution on the basis of their efficacy. For the rat, the SSDR repertoire includes fighting, fleeing, freezing and hiding. The actual avoidance response that the subject has to learn will be acquired quickly if and only if it is part of the SSDR repertoire and it is functionally effective in the sense that it allows the subject to protect himself physically from the danger.

In a related manner, aggressive behavior can be better understood if, instead of describing the botanic-like diversity of different aggressive behaviours observed in different eliciting situations, one realizes that aggression is organized along two requirements, the attacker must reach target areas for bites and the defender must protect these areas from injury (Blanchard and Blanchard, 1981). Two main strategies can therefore be distinguished, offensive and defensive behaviors. There is now a wealth of evidence documenting the fact that these strategies are differentially organized in the brain and are associated to different autonomic and neuro-endocrine patterns.

Nociceptive stimuli have long been considered only as sources of SSDR. The observation that stressful stimuli activate endogenous analgesic systems even when they are not painful has prompted the search for possible functions of stress-induced analgesia (SIA). Based once more on evolutionary considerations, Bolles and Fanselow (1980) have suggested that SIA might play a critical role in modulating the behavioral responses that evolved as antipredator defense. The basis for their hypothesis is very simple. In order to quickly and efficiently respond to innate or acquired danger signals, animal must ignore injurious pain and concentrate their attention on the best way to escape danger. For example, licking an injured limb is better carried out in a safe and remote place than in front of the predator. The concept is that endogenous analgesic mechanisms are activated by the same stimuli that activate defensive behavior, so that analgesia can prevent the disruptive influences of pain on coordinated defense activities. Stated in psychological terms, the fear-motivated defensive system inhibits the pain-motivated system.

A clear demonstration of this inhibitory influence of fear on pain is given by an experiment by Fanselow (1985) in which rats are injected with a dilute formalin solution beneath the dorsal surface of their hind paw. Animals respond to this injection by engaging in stereotypical pawlicking and pawlifting responses. These responses disappear or take longer to appear if rats are placed individually in a cage containing the odor of a stressed donor, in this case another rat which has received a series of electric shocks.

That this fear-induced analgesia is mediated by the release of endogenous opioids is indicated by the observation that pretreatment with naltrexone blocks its development.

SIA is an heterogenous phenomenon since it is not always blocked by opiate receptor antagonists. Different forms of SIA appear to be associated with different defensive reactions. Mice that are exposed to a highly aggressive conspecific initially exhibit a non-opioid form of analgesia that is blocked by benzodiazepines. Opioid analgesia occurs later in the encounter, when, the attacked animal does no longer tries to fight back or to flee, and when these responses are replaced by passive defense or submissive behavior. Based on these observations and other data from the literature relating SIA to the uncontrolability of stressors (cf. bellow) Rodgers and Randall (1986) have proposed that non-opioid analgesia is typically associated with active defensive behavior initiated in the face of a still uncertain and remote danger. The function of analgesia in this context is to facilitate the shift between strategies depending on their respective outcomes. In contrast, prolonged contact with the threatening stimulus induces an opioid form of analgesia. The function of this analgesia is to strengthen the immobility and loss of reflexive movements, so that the attacker loses interest in its prey.

This interpretation has two important aspects. First, it emphasizes the fact that a strong coupling must exist between behavioral responses and endogenous analgesic systems. Second, it makes clear that the reaction to stressors can take different forms depending on the strategy that is selected.

The first point is not new and has received much attention in the modern stress literature. Systematic experiments on animals exposed to various forms of stressors have demonstrated that the effects of a given stressor on the organism do not depend on its physical characteristics but on the subject's ability to predict and control its occurrence and termination (Dantzer, 1989). Although most experiments use electric shocks as stressors, similar results have been obtained using other stressors. For example, rats exposed to signaled intermittent food show less of an elevation in tail-flick latencies than rats exposed to unsignalled food (Tazi et al., 1987). In the same manner, rats that get their food by pressing a lever in a Skinner box, display little or no elevation in tail-flick latencies, as compared to yoked rats which receive food independently of their behavior.

The effects of controlability and predictability on stress hormones and other physiological indexes have usually been interpreted within the context of the concept of activation. Stress is claimed to be equivalent to arousal and since coping behavior is supposed to be effective in attenuating the consequences of stress, it is by definition de-arousing. Using a single measure such as plasma levels of corticosterone, results that appear to be in agreement with this hypothesis have been obtaine. However, when several measures of activation are considered at the same time, a more complex picture emerges (Dantzer, 1989). The present concept is that the stress reaction is not unidimensional, with the organism being more or less activated depending on the selected strategies. Actually, the stress reaction can be described in a two-dimensional space opposing an effort axis coupled with activation of the sympathetic and adrenal medullary system to a distress axis coupled with activation of the pituitary-adrenal system (Henry and Stephens, 1977). Typically, active efforts to control the aversive situation are associated with release of catecholamines and, if successful, with little activation of the pituitary-adrenal axis. In contrast, loss of control and tense immobility are associated with release of catecholamines and, if successful, with little activation of the pituitary-adrenal axis. In contrast, loss of control and tense immobility are associated with an increase in plasma levels of cortisol. Once again, these physiological responses are not just consequences of behavior, they can themselves influence the mode of behavioral responding to a given threat: a subject with a high sympathetic tone is more likely to try to respond to danger in an active way than a subject with high levels of cortisol. A third dimension involving sex hormones could also play a role, but its exact contribution remains to be determined.

II. THE GUT DEFENSE SYSTEM

Water-deprived rats that are poisoned after having ingested a new taste solution (e.g. a 0.10% saccharin solution) avoid drinking this solution in the future.

First demonstrated by Garcia and his colleagues, taste aversion learning is a very general adaptive phenomenon for species that are eclectic in their gastronomic choices (Garcia et al., 1974). Taste aversion learning works at its best when it is coupled with neophobia since it allows the subject to assess whether ingestion of a small sample of the new food item leads to unfavorable consequences (sickness) or not.

Taste aversion learning has first attracted the attention of learning theorists because of its rather unusual properties (the long delay between the conditioned stimulus, the new taste solution, and the unconditioned stimulus, illness resulting from poisoning; preparedness, i.e. the fact that rats tend to attribute gastro-intestinal sickness to alimentary events rather than to exteroceptive events). Taste aversion learning appears to be part of a more general defense system, called by Garcia et al. (1985) the gut defense system. The gut defense system is associated with nausea, conditioned taste aversion (CTA) and emesis. This defense system is activated by ingested toxins. In the case of CTA, its output consists of a set of orofacial movements and whole body movements enabling the expulsion of the unpalatable food. Although this defense system is highly effective for feeds that can easily be recognized by their flavor, it is likely to play little or no role for other nutriments which are recognized as toxic only when they have already been ingested. In this case, active rejection of the incriminated food is necessary. This can be achieved either by emesis or by a combination of increased intestinal emptying and decreased absorption (e.g., diarrhea). Species like rats which do not vomit might have developed other ways of dealing with ingested toxins such as ingestion of absorbent material (geophagia).

It is interesting to note that hormones released during nausea differ according to the presence or absence of emesis as a defense mechanism. Primates which vomit release vasopressin during nausea and this hormonal response might be adaptive in helping to decrease water loss. In contrast, rodents which do not vomit display a striking increase in plasma levels of oxytocin but no change in vasopressin levels (Verbalis et al., 1986). The function of this nausea-induced oxytocin secretion is not understood.

In hormonal terms, all CTA-inducing treatments activate the pituitary-adrenal axis, although the effect is more likely due to the novelty of the changes in internal state induced by the treatment than to a direct effect of this treatment on the pituitary-adrenal axis. Reexposure to the taste solution paired with sickness also increases pituitary-adrenal hormones, but only if the subject is forced to ingest the aversive solution (Hennessy et al., 1976).

The diversity of treatments that can give rise to CTA suggest that this phenomenon is unlikely to be induced only through the receptors and neural pathways that mediate emesis (Grant, 1987). There is even some controversy about the role of sickness in CTA. Within the framework of this paper, it is not possible, however, to enter into the details of this controversy and the reader is referred to Goudie (1987) for further information.

A relatively neglected phenomenon in the field of CTA is the ability of animals to associate not only taste stimuli but also contextual stimuli to sickness (Krane, 1980). It makes sense for an animal to learn at the same time which food is poisonous and where it is located. There has been, however, little study of the physiological mechanisms underlying this contextual learning.

III. BEHAVIORAL RESPONSES TO PATHOGENS

At the onset of infectious diseases, sick individuals are often lethargic, depressed and aphagic. They do not feel well and in the case of fur bearing animals, their coat is often rough, as if they were less actively grooming themselves.

Since most scientists do not like to work with sick animals except for studying the pathophysiological mechanisms of specific diseases, it is not surprising that these non-specific symptoms of disease have been neglected. However, this situation is now changing rapidly with the identification of chemical messengers from the immune system to the brain.

Regulation within the immune system in response to pathogens is dependent on cytokines which are released by lymphoid cells and activate the metabolism and proliferation of other lymphoid cells. Besides their role within the immune system, some of these cytokines can also act at a distance to coordinate metabolic, hematologic and hormonal responses to infection. A typical example is interleukine-1 (Il-1), a polypeptide that is produced by activated macrophages. Il-1 enters the general circulation to reach several target organs at the level of which it acts like a hormone. Il-1 can be described as a mediator of fever and inflammation (Dinarello, 1988). On hepatocytes, Il-1 stimulates the synthesis and release of acute phase proteins. On vascular endothelial cells, it increases leukocyte adherence and also orchestrates a cascade of cellular and biochemical events that lead to vascular congestion, clot formation, cellular infiltration and endothelial leakage. Il-1 also acts on the thermosensitive neurons of the hypothalamus to initiate fever. It induces the release of pituitary-adrenal hormones, although its exact site of action is still disputed. In addition, central and peripheral injections of Il-1 have demonstrated that Il-1 is able to induce other non-specific symptoms of disease such as general malaise (Tazi et al., 1988), increase in slow-wave sleep (Shoham et al., 1987), decreased food consumption (McCarthy et al., 1986) and decreased interest for social activities (unpublished observations).

These neurophysiological and behavioral effects of Il-1 are shared by many other cytokines such as interferons, tumor-necrosis factor and interleukin-6. The present concept is that sickness behavior is not an artifact but a part of a more global adaptive response to pathogens (Hart, 1988). Sick individuals that respond to infection by a febrile response must invest all their available resources in trying to get rid of the pathogens. To engage in foraging behavior would be counter-productive for a weakened organism. The best way to ensure that this is not the case is to turn off motivation for food, water and social contacts. Fever is adaptive because it stimulates immune defenses and lowers the ability of many pathogens to grow and proliferate. Fever has a high metabolic cost that can only be achieved if the organism does not engage in other physically-demanding activities. If an animals stays at the same place and lies down, it saves on body energy resources and, in addition, reduces heat losses. Reduction of grooming serves the same purposes.

IV. CONCLUSION

These different defense systems are not simply juxtaposed. They share common pathways and can interact with each other. Activation of the pituitary-adrenal axis is a common feature of the skin defense system, the gut defense system and the reaction to pathogens. Our understanding of the functional meaning of these responses cannot be based on the recognition of this non-specificity since it is likely that the release of glucocorticoids serve different purposes within each defense system, depending on the other neuro-endocrine and autonomic components of the response. There has been little or no study of possible interactions between defense systems, besides the mutual inhibition between fear and pain already noted in section I. It is likely that behavioral responses to external stressors can affect sickness behavior and vice-versa, but the evidence is clinical rather than experimental. Depressed patients report more intense subjective symptoms of influenza in spite of similar biological symptoms. Conversely, chronically-ill patients are less able to cope with stressful life events than control populations.

In this paper, we have argued for the existence of adaptive specializations in response to dangers threatening the physical and psychological integrity of the organism. The search for generalities (the stress concept) has resulted in the relative neglect of the diversity of the different defense systems and there is still much to be done to be able to understand this diversity and the common elements in it.

REFERENCES

Blanchard, R.J. & Blanchard, D.C. (1981): The organization and modeling of animal aggression. In *The Biology of Aggression*, eds. P.F. Brain & D. Benton, pp.529-561. Alphen aan den Rijn: Sijthoff & Noordhoff.

Bolles, R.C. (1970): Species-specific defense reactions and avoidance learning. *Psychol. Rev.* 77: 32-48.

Bolles, R.C. & Fanselow, M.S. (1980): A perceptual defensive recuperative model of fear and pain. *Behav. Brain Sci.* 3: 291-323.

Dantzer, R. (1989): Neuroendocrine correlates of control and coping. In *Stress, Personal Control and Health*, eds. A. Steptoe & A.D. Appels, London: Wiley, in press.

Dinarello, C.A. (1988): Biology of interleukin-1. *FASEB J.* 2 : 108-115.

Fanselow, M.S. (1985): Odors released by stressed rats produce opioid analgesia in unstressed rats. *Behav. Neurosci.* 99: 589-592.

Garcia, J., Hankins, W.G. & Rusiniak, K.W. (1974): Behavioral regulation of the milieu interne in Man and Rat. *Science* 185: 824-831.

Garcia, J., Lassiter, P.S., Bermudez-Rattoni, F. & Deems, D.A. (1985): A general theory of aversion learning. *Ann. N.Y. Acad. Sci.* 443: 8-21.

Goudie, A.J. (1987): Aversive stimulus properties of drugs. In *Experimental Psychopharmacology*, eds. A.J. Greenshaw & C.T. Dourish, pp. 341-392. Clifton: Humana Press.

Grant, V. (1987): Do conditioned taste aversions result from activation of emetic mechanisms? *Psychopharmacology* 93: 405-415.

Hart, B.L. (1988): Biological basis of the behavior of sick animals. *Neurosci. Biobehav. Rev.* 12: 123-137.

Henry, J.P. & Stephens, P.M. (1977): *Stress, Health and the Social Environment: A Sociobiologic Approach to Medicine.* New York: Springer.

Hennessy, J.W., Smotherman, W.P., & Levine, S. (1976): Conditioned taste aversion and the pituitary-adrenal system. *Behav. Biol.* 16: 413-424.

Krane, R.V. (1980): Toxicophobia conditioning with exteroceptive cues. *Anim. Learn. Behav.* 8: 513-523.

McCarthy, D.O., Kluger, M.J. & Vander, A.J. (1986): Effects of centrally-administered interleukin-1 and endotoxin on food intake of fasted rats. *Physiol. Behav.* 36: 745-749.

Rodgers, R.J. & Randall, J.I.. (1986): Acute non-opioid analgesia in defeated male mice. *Physiol. Behav.* 36: 947-950.

Rodgers, R.J. & Randall, J.I. (1986): Extended attack from a resident conspecific is critical to the development of long-lasting analgesia in male intruder mice. *Physiol. Behav.* 38: 427-430.

Shoham, S., Davenne, D., Cady, A.B., Dinarello, C.A. & Krueger, J.M. (1987): Recombinant tumor necrosis factor and interleukin-1 enhance slow-wave-sleep. *Amer J. Physiol. Regul. Integr. Comp. Physiol.* 253: R142-R149.

Tazi, A., Dantzer, R. & Le Moal, M. (1987): Prediction and control of non-nociceptive stimuli modulate endogenous pain inhibitory systems. *Behav. Brain Res.* 23: 107-124.

Verbalis, J.G., McHale, C.M., Gardiner, T.W. & Stricker E.M. (1986): Oxytocin and vasopressin secretion in response to stimuli producing learned taste aversion in rats. *Behav. Neurosci.* 100: 466-475.

Assessing life events in stress-related disease

Siegfried Geyer and Johannes Siegrist

Department of Medical Sociology, Medical School,
University of Marburg, Bunsenstrasse 2, D-3550 Marburg, FRG.

ABSTRACT

Critical life events (LE) have been related to disease onset in many studies, but only a minority of these was based on appropriate, i.e. valid and reliable measurement. We present findings from three independent studies using two alternative approaches of assessing LE, contextual rating and subjective evaluation. Both approaches have documented validity and reliability.

The first study, based on a retrospective case-control design, explores psycho-social, behavioral and medical characteristics of 380 male survivors of a first acute myocardial infarction and of matched controls. Number and subjective impact of LE turn out to be strong discriminators between patients and controls, and a series of additional findings supporting the hypothesis is presented. In study II, recurrence of disease is associated with frequency of LE in recent past in a group of 75 patients with defined duodenal ulcer. A semi-prospective design is used in study III where LE are explored in 92 women undergoing breast biopsy at hospital. Very severe LE are significantly more frequent in women whose diagnosis turns out to be malign.

In conclusion, LE, assessed in a valid and reliable way, play an important role in triggering onset of stress-related diseases.

INTRODUCTION

It is by now widely recognized that higher nervous activity due to socio-emotional distress has a direct impact on the development of distinct patterns of bodily dysfunction and, eventually, on their precipitation into overt clinical disease (Cullen et al., 1984; Weiner et al.,1989).

The role of neurotransmitters and neuromodulators in coordinating adaptive endocrine, autonomic and immune responses to stressors has been elucidated to a considerable degree. However, few studies so far have been conducted to demonstrate clear time-dependent associations between duration and intensity of socio-emotional distress and subsequent bodily dysfunction or overt disease in humans. This lack of information is due to the many conceptual and methodological difficulties inherent in the study of human behavior. Life event research is one promising approach to overcome some of these difficulties (Dohrenwend & Dohrenwend, 1981).

Main propositions of life event (LE) research are as follows:

1. The level of socio-emotional distress in an individual is considered the net effect of duration and intensity of chronic socio-environmental stressors and of individual or interpersonal coping resources.
2. Individual coping failure, i.e. high level of distress and of subsequent adaptive breakdown is more likely if severe subacute socio-environmental stressors aggravate the conditions mentioned above.
3. Life events, or more precisely, critical life events, are defined as those subacute socio-environmental stressors which most probably evoke sustained negative feelings such as anxiety, irritation, grief, or helplessness.
4. In order to be critical a life event must be 1.) subjectively important, 2.) disruptive or threatening, 3.) unpredicted or uncontrollable, 4.) demanding high costs of adaptation.

The following main hypothesis is derived from these propositions in terms of a prospective study design: After adjusting for biobehavioral risk factors and for level of chronic socio- en-

vironmental stressors experienced those individuals who have been exposed to critical life events are at higher risk of suffering from subsequent disease manifestation as compared to those individuals who have not been exposed to critical life events.
In terms of a retrospective case-control- design the main hypothesis can be stated as: After adjusting for biobehavioral risk factors and for level of chronic socio-environmental stressors experienced, significantly more patients versus matched controls are expected to have experienced critical life events in their recent past.
This paper presents evidence on these main hypotheses both from semi-prospective and from retrospective studies conducted in our research group. Those studies focus on different clinical conditions, namely ischemic heart disease in men, breast cancer in women, and gastro-intestinal disorders in men and women.

METHODS

Currently, there are two major different methods established in LE research. One method, called subjective evaluation, focusses on information provided by the subject. A structured interview collecting descriptive information about LE is combined with a scaling procedure where the subjective evaluation of every single event is rated. The second method, called contextual rating, uses a semi- structured interview approach. Events are evaluated by the interviewer. Judgements about severity and impact of an event are based on a systematic analysis of an individual's living contexts.
Both approaches have their strengths and limits. Subjective evaluation relates to the cognitive theory of stress, it is an efficiently applicable and considerably reliable method. However, the time span of retrospective inquiry is restricted to a maximum of two years, and under specific clinical conditions, e.g. in psychiatry, subjective evaluation may not serve as valid information. Contextual rating, on the other hand, gives more detailed information about experienced LE, it covers a longer time interval, and it is thought to be applicable in a variety of clinical

conditions. Yet contextual rating disregards subjective evaluation and, in addition, demands a great deal of time and training.

The Life Events and Difficulties Scale (LEDS), developed by G. W. Brown et al. (Brown & Harris, 1978), consists of a set of rules for rating LE along several dimensions considered to be important. Event examples ordered according to the severity of threat serve as reference points for raters. The LE are assessed by a semi-structured, usually tape-recorded interview.

A method of subjective evaluation called Inventory of Life Events (ILE) was developed in our group and was applied in several epidemiologic and clinical studies (Siegrist & Dittmann, 1984). It is based on a structured interview exploring the prevalence of 34 defined negative LE over the past two years in the interviewee and his/her closest family members. Each event, once experienced, is evaluated in terms of eight theoretically meaningful dimensions of stress and coping by a Likert-scale procedure and is given a sum score ranging from 2 (no subjective impact) to 44 (extremely high subjective impact). Thus, information is obtained on number, type, timing, and stress-related scoring of LE.

In a comparison of both methods we have shown high correlations between ILE scores and LEDS-threat-ratings of events ($r=.80$ ($p=.001$) for events with short-term threat and $r=.73$ ($p=.01$) for events with long-term threat). Thus, it is indicated that both approaches provide reliable, well comparable information.

In study I, the ILE was applied, among others, in a large retrospective case-control study on 380 male patients (age 30 to 55 yrs.) with documented first acute myocardial infarction and a healthy control group matched by age, sex, and occupation with the sample half (Siegrist et al.,1980; Siegrist et al., 1982). Study II involves a group of 75 patients (age 26-59 yrs.) (84 per cent men, 16 per cent women) with endoscopically documented duodenal ulcer who did (57 per cent) or did not (43 per cent) suffer from recurrent ulcers during the past 12 months (Haltenhof, 1981).

Study III is a semi-prospective research on 92 women undergoing breast biopsy at hospital (age 25 to 60 yrs.). Here, the LEDS method was applied: The interview was performed at the day of hospital admission before biopsy and LE were rated immediately after interview but before information about diagnosis was obtained. This enabled us to estimate the predictive effect of LE for respondents with malign vs. benign diagnosis (Geyer, 1989).

RESULTS

In study I, significantly more patients with myocardial infarction (MI) than healthy controls experienced LE over the past two years. Respective results are displayed in Table 1: 31 per cent of patients vs. 14 per cent of controls suffer from three or more events, only 19 per cent of patients vs. 36 per cent of controls report no negative events. Futhermore, mean number of LE per person is twice as high in patients as compared to controls (T=5,6; p<.001). The relative risk of experiencing a LE during the past twelve weeks before infarction or before interview is 2,8 for MI-patients (U=2.60; p<.01). Also, more severe events occur in the patient group: events which threaten the social status of an individual (job, finances, family cohesion etc.) occur 2.8 times as often in MI-patients than in controls (U=5.62; p<.001).

Table 1: Cumulation of life events in patients with myocardial infarction (MI- group; n= 190) and in matched healthy controls (H- group; n=190) over the past two years

	per cent of individuals reporting			
	no event	1 event	2 events	3 or more events
MI- group	19.0	26.5	23.3	31.2
H- group	36.4	36.4	13.6	13.6

U= 2.60 p < .01

Mean score of stress-related impact is significantly higher in patients as well, but after adjusting for number of events experienced the difference is clearly reduced. This indicates: the more events a person experiences the higher the subjective impact of every single event.
All associations reported so far remain statistically significant after adjusting for the effects of neuroticism, age, and socio-economic status. Finally, the LE score turns out to be the strongest predictor in terms of correct classification of patient status.
In sum, there is a clear statistical association between number, severity, time pattern and subjective impact of LE and group membership (MI-patients vs. healthy controls).

In study II, number and score of LE in respondents' recent past are compared between subgroups of gastro-intestinal patients with and without recurrent duodenal ulcer. Again, significantly more events per person are found in the recurrence group as compared to the control group ($p<.05$). Of all respondents with at least one event, every second in the recurrence group, but only every fourth in the control group, suffers from two or more events. Furthermore, mean sum score of experienced events is higher in the recurrence group, and it does not vary significantly according to age, sex, or occupational status. Again, the results strongly support the main hypothesis mentioned above.

In study III, LE as assessed by the LEDS approach were rated according to severity of threat (6 categories). Events of the severest category (category 6 vs. categories 1-5) were expected to be more frequent in the prospective breast cancer group. No difference was expected between the two groups with respect to less severe events. Table 2 shows the distribution of LE rated as most severe among the two groups of women with benign vs. malign diagnosis. The 14 critical LE experienced cover a time interval of four years. As can be seen from Table 2, significantly more severe events occur in the malign group ($chi2= 7.35$; $p<.01$). This result remains basically stable after adjusting for possible confounders such as family history of breast cancer, age, and socio-economic status.

Table 2: Distribution of most severe life events in women undergoing breast biopsy with a malign (n= 33) and a benign (n= 59) diagnosis

obs. / exp. / res.	life events: yes	life events: no	
benign group	23 28.0 -5.0	10 5.0 5.0	33 35.9%
malign group	55 50.0 5.0	4 9.0 -5.0	59 64.1%
	78 84.8%	14 15.2%	92 100%

chi- sq.: 7.34; df= 1; p=.007

DISCUSSION

Results from all three studies support the hypothesis that LE are more frequent and/or more severe in persons who recently experienced onset or recurrence of a somatic disease (myocardial infarction, duodenal ulcer) or in persons who were diagnosed as having cancer. Two types of study designs (retrospective and semi-prospective) and two different methodological approaches (subjective evaluation and contextual rating) were used. In every study, a number of confounding variables was taken into account. While these results are generally encouraging, several points need further clarification. For instance, in cardiovascular and gastro- intestinal patients, both, frequency and severity of events were important variables, whereas in the breast biopsy group only severity discriminated between benign and malign diagnosis. Apart from different time interval, type of event and quality of socio-emotional distress might differ considerably between the respective disease conditions. Several studies suggest that LE which induce loss of control and helplessness selectively stimulate the hypothalamic-adrenocortical stress axis with increased ACTH release and impact on immunocompetence (Fox & Newberry, 1984; Cullen et al., 1984; Weiner et al., 1984). A single, extremely severe event inducing loss of control may override the significance of minor life changes in prospective cancer patients. Sustained states of impaired immunity due to experience of loss of control can contribute to tumor promotion in individuals who are already susceptible to this type of disease. On the other hand, in disease pathologies related to excessive sympatho-adrenergic activation such as cardiovascular and possibly gastro-intestinal disorders, frequency of challenging and effort-stimulating events might be an important mechanism. An answer to this intriguing question can be expected from studies which combine endocrine/immunologic and psychosociological parameters in a prospective design.

A second point of discussion relates to attributional processes in sick people which might create a systematic bias, especially so in retrospective case-control studies. Although such effects cannot be ruled out completely we analyzed a variety of variables in this context, such as neuroticism, denial, lay aetiology about disease, educational level, level of psychological well-being. From our analyses, no striking evidence was found that these effects were major determinants number or severity of reported events.

On the other hand, additional evidence in favour of our conclusion can be found. As stated in proposition 2 in the introductory section, LE are postulated to aggravate the impact of chronic socio-environmental stressors. In all three studies, we found highly significant associations between LE and indicators of chronic socio-emotional distress (work, family, private life, lack of social support). These findings are in line with the assumption of cumulative intensity of sustained distress as a trigger of adaptive breakdown. Again, prospective studies in highly distressed groups using combined endocrine-immunologic and psycho-sociological information will be useful in elucidating the biologi cal basis of "stressfulness" of critical life events.

In conclusion, our studies provide additional empirical evidence that critical life events contribute to the onset and recurrence of a variety of stress-related bodily dysfunctions and overt clinical diseases. Due to recent advancements in concepts and methods, life events by now can be assessed with considerably reliable and valid measures. It is hoped that transdisciplinary research in the near future makes more use of these recent developments.

REFERENCES:

Brown, G.W. & Harris T. (1978): Social Origins of Depression. London: Tavistock Publications.

Cullen, J. & Siegrist, J., eds. (1984):Breakdown in Human Adaptation to Stress, Volume 1: Psychological and Sociological Parameters for Studies of Breakdown in Human Adaptation. Boston/ The Hague/ Dordrecht/ Lancaster: Martinus Nijhoff Publishers.

Dohrenwend, B.P. & Dohrenwend, B.S., Eds.(1974):Stressful Life Events and their Contexts. New York: Prodist.

Fox, B.H. & Newberry, B.H. (1984): Impact of Psychoendocrine Systems in Cancer and Immunity. Göttingen, New York, Toronto: Hogrefe.

Haltenhof, H. (1981): Lebensverändernde Ereignisse und Rezidive beim Ulcus Duodeni. Marburg. (Unpublished doctoral dissertation.

Geyer, S. (1989, in preparation): Lebensereignisse und Brustkrebs- eine Untersuchung ihrer Bedeutung und des Designs.

Siegrist, J.,Dittmann, K., Rittner, K. & Weber, I. (1980): Soziale Belastungen und Herzinfarkt. Stuttgart: Enke.

Siegrist, J., Dittmann, K., Rittner, K., & Weber, I. (1982): The Social Context of Active Distress in Patients with Early Myocardial Infarction. *Social Science and Medicine, 16:* 443- 453.

Siegrist, J. & Dittmann, K.(1984): Inventory of Stressful Life Events. In: *Breakdown in Human Adaptation to Stress, Vol.1,* Psychological and Sociological Parameters for Studies of breakdown in Human Adaptation. Eds. J. Cullen & Siegrist, J. Boston/ The Hague/ Dordrecht/Lancaster: Martinus Nijhoff Publishers.

Weiner, H., Florin, I., Murison, R. & Hellhammer, D., Eds.(1989): Frontiers of Stress Research. Bern, Toronto, Lexington, Stuttgart: Huber.

Clinical identification of stress related disorders of the gastrointestinal tract in adults

John F. Fielding

Department of Medicine and Gastroenterology, Beaumont Hospital, Dublin 9, Ireland

Stress related motility disorders of the gastrointestinal tract have been described in the medical literature for at least 170 years (Fielding 1977(a)), although from interpretation of paintings such as Botticheli's 'The Birth of Venus' (1485) they have been recognised for a far longer time. In passing I would point out that I consider the term coping related bowel bowel dysfunction a more accurate and comprehensive one than stress related motility disorders of the gastrointestinal tract but will not insist on altering the title of the work-shop. To the Clinician the entire length of every gastrointestinal tract is, by nature irritable. When such irritability disturbs any combination of gastrointestinal motility, sensation and or secretion leading to perceived abnormality of such functions then an irritable bowel syndrome exists. When medical advice is sought as a consequence of such perception then that patient suffers from one of the irritable bowel syndromes. Such patients account for more than half the new referrals seen by Gastroenterologists on both sides of the Atlantic. The irritable bowel syndrome has been known by numerous names over years (Fielding 1977(b)); each name shows insight into a facet or facets of the condition. To most Gastroenterologists the term irritable bowel syndrome is synonymous to the irritable gut syndrome; both being synonymous and superior to the irritable colon syndrome. I well recognise that in this condition the entire gut is involved (this ubiqitous involvement in a well patient is one of the great clinical clues to the diagnosis) but a given patient at a given point in time complains of abnormality predominantly referable to one of three regions: Oro-pharynx and/or upper oesophageal sphincter; the oesophagus, stomach and/or duodenal region, and, most frequently, the colon. I refer to these clinical entities as upper, middle and lower irritable bowel syndrome: Globus sensation is a typical presentation of the first, the second is often referred to as nervous dyspepsia or Xray negative dyspepsia and the third can correctly be referred to as the irritable colon syndrome. It must be stressed that the title I give these syndromes relates to the predominant symptoms at that point in time and that the title is a clinical one. It is nonetheless a useful one in that it conveys that part of the gastrointestinal tract which is giving rise to most symptoms whilst at the same time recognising panintestinal nature of the abnormality. Upper IBS is the least common varient accounting for but 2.5% of cases, middle IBS is present in 40% and lower IBS in 57.5% (Fielding 1984). The panintestinal nature of the syndrome is readily recognised in that middle and lower IBS symptoms are present in upper IBS, upper and lower symptoms in middle IBS and upper and middle symptoms in lower IBS. Indeed, no patient has symptoms confined to one site. Moreover, the major symptomatology may change from one sub-group to another. This diffuse or panintestinal nature of symptoms in the given clinical setting is virtually diagnostic of the irritable bowel syndrome. What other gastrointestinal abnormality can produce such diffuse symptomatology in the presence of well-being?.

Lower IBS or the irritable colon syndrome in my terminology is what other Gastroenterologists refer to as the irritable bowel syndrome. From what I have said earlier it can be seen that the difference is one of terminology rather than in a difference in appreciation of the diffuse nature of the syndrome. Initially I supported the view that one needed to exclude organic disease to make a diagnosis of irritable colon syndrome (Fielding 1977(b)) but increasing experience enabled me to state; 'a diagnosis of the irritable bowel syndrome is justified in the presence of typical symptoms and signs; it can be substantiated by minimal investigation' (Fielding 1982). It is my firm belief that a positive clinical diagnosis of the irritable bowel syndrome can be made; indeed if other pathology is found on investigation it is my contention that more often than not it is an 'incidental' finding and does not invalidate the IBS diagnosis. This point is often missed even by doctors and false symptoms are thus attributed to such conditions as gall stones, duodenal ulceration and even cancer of the colon.

What are the characteristic features of the irritable colon syndrome. The patient is more likely to be female, may well be the youngest or oldest child, and may have no siblings of the same sex. She is likely to be in the third or fourth decade but symptoms may well have been present for many years. Symptoms in childhood may be recalled on detailed questioning and it is extremely rare for symptoms to begin after the age of forty years. True onset of symptoms after the age of forty years virtually excludes the diagnosis of IBS.

A detailed history and examination will show that IBS is a much more homogeneous condition than many realise. The clinician who only determines 'what the patient complains of' is no true clinician; the latter will not be satisfied until he knows 'of what the patient complains'. A detailed history and examination may be performed in five phases (Fielding 1983(a)): Phase 1 records and enquires into the patient's complaints; Phase 2 enquires if the patient has any further complaints; Phase 3 enquires directly concerning bowel habit, abdominal pain, the passage of mucus per rectum and flatulence if these symptoms have not been previously mentioned; Phase 4 makes a detailed enquiry into those parts of the history where no abnormality has been previously detected; e.g. if a patient has a normal bowel habit the frequency and nature of stool passed is determined. Phase 5 involves examination. With this approach it can be seen that whereas at presentation 75% complain of abdominal pain, 22% of constipation and 30% of diarrhoea by phase 5 no less than 92% have abdominal pain, 90% constipation and 92% diarrhoea. It is of interest that by phase 3 84% have abdominal pain, 70% constipation and 57% diarrhoea, the figures given in many articles on IBS. Yet when one looks at which phase full clinical information is available it can be seen that it is only present in 43% of patients by phase 3.

These findings support the views that patients symptoms change from time to time, that most doctors do not perform a sufficiently detailed history and examination with regard to IBS and that IBS is much more homogeneous than superficial enquiry and examination would suggest. Further enquiry shows that IBS patients have symptoms outside the gastrointestinal tract; most often related to the genito-urinary systems (Fielding 1977(c)). In addition over half the patients have a cancer phobia. One fifth of patients will have lost weight at presentation but such weight loss is not associated with true anorexia (again detailed questioning may be required on this point) but rather with a diminished food intake, either because of the symptoms which follow such intake or as part of a physiological or psychological desire to lose weight.

On examination these patients have a well being out of all proportion to their symptoms. They also demonstrate many signs supportive of the diagnosis of IBS to varying degrees. These signs are most conveniently divided into; general, abdominal, perianal and rectal. The general signs include cool clammy hands, neurodermatitis and brisk neurological jerks. There is objective evidence that the skin is cooler in IBS patients than in controls. These signs have a sensitivity of over 80% but a very low specificity. Another interesting sign is the sudden slowing of the pulse rate when taken (Fielding 1977(c)): This slowing which occurs within three pulse beats following palpation is of the order of 10% in all IBS sub-groups; it occurs later and to a lesser degree in controls. IBS patients also have excessive cold pressor responses (Fielding and Regan 1984). They also have increased muscle tension as measured electromyographically. The abdominal signs are an excessively tender and excessively palpable colon, a right iliac fossa squelch sign and the presence of abdominal scars from previous surgery. The colon signs, the best markers of IBS, have very high sensitivities and specificities; the right iliac fossa squelch sign has low sensitivity but high specificity. It is of interest that these patients have excess extra abdominal surgery as well as excess abdominal surgery (Fielding 1983(b)). Of the perianal signs clinically assessed increased sphincteric tone has a high sensitivity but low specificity. The four rectal signs; painful digital insertion, positive mucosal tap, empty or nearly empty rectum and when present hard or firm faeces, all have high specificities. The positive mucosal tap sign is also a sensitive sign. The three best clinical markers are an excessively palpable colon (sensitivity 86%, specificity 84%), an excessively tender colon (78% and 94%) and a positive rectal mucosal tap sign (70% and 95%).

Sigmoidoscopy may be useful in several ways. There is often evidence of excess muscular spasm, evidence of excess mucus production and the patient's pain may be reproduced both in nature and site on the insufflation of air. Biopsy may confirm excess mucus production.

Radiology, when deemed necessary shows evidence of both excessive and uncoordinated muscular activity.

There is one condition I wish to make brief reference to because I believe it is not sufficiently recognised and that its non recognition leads to patient mismanagement. I refer to a proctitis which on occasions is associated with IBS. I believe it to be different from the proctitis of inflammatory bowel disease; to me these patients have a proctitis which is part of their IBS rather than a limited form of ulcerative colitis with superimposed IBS. They are often labelled as suffering from ulcerative colitis and because of their symptoms they are deemed to have an aggressive form of that disease and consequently grossly over treated with cortico-steroids, and sometimes surgery is even contemplated. This diagnostic mix-up probably accounted in the past to the erroneous ascribing of severe abdominal pain and constipation together with certain personality traits to patients with ulcerative colitis confined to the rectum.

How may one recognise such patients?. They have all the hallmarks of IBS with superimposed episodes of bleeding per rectum. These bleeding episodes are almost always associated with episodes of constipation. On sigmoidoscopy there is a sharp cut off point(usually at 15cms sometimes at 22cms) between inflammed and normal mucosa. Biopsy of the inflammed mucosa does not show distortion or shortening of the glands and there is excess or normal rather than normal or diminished mucus. Despite severe symptoms these patients laboratory indices are normal apart from an occasional patient who has a low haemaglobin level; serum albumin, α_1 acid glycoprotein, C reactive protein, ESR and platelet count all remain normal-excluding symptomatic inflammatory bowel disease.

A proper attention to history and examination lessens the liklihood of missing this important clinical entity.

REFERENCES

Fielding, J.F. (1977(a)). The irritable bowel syndrome: An historical view. Jour Irish Colls Phys Surgs 6, 133-140.
Fielding J.F. (1977(b)). The irritable bowel syndrome. Clinical Spectrum. In Clinics in Gastroenterology: The GI tract in Stress and Psychosocial Disorder. T.P. Almy and J.F. Fielding Eds. London Saunders pp 607-622.
Fielding J.F. (1977(c)) A year in out-patients with the irritable bowel syndrome. Irish Jour Med Sci 146, 162-166.
Fielding,J.F. (1982) The Irritable Colon Syndrome. Acta Gastro-ent Belg 45,477-484.
Fielding, J.F. (1983(a)) Detailed history and examination assist positive clinical diagnosis of the Irritable Bowel Syndrome. J Clin Gastroenterol 5, 495-497.
Fielding, J.F. (1983(b)) Surgery and the Irritable Bowel Syndrome: The Singer as well as the Song. Irish Med Jour 76,33-34.
Fielding, J.F. (1984) The Irritable Bowel Syndromes. Acta Gastro-ent Belg 47, 64-66.
Fielding, J.F. and Regan R (1984). Excessive Cold Pressor Responses in the Irritable Bowel Syndrome. Irish Jour Med Sci 153,348-350.

Hormone levels and personality in individuals with functional disorders of the gastrointestinal tract

Kerstin Uvnäs-Moberg

Department of Pharmacology, Karolinska Institute, S-104 01 Stockholm, Sweden

ABSTRACT

The aim of the present study was to investigate whether individuals with functional disorders of the gastrointestinal tract had a hormonal pattern and a personality pattern that differed from controls. 27 individuals having received a diagnosis of nonulcer dyspepsia (NUD) and/or irritable bowel syndrome (IBS) at a primary health care centre were included in the study. 24 blood samples were drawn during an experiment in which various provocations such as a friendly greeting, a light meal and a stressful conversation were performed. Gastrin, somatostatin and oxytocin levels were measured with radioimmunoassay. The subjects' personality profile was described with personality inventories such as the Karolinska Scales of Personality and the Bergman Scale and their symptom levels were scored.

Basal gastrin and in particular somatostatin levels were significantly higher in the patients whereas oxytocin levels were lower than in controls. In addition, a different reaction pattern in response to the provocation tests was seen. Gastrin and oxytocin levels correlated positively and somatostatin negatively with the level of reported symptoms.

In the KSP scales the patients were found to score higher in two anxiety items (somatic anxiety and muscular tension) and lower in socialization. Interestingly, gastrin levels correlated significantly and positively with the scores of the anxiety items discussed above and inversely with socialization. Somatostatin levels correlated inversely with social dependence (Bergman) and psychic anxiety (KSP) and positively with self-confidence. An opposite correlation pattern was seen in the case of oxytocin.

In conclusion, we have found that individuals with NUD and IBS seem to be a heterogeneous group with regard to the levels of gastrointestinal hormones. One subgroup of individuals has high gastrin levels and a second one has high somatostatin levels. Furthermore, the peptides seem to be associated with different personality profiles.

INTRODUCTION

Individuals with peptic ulcer disease have been shown to have certain physiological as well as psychological characteristics. As a group, they have an elevated vagal tone as reflected by e.g. an increased rate of HCl secretion, by an exaggerated gastrin response to feeding etc. (Uvnäs-Moberg, 1987). Weiner et al. (1957) reported that young men that developed peptic ulcer when draughted into the army were not only hypersecretors of gastric acid as evidenced by elevated levels of serum pepsinogen, they also had a psyche characterized by dependence and great demands for care and nurturance.

Little is known about possible physiological and psychological traits characteristics of individuals having nonulcer dyspepsia (NUD) or irritable bowel syndrome (IBS), However, they were recently found to have elevated levels of gastrin during basal conditions (Nyrén et al., 1986). The present study was undertaken in order to show whether a group of patients having received a diagnosis of NUD or IBS had any physiological and psychological characteristics. Therefore a large number of hormones was measured in patients as well as in controls during basal conditions and following provocations aimed at influencing the activity of the autonomic nervous system. The personality profile of the patients was determined with established personality inventories such as the Karolinska Scales of Personality and the Bergman scale. In this paper gastrin, somatostatin and oxytocin levels will be discussed and their relation to symptom levels and to the scores obtained in the various dimensions of the personality inventories. A more detailed description of the results is given in three original papers (Arn et al., 1989; Uvnäs-Moberg et al., 1989a, b).

MATERIAL AND METHODS

The patients were recruited from the patient register in one of the primary health care centres in the southern suburbs of Stockholm. 27 patients who had received a diagnos of nonulcer dyspepsia (NUD) or irritable bowel syndrome (IBS) were included in the study. Gastroscopy or X-ray examination was not performed routinely. Such examinations were performed when needed as revealed by a thorough medical history. Patients with cancer, ulcer, advanced alcohol abuse or who were not speaking Swedish were excluded from the study. The patients, 20 females and 7 males, were 40 (range 21-55) and 50 (range 40-59) years of age. (10 individuals of the same age and with a similar sex distribution but without gastrointestinal symptoms served as a control group). At the time of the study, no patients were on drugs such as anticholinergic agents, which might influence the symptom level or hormonal secretion rate.

Patients and controls had group therapy (10 sessions in 3 months) with the same group therapist. In both groups of patients, the aim of the therapy was a better understanding of symptoms and the psychological background of the disease.

The intensity of the symptoms was evaluated by means of a self-administered questionnaire before, 3 months and 3 years after therapy. Gastrointestinal symptoms were recorded by means of a list of 13 symptoms from the upper and lower abdomen. For each symptom, the subject was asked whether he/she had had the symptom during the last 3 months and, if so, how often. For each symptom, a five-graded response was to be given ranging from "never" = 0 to "almost always, sometimes even at night" = 4. All these symptom items were added to one another. This resulted in a total score which could range from 0-52. In addition, separate scores for abdominal and intestinal complaints were formed.

The effects of therapy on the patients is reported in another paper. In short, the symptom level decreased immediately after therapy but had returned to pretherapy levels after 3 years (Arn et al., 1989).

Three years after group therapy, patients were subjected to a blood sampling experiment.

Experimental protocol

On the day of experiment, the patients were allowed to eat a light lunch at 12 o'clock. The patients came to the medical ward at 5 o'clock p.m. and an indwelling cannula was inserted into an antecubital vein to allow sampling of blood. Blood samples were collected by a nurse who stayed with the patients during the entire experimental period. After 15 min, 5 blood samples were drawn with 1 min intervals. Then the group therapist entered the room, greeted the patient and talked to him/her about a neutral subject, while 5 new samples were drawn with 1 min intervals. The group therapist left the room and reentered within 20 min. Just before reentering, 2 blood samples were drawn with 1 min intervals. After entering, 5 blood samples were drawn when the patient received a snack consisting of juice and a piece of chocolate (food stimulus). The group therapist entered a third time after another 20 min and now the therapist started to discuss a subject known to be a problem with the patient (stress stimulus), while 5 blood samples were drawn with 1 min intervals.

24 blood samples of 5 ml were drawn into ice-chilled tubes containing heparin (10 IU ml^{-1}) and Trasylol (500 IU ml^{-1}). The samples were centrifuged and plasma was taken off and frozen for later analyses of gastrin, somatostatin and oxytocin. All the determinations were performed by radioimmunoassays as described earlier. Somatostatin and oxytocin determinations were performed after prior SEP-PAK purification of the plasma samples (Nilsson, 1975; Efendic et al., 1980; Stock and Uvnäs-Moberg, 1988).

Gastrin, somatostatin and oxytocin levels were approximately normally distributed and therefore no logarithmic transformations were performed.

First of all, for each occasion and endocrine parameter during the provocation test, patients and control persons were compared using an unpaired two-tailed t-test. Secondly, using individuals who had valid observations for all occasions during the provocation test, a two-way analyses of variance (mixed model) was performed for each parameter. The two-way analyses of variance tests show whether there are significant differences in average level between the two groups during all the observations, whether the different stimuli cause significant effects within the experiment and finally whether these effects differ between the two groups (two-way interaction).

Mean values of samples 1-24 were formed for each hormone and individual in the patient group.

Relationships between the mean hormone levels described above and scores of symptoms total as well as abdominal and intestinal obtained before, 3 months and 3 years after therapy were calculated using the Pearson correlation coefficient.

Determination of personality traits were studied by means of the Karolinska Scales of Personality (KSP) which is an inventory by Schalling and coworkers, consisting of several self-report scales. The KSP scales have been grouped into three main groups; 1) Anxiety proneness scales. The Psychic anxiety scale concerns cognitive-social anxiety and insecurity, worrying and having slow recovery after stress. Psychiatric and psychosomatic patients have consistently higher scores than controls. The Somatic anxiety concerns self-reported autonomic disturbances, diffuse distress and panic attacks. The Muscular tension scale concerns subjective muscular tenseness and aches and difficulty in relaxing. 2) Extraversion-related scales. Two of the scales, Impulsiveness and Monotony avoidance, represent extraversion-related dimensions. 3) Aggression-Hostility scales. The subscales Indirect aggression (undirected expressive aggression, e.g. slamming doors), the Irritability (readiness to explode with negative affect at the slightest provocation, feelings of irritation) and Verbal aggression (aggressive feelings expressed in style and content of speech) form a composite scale for Aggression. The subscales Suspicion (being distrustful, projecting hostility on others) and Guilt (feelings of remorse and shame) form a composite scale for Hostility. Remaining scales. The Psychasthenia ('subvalidity') scale comprises items, implying a low degree of mental 'energy' and difficulty to compensate for energy consumption. The Detachment 'superstability' scale is related to schizoid traits such as needs for distance to other people. The Inhibition of aggression scale comprised items from Assertiveness training scales and refers to unexpressed anger and lack of ability to speak up and assert oneself in social situations. Finally, the Socialization scale has been adapted from a Swedish translation and psychometric analyses of the CPI Socialization scale. The KSP items have a four point response format. Most scales consist of ten items. Exceptions are the Socialization (20 items) and Aggression scales (15 items). The items explicitly refer to habitual behaviour or feelings (Björvell et al., 1985).

In addition, some of the items from the Bergman scale, reflecting the levels of social dependence and self-confidence were filled in by the patients before and after therapy.

RESULTS

<u>Hormone levels</u>
Gastrin levels tended to be higher in patients than in controls ($p=0.11$, Anova) and several individual time points obtained during the first and the second provocations were significantly different on the 10% confidence level. Significant changes of gastrin levels occurred during the experiment in both the patients and controls. Thus, gastrin levels were higher in the beginning of the experiments and rose again towards the end of the experiment in response to the stress stimulus ($p<0.0001$, Anova) (Fig. 1).

Somatostatin levels were significantly higher in patients than in controls in the beginning of the experiment and in response to the food stimulus. In addition, the effect caused by the provocations on somatostatin levels differed significantly between patients and controls ($p<0.01$, Anova). Thus, controls decreased their somatostatin levels, whereas in patients small rises of somatostatin levels were seen in response to the stimuli (Fig. 1).

Oxytocin levels were lower in patients than in controls ($p<0.05$, Anova) although the response pattern did not differ between the two groups (Fig. 1). Women had significantly higher oxytocin levels than men ($p<0.01$).

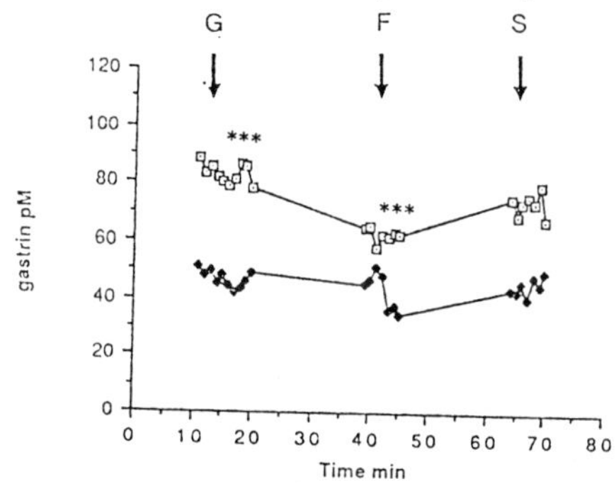

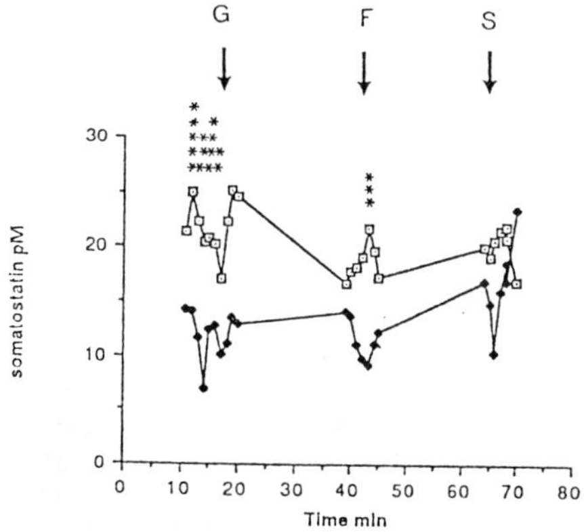

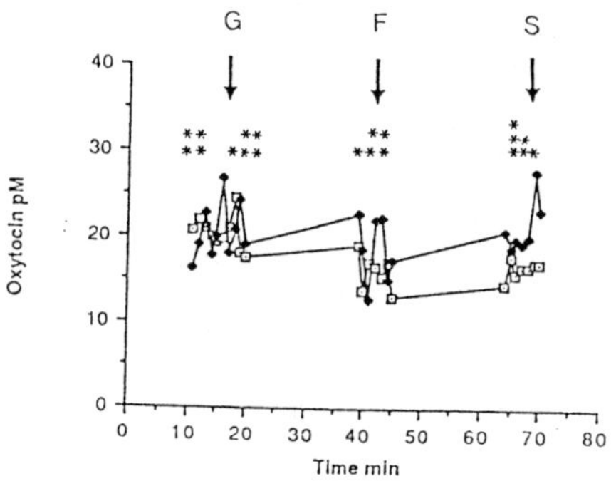

<u>Fig. 1</u>.
Gastrin, somatostatin and oxytocin levels during the provocation experiment in patients (□—□) and controls (◆—◆). G, F and S denote the timing of the friendly greeting, the food and the stress stimulus, respectively. * $p<0.1$, ** $p<0.05$, *** $p<0.01$, **** $p<0.001$, ***** $p<0.0001$.

When individual patients were studied, very different response patterns were seen. In Fig. 2 one patient who reacts with clearcut rises of gastrin levels in response to the initial greeting and to the stress stimulus - but not in response to the food stimulus - is illustrated.

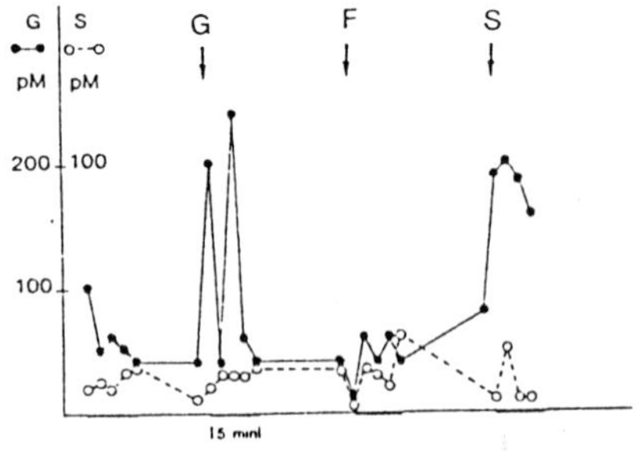

Fig. 2.
Gastrin and somatostatin levels during the provocation experiment in one individual. G, F and S denote the timing of the friendly greeting, the food and the stress stimulus, respectively.

Correlation between hormone levels and symptom scores
Immediately after therapy, gastrin and oxytocin levels correlated positively with symptom levels (total as well as abdominal and intestinal). In contrast, negative correlations between symptom scores and somatostatin levels were seen (Table 1).

Table 1. Correlation coefficients hormone/symptom level.

	Symptom level total	intestinal	abdominal
Gastrin	0.52 ***	0.38	0.20
Somatostatin	-0.22	-0.53 **	0.15
Oxytocin	0.27	0.35	0.12

** $p<0.05$, *** $p<0.01$

Personality inventories
The whole group of individuals scored significantly higher in some anxiety variables such as somatic anxiety ($p<0.05$) and muscular tension ($p<0.05$) than a reference group and significantly lower in socialization ($p<0.001$) in the Karolinska Scales of Personality. No difference between patients and a reference group was found in the Bergman scale.
Gastrin levels correlated positively with socialization R=-0.49 ($p<0.05$) in the whole group and R=-0.69 ($p<0.01$) in women alone. In the group of women alone, significant correlations were obtained with somatic anxiety R=0.57 ($p<0.05$), muscular tension R=0.51 ($p<0.05$) and self-confidence R=-0.57 ($p<0.01$).
Somatostatin levels correlated negatively with psychic anxiety R=-0.58 ($p<0.05$), guilt R=-0.595 ($p<0.05$) and social dependence R=-0.62 ($p<0.01$) and positively with self-confidence R=0.73 ($p<0.001$).

Oxytocin levels correlated with psychic anxiety R=0.66 ($p<0.05$), indirect aggression R=0.86 ($p<0.001$), verbal aggression R=0.72

$p<0.01$), guilt $R=0.77$ ($p<0.01$), social dependence $R=0.77$ ($p<0.00$).

DISCUSSION

In the present study 27 patients, having received a diagnosis of nonulcer dyspepsia (NUD) and/or the irritable bowel syndrome (IBS) at a primary health care centre, participated. However, when reporting symptom levels in the questionnaire, it was found that most individuals had both abdominal and intestinal symptoms irrespective of the diagnosis received, suggesting that the two diseases may represent variants of the same functional disease.

In a recent study, basal gastrin levels were found to be higher in NUD patients than in healthy controls (Nyrén et al., 1986), which is in agreement with the finding of elevated gastrin levels in our patient group. Additional aberrations of basal hormone levels were found in our study (Uvnäs-Moberg et al., 1989 a), some of which will be discussed below. Thus basal gastrin and somatostatin levels were significantly higher in patients than in controls and oxytocin levels were lower.

The mechanism behind the elevated gastrin levels can only be speculated upon. Duodenal ulcer patients known to have an enhanced vagal tone have a different gastrin profile with normal basal gastrin levels and elevated levels in response to feeding (Uvnäs-Moberg, 1987). Some studies indicate a very close relationship between an individual's gastric acid secretory capacity and plasma gastrin levels, individuals with atrophic gastritis forming an extreme group with very high gastrin levels. Acid secretory capacity was not measured in our patients, but the most likely explanation to the high gastrin levels observed ought to be a low rate of acid production due to a low vagal nerve tone or to a reduced capacity for production of HCl in the parietal cells.

Somatostatin in the circulation derives from the gastrointestinal tract. It inhibits gastrointestinal secretion and motility. The release of the peptide is controlled by intragastric factors such as food constitutents and pH and by nervous mechanisms. Since somatostatin secretion is inhibited by vagal nerve activation and stimulated by the sympathetic nervous system, basal levels of somatostatin represent a net effect of vagal and sympathetic nervous tone (Uvnäs-Moberg, 1987). If so, the data would indicate that our patient group having higher somatostatin levels than the control group has an elevated sympathetic nervous tone.

The individuals having high gastrin and somatostatin levels, respectively, did not appear to be the same ones since gastrin and somatostatin levels did not correlate, supporting the assumption that different mechanisms lie behind the hypersecretion of the respective hormones.

It can of course not be excluded that a disturbed gastric motility and rate of gastric emptying shown to be present in NUD and IBS patients may also contribute to differences in gastrin and somatostatin levels between patients and controls.

Oxytocin is produced in neurons of the paraventricular and

supraoptical nuclei of the hypothalamus. Axons project to the neurohypophysis from which it is secreted into the circulation and to many brain regions including the autonomic centra in the brain stem (Sawchenko, 1983). Oxytocin is responsible for milk ejection during lactation and also for certain components of maternal behavior as well as in the bonding occurring between mother and infant (Numan, 1988). The reason for measuring oxytocin levels in the present study was that an inverse relationship between plasma levels of oxytocin and somatostatin has been shown to occur in previous studies. Thus, individuals with low somatostatin levels tend to have high oxytocin levels and vice versa (Uvnäs-Moberg, 1989). The mechanism behind the relationship could be that oxytocinergic neurons projecting from the paraventricular nucleus to the vagal motor nuclei stimulate efferent vagal nerve activity. Consequently, when the activity of the hypothalamic oxytocin neurons are high, elevated circulating levels of oxytocin may be seen together with low somatostatin levels as a reflection of a high vagal nerve tone since oxytocin is released in parallel into the brain and into the circulation (Kendrick et al., 1988). The fact that the sick individuals as a group had significantly lower oxytocin levels than controls is therefore consistent with the suggestion that the patients have low vagal tone and a high sympathetic nervous tone.

Both patients and controls were exposed to three provocations aimed at influencing the activity of the autonomic nervous system. Gastrin and somatostatin levels but not oxytocin levels were significantly influenced by the food and the stress stimuli. In the case of somatostatin, different effects were seen in patients and controls. Thus, somatostatin levels increased in the former group and decreased in the latter. Since somatostatin levels decrease in response to vagal stimulation, controls may have reacted with a more parasympathetic type of response than did the sick individuals - an interpretation which is in line with the assumption that patients have high basal somatostatin levels due to an increased sympathetic tone. However, it is of importance to mention that the variation in the response patterns between individuals was considerable.

The influence on hormone levels caused by the provocations is interesting from another point of view. Since similar in vivo situations occur repeatedly during day-time, the levels of the above-mentioned peptides fluctuate also in between meals. Since gastrin and somatostatin influence gastrointestinal motility and secretion, the abnormal hormonal reaction pattern seen in the patients could hypothetically together with other neuroendocrine factors be related to their gastrointestinal symptoms. But since average gastrin and oxytocin levels correlated positively and somatostatin levels negatively with the symptom scores total as well as abdominal and intestinal, there seemed to be no clear association between a specific hormone and abdominal or intestinal symptoms.

When the personality of the patients included in the study was assessed by means of the personality inventory KSP, they were found to score higher in certain anxiety dimensions and lower in socialization than a reference group.

In addition, the scores obtained in some of the personality

dimensions were found to correlate with hormone levels measured in the patients. We are aware that the meaning of correlations may be difficult to interpret. It should be stated that the relationships discussed here have been further validated by statistical methods described elsewhere (Uvnäs-Moberg et al., 1989b). Furthermore, it may be of interest to mention that other hormones which were also measured in the study, e.g. insulin, glucagon, prolactin and VIP, showed absolutely no correlations with the scores of the personality dimensions.

In the present material gastrin levels correlated with the scores of somatic anxiety and muscular tension of the KSP scale and an inverse correlation between gastrin levels and the KSP dimension socialization was found. Since gastrin and anxiety levels were higher and the level of socialization lower in our patients than in a reference group, there appears to be a subgroup of individuals characterized by abnormally high gastrin levels, high levels of anxiety and low levels of socialization in our group of patients.

Somatostatin correlated inversely with the personality dimensions psychic anxiety, guilt and social dependence and positively with self-confidence. Thus, the person having low somatostatin levels appears to be an anxious, dependent individual with a low self-confidence, perhaps a personality related to the one described by Weiner et al. (1957) characterized by dependence and vagal hyperactivity as reflected by high plasma levels of serum-pepsinogen.

Since oxytocin is a widely distributed brain peptide which is released in parallel to the brain and the circulation (Kendrick et al., 1988), the relationship seen between oxytocin and the above described psychological dimensions could be caused by oxytocin influencing neurotransmission in the brain. As described above, oxytocin is related to maternal behavior (Numan, 1988) and therefore the relationship with social dependence is particularly interesting since this could be a personality trait related to maternal characteristics such as caring, interaction and bonding. Interestingly, oxytocin correlated with the same personality items as did somatostatin but in the opposite direction. It is likely that the correlations with somatostatin are indirect reflecting the inverse relationship between oxytocin and somatostatin levels described above.

The data discussed above indicate that certain psychological and physiological characteristics occur together and that these combinations of certain psychological traits and physiological characteristics are small reflections of some 'life strategy' patterns? Such patterns could be inborn or imprinted early in life. One such pattern the 'archetypal mother', having a caring and dependent personality and a soma adapted for nutrient assimilation and growth, hormonally characterized by high oxytocin and low somatostatin levels, has described elsewhere (Uvnäs-Moberg, 1989).

REFERENCES

Arn, I., Theorell, T., Uvnäs-Moberg, K., and Johnsson, C.-O. (1989): Psychodrama group therapy for patients with functional gastrointestinal disorders- a controlled long-term follow up study. J. Psychosom. Res. (Submitted).

Björwell, H., Edman, G., Rössner, S., and Schalling, D. (1985): Personality traits in a group of severely obese patients: a study of patients in two self-chosen weight reducing programs. Int. J. Ibes. 9: 257-266.

Efendic, S., Enzman, F., Nylén, A., Uvnäs-Wallensten, K., and Luft, R. (1980): Sulphonylurea (Glibenclamide) enhances somatostatin and inhibits glucagon release induced by arginine. Acta Physiol. Scand. 108: 231-233.

Kendrick, K.M., Keverne, E.B., Chapman, C., and Baldwin, B.A. (1988): Microdialysis measurement of oxytocin, aspartate, gamma-aminobutyric acid and glutamate release from the olfactory bulb of the sheep during vaginocervical stimulation. Brain Res. 442: 171-174.

Nilsson, G. (1975): Increased plasma gastrin levels in connection with inhibition of gastric acid in response to sham feeding following bulbar perfusion with acid in dogs. Scand. J. Gastroenterol. 10: 273-277.

Numan, M. (1988): Maternal behaviour. In The Physiology of Reproduction, eds E. Knobil, J. Neill et al., pp. 1569-1644. New York: Raven Press Ltd.

Nyrén, O., Adami, H.-O., Bergström, R., Gustavsson, S., Lööf, L., and Lundqvist, G. (1986): Basal and food-stimulated levels of gastrin and pancreatic polypeptide in non-ulcer dyspepsia and duodenal ulcer. Scand. J. Gastroenterol. 21: 471-477.

Sawchenko, P.E. (1983): Central connections of the sensory and motor nuclei of the vagus nerve. In Vagal Nerve Function: Behavioral and Methodological Considerations, eds J.G. Kral, T.L. Powley & C.McC. Brooks, pp. 13-26. Elsevier Science Publishers B.V.

Stock, S., and Uvnäs-Moberg, K. (1988): Increased plasma levels of oxytocin in response to afferent electrical stimulation of the sciatic and vagal nerves and in response to touch and pinch in anaesthetized rats. Acta Physiol. Scand. 132: 29-34.

Uvnäs-Moberg, K. (1987): Gastrointestinal hormones and pathophysiology of functional gastrointestinal disorder. Scand. J. Gastroenterol. 22 (suppl. 128): 138-146.

Uvnäs-Moberg, K. (1989): Neuroendocrine regulation of hunger and satiety. In Obesity in Europe: I, eds P. Björntorp and S. Rössner, pp. 1-13. London: John Libbey & Company Ltd.

Uvnäs-Moberg, K., Arn, I., Jonsson, C.O., and Theorell, T. (1989a): Gastrin, somatostatin and VIP levels in patients with functional disorders of the gastrointestinal tract. Scand. J. Gastroenterol. (Submitted).

Uvnäs-Moberg, K., Arn, I., Jonsson, C.O., and Theorell, T. (1989b): Personality traits in a group of individuals with functional disorders of the gastrointestinal tract - and their correlations with gastrin, somatostatin and oxytocin levels. J. Psychosom. Med. (Submitted).

Weiner, H., Thaler, M., Reiser, M.F., and Mirsky, I.A. (1957): Etiology of duodenal ulcer. I. Relation of specific psychological characteristics to rate of gastric secretion (serum pepsinogen). Psychosom. Med. XIX: 1-10.

Constipation, anxiety and personality : what comes first ?

Ghislain Devroede, Michel Bouchoucha, Gilles Girard

Départements de chirurgie et de psychologie, Faculté de Médecine, Université de Sherbrooke, Québec, Canada; Département de physiologie, CHU Necker, Paris, France

The term "chronic idiopathic constipation" is used when no organic disease is found in constipated people. Colonic inertia and constipation by delayed colonic transit are two underlying mechanisms, where the transit of radiopaque markers is delayed in the ascending colon. In the first situation, this is due to a lack of contractile activity in the bowel. In the second, it is due to distal excessive activity of the colon, as evidenced by back and forth movement of the markers from right to left colon. Patients affected by one of these two motor dysfunctions also have motor abnormalities in the esophagus and bladder. Other abnormalities such as idiopathic galactorrhea, migraine headaches, and orthostatic dizziness point out to a systemic disorder(5). In the present study, an attempt was made to see if the functional symptoms could be considered as body clues, reflecting emotional overload.

METHODS AND RESULTS

We have compared the personality of severely constipated patients to that of arthritic subjects, two groups of chronic pain sufferers. All personality data have been compared to a background of normal subjects. A sample of 90 female subjects seen consecutively, was divided into four different groups: 19 patients with constipation by delayed colonic transit, 19 with constipation by colonic inertia, 29 with rheumatoid arthritis and 23 with degenerative arthritis. Segmental large bowel transit time (1) was measured in constipated patients, who were selected, if extensive clinical assessment had failed to uncover an organic disorder, and if they had failed to respond to a high residue diet, ingested for at least one month. The personality of patients was measured with the Minnesota Multiphasic Personality Inventory (MMPI). T scores with K corrections are used throughout the text. Results are expressed with regards to the normal range in a healthy population.

Constipated women were found to have significantly higher scores on the Hypochondria (Hs), Hysteria (Hy), (Figure 1)

PERSONALITY OF WOMEN WITH CONSTIPATION AND ARTHRITIS ($\bar{X} \pm SE$)

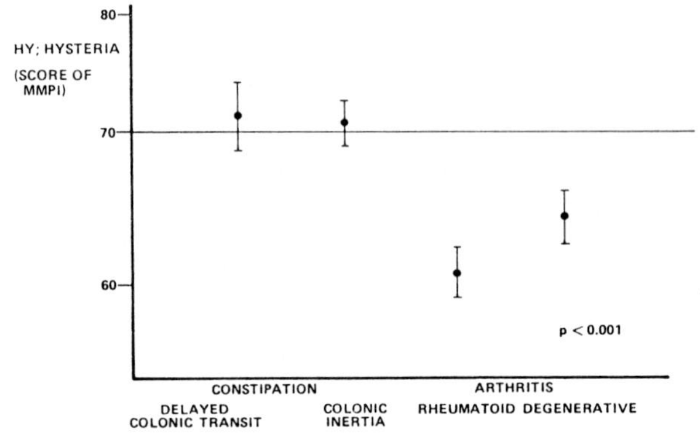

Control (CN) and Low Back Pain (LB) scales and a lower score on the Masculinity - Femininity (MF) scale ($p < 0.001$). Hypochondria and Hysteria scores are greater than the score of Depression in constipation, giving a "V" configuration to the first three scales. This was not so in arthritis ($p < 0.01$). Discriminant analysis permitted to sort out constipated from arthritic patients in 83% of cases, relating only to the personality data. Constipation begins usually at a slightly younger age than arthritis. If discriminant analysis was performed with the MMPI data and age, the computer recognized correctly 97% of the subjects as either constipated or arthritic: it erroneously made a diagnosis of constipation in 3 arthritic women (Figure 2).

DISCRIMINANT ANALYSIS OF CONSTIPATED AND ARTHRITIC WOMEN
(MMPI DATA AND AGE)

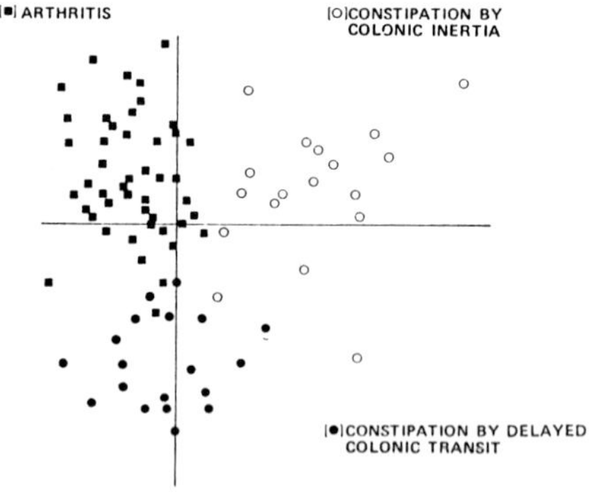

Details of the methodology and results are published elsewhere (2).

In women with constipation by delayed colonic transit, multiple regression analysis demonstrated a close link ($r=0.90$; $p < 0.001$) between transit time in the ascending colon and levels of anxiety, corrected for scales reflecting the self control of patients. The simple correlation between mean transit time and the anxiety/repression scores ratio is 0.75 ($p < 0.001$) and indicates that constipation is, in a way, a mirror of anxiety. Because of the multiplicity of variables, a simple correlation is meaningless. Yet, both the regression analysis and the partial correlations coefficients confirm the finding. Figure 3 shows a "skeleton" of personality, made of partial correlations. It confirms that transit time is really part of the personality of women with delayed colonic transit.

Principal component analysis is a statistical method which permits to recognize variables which are important to characterize a group. Variables are projected on the planes defined by the principal axes: the closer they are of one another, the more they are alike and correlated. The normalized variables are shown on a circle with a radius equal to 1. The more peripheric the variable, the more its importance in the constitution of the axis in terms of variance: this means that there is a wider spectrum in individual data for this given variable, than if it was close to the center. The analysis confirmed

PERSONALITY AND PHYSIOLOGIC CHARACTERISTICS OF CONSTIPATED WOMEN

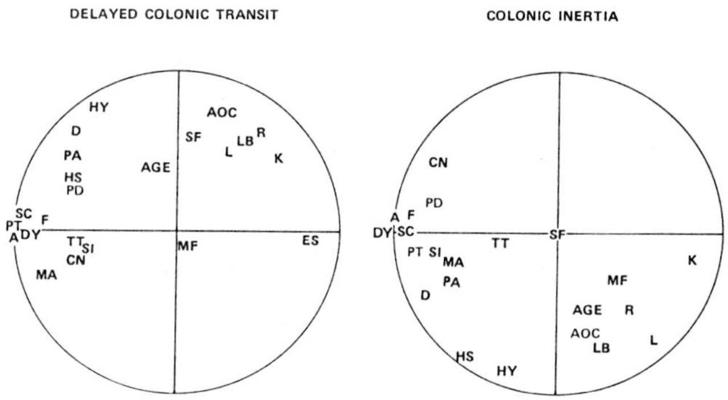

PERSONALITY STRUCTURE OF CONSTIPATED WOMEN (1)

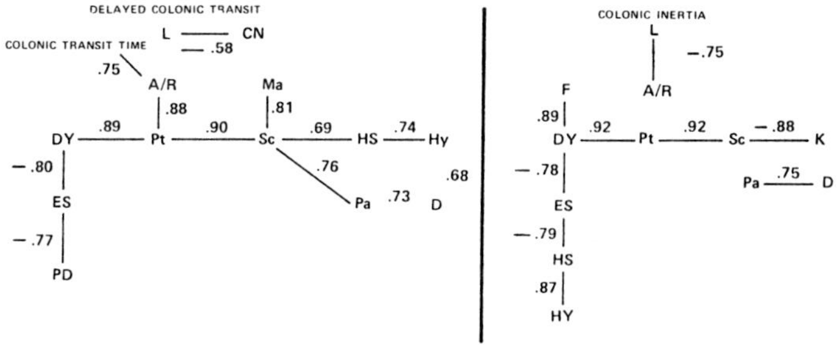

(1) ITEMS OF MMPI
A/R: RATIO OF ANXIETY/REPRESSION SCORE
ALL PARTIAL CORRELATION COEFFICIENTS ARE SIGNIFIANT AT THE $p < 0.001$ LEVEL

conclusions obtained from partial correlations and multiple regression analysis. In women with colonic inertia, mean ascending colon transit time stands relatively alone, irrespective to personality data, in contrast to subjects with constipation by delayed colonic transit (Figure 4).

DISCUSSION

This study demonstrates marked differences between the personality of constipated and arthritic women. The "V" shape configuration of the first three scales, in patients with constipation, is classically attributed to psychosomatic disorders. Some constipated patients may thus be prone to demonstrate psychophysiologic responses to life stresses. Said in simple terms, constipation protects patients from more free-floating anxiety and thus they are less depressed because they are constipated.

Does constipation induce personality changes? Is it the reverse? Do both reflect something else? This study cannot answer that question. However, preliminary studies have confirmed that during psychotherapy, colonic transit time accelerates (3,4). The following anecdote demonstrates that colonic transit time may normalize suddenly, while the change in personality occurs more slowly prior to cure. If more such reports could be produced, it would demonstrate that the type of personality described in this paper is not the consequence of constipation.

A CASE REPORT

Life of Martha

When she consulted at the age of 35 she only had a bowel movement every two months, and she told us at first visit that she was going to commit suicide if we did not cure her. She also said she had been raped by her father at the age of 16.

Her past medical history was heavy. She had been hospitalized at least once a year, each time from 1 to 30 days, for the past 10 previous years. She had undergone multiple abdominal operations, including a hysterectomy for functional problems, the specimen being normal. On two occasions, she had had evidence of self-inflicted injury, in the vagina and in the rectum.

Recorded stool frequency was indeed 1 per 1-2 months, despite the fact she was placed on a high fiber diet. A transit study of radiopaque markers provided objective evidence of the constipation (Figure 5).

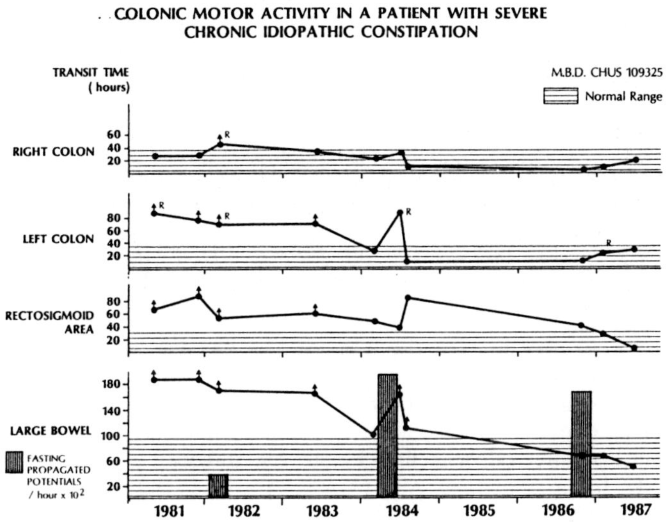

Electromyography of the colon showed little propagating electrical activity at rest (0.42 propagating potentials/hour), and no postprandial increase (0.50/hour), as normally expected.

A diagnosis of Munchhausen's syndrome with psychogenic constipation and depression, was made. Objective evidence of the depression was provided by an MMPI study (Minnesota Multiphasic Personality Inventory) (Figure 6).

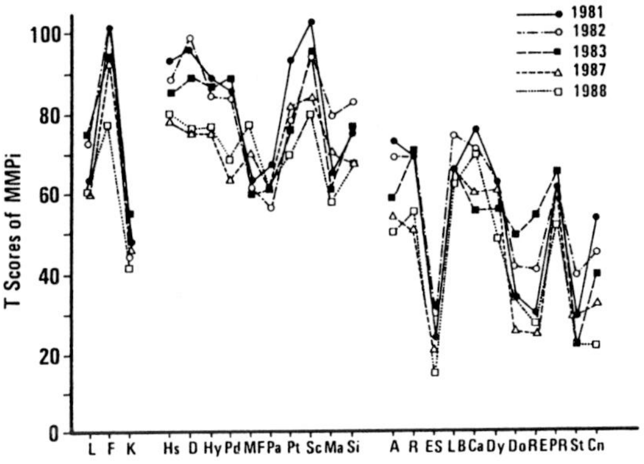

The constipation was managed symptomatically. She was given a lot of time and attention, and was seen 50 times, on an outpatient basis, between the 28 of March 1981 and the 28 of October 1986, at which time she reported normal bowel habits. During the follow-up, we learned that the rape by the father had been a sodomy. The change towards normal bowel habits occurred quite suddenly. When her father died in October 1986, she was encouraged to pursue her own idea to ventilate her rage at him. She did so by writing a six pages long letter which she placed in his suit, prior to the burial: change in bowel habits was instantaneous (Figure 5).

In December 1986, she recorded 26 stools over 34 days. There was a concomitant improvement in propagating electrical activity at rest.

There was also a marked improvement in the MMPI. Figure 6 shows the change from an almost psychotic depression to an anxiodepressive reaction. Improvement had occurred already before 1986, when constipation disappeared. Over the years, the scores on Hypochondriasis (Hs), Hysteria (Hy) and Control (CN) decreased progressively. In this particular situation, a high score on Depression (D) progressively diminished, so that by 1988, a "V" shape began to appear on the first three scales. Of note, the patient initially had a very poor self-esteem, and over the years the F scale (autodepreciation and/or distorted perception) progressively decreased in score.

CONCLUSION

Women with constipation of colonic origin have a different personality than arthritic women. In some subjects, constipation reflects repressed affect and they may be more prone to demonstrate psychophysiologic responses to life stresses than emotional responses.

BIBLIOGRAPHY

1- Arhan, P. et al., (1981): Segmental colonic transit time. Dis. Col. & Rectum 25, 625-629.
2- Devroede, G. (1989): Idiopathic constipation by colonic dysfunction: Relationship with personality and anxiety. Dig Dis Sci (in press).
3- Devroede, G. (1985): The irritable bowel syndrome: clinical and therapeutical aspects. In Small Intestinal and Colonic Motility, ed. P. Poitras, pp. 129-139. Montreal: Jouveinal Laboratories.
4- Devroede, G. (1985): La constipation: du symptôme à la personne. Psychologie Médicale 17, (10), 1515-1524.
5- Watier, A. et al., (1983): Constipation with colonic inertia: a manifestation of systemic disease. Dig Dis & Sci, 28, (1) 1025-1033.

2nd SESSION :

Experimental approach in humans

Moderators : *J. Malagelada, M. Wienbeck*

Disturbances of gastric myoelectrical and neuroendocrine activity and the stress of motion sickness

Kenneth L. Koch, M.D., Robert M. Stern, Ph.D., Timothy S. Harrison, John F. Seton and Lawrence M. Demers

From the Departments of Medicine, Pathology, Psychology and Surgery, The Pennsylvania State University, Hershey and University Park, Pennsylvania, U.S.A.

Vection is a central nervous system stimulus which produces visual - vestibular - proprioceptive neurosensory mismatch (Dichgans, 1973). The visual stimulus creates the illusion of self-motion, while simultaneous vestibular and proprioceptive sensory inputs to the central nervous system indicate the subject is not moving, a stressful situation producing nausea and other symptoms of motion sickness in healthy susceptible individuals. Thus, vection provides a novel and stressful environment for the study of nausea in man.

Nausea is often experienced as an unpleasant discomfort in the epigastrium. Thus, it is not surprising that stomach function is altered during the nausea accompanying motion sickness. Studies performed almost 50 years ago showed that gastric peristalsis and gastric tone diminished in subjects who developed nausea in response to parachute training exercises and other movement devices (Wolf, 1943; Mcdonough and Schneider, 1944).

Gastric peristalses are coordinated normally by gastric slow waves. Slow waves are produced by the spontaneous depolarizations of longitudinal muscle, outer circular muscle layers and/or interstial cells of Cajal along the greater curvature of the stomach near the juncture of fundus and body. The normal slow wave propagates circumferentially and migrates distally to the pyloris at a frequency of 3 cpm in man (Meyer, 1987).

Abnormal slow wave frequencies termed tachygastrias and bradygastrias have been recorded in patients with idiopathic nausea and vomiting (You et al, 1980; You et al, 1983). Normal 3 cpm gastric myoelectrical activity and gastric dysrhythmias are recorded accurately by mucosal, serosal and cutaneous electrodes (Smout et al, 1980; Abell and Malagelada, 1985; Hamilton et al, 1986). Gastric dysrhythmias are described in patients with chronic dyspepsia (Geldof et al, 1986), nausea of pregnancy (Koch et al, 1987), anorexia nervosa (Abell et al, 1987) and diabetes mellitus (Koch et al, 1986). Healthy subjects develop nausea and gastric dysrhythmias after glucagon infusions (Abell and Malagelada, 1985). We have reported previously that gastric dysrhythmias also develop in healthy subjects who report nausea and motion sickness during vection (Stern et al, 1987).

In the studies to be described below, we combined optokinetic stimuli which produces illusory self-motion or vection, electrogastrographic techniques which provide non-invasive measures of gastric myoelectrical activity and neuroendocrine assays in order to investigate gastric myoelectrical activity and neuroendocrine responses to vection-induced nausea in man.

METHODS

Subjects

Thirty-four healthy volunteers (19 men, 15 women, 22-39 years) were studied. Subjects had no histories of gastrointestinal, vestibular or central nervous system disorders.

Vection

Vection (illusory self-motion) was created by rotating a drum counterclockwise around the stationary, seated subject at a rate of 60 degrees per second. The inner surface of the drug was painted with alternating black and white vertical stripes subtending 5.7 and 9.3 degrees, respectively. Descriptions of the drum have been published previously (Stern et al, 1985). The subjects sat upright with the head supported by a chin rest and positioned in the center of the drum.

Electrogastrography

Miniature Skin Electrodes (SensorMedics Corp., Anaheim CA) were positioned on the abdomen of the subjects to record the electrogastrogram. Three electrodes were placed in the left upper quadrant and epigastric regions. The fourth electrode served as a reference electrode and was positioned in the right upper quadrant along the line formed by the other three electrodes. The electrodes were connected to a rectilinear recorder (R611, SensorMedics) through direct nystagmus couplers (9859, SensorMedics). The low frequency cutoff was 0.016 Hz (time constant 10 sec) and the high frequency cut off was 0.30 Hz. The EGG signals were recorded simultaneously on magnetic tape (Honeywell 101, Honeywell Instruments, Denver CO) for computer analysis.

Neuroendocrine Studies

An indwelling venous catheter was placed in an antecubital vein and kept open with (1/10,000) heparin solution. The subjects reclined in a comfortable chair for 45-60 minutes after needle insertion and before beginning the protocol described below. Venous samples were placed in ice and centrifuged 20 minutes at 1500 rpm and 4 degrees Centigrade. Plasma was frozen at -20 degrees Centigrade and analyzed subsequently with standard and specific assays for norepinephrine, epinephrine, dopamine, cortisol, beta-endorphin, vasopressin and oxytocin.

Symptoms During Vection

Subjects reported spontaneously any symptoms during vection. Symptoms were recorded on the EGG chart paper; in addition, every two minutes inquiries were made concerning the subject's sense of well-being. Motion sickness was considered present if nausea was reported.

Design of Studies

The study comprised three 15 minute periods. Baseline - during which the subject sat in the drum; Drum Rotation - during which rotation of the drum produced illusory self-motion; and Recovery - during which the subject remained seated in the drum. Subjects were allowed to stop the drum at any time during drum rotation if symptoms became intolerable. Venous samples were obtained at the beginning and at the end of the 15 minute Baseline period (-15 minute and -1 minute) and in the Recovery period +1, +10 and +20 minutes after drum rotation had stopped. The -15 minute sample was drawn just before the subject entered the drum whereas the -1 minute sample was drawn while the subject sat within the drum and awaited the onset of drum rotation. Subjects fasted at least two hours before the protocol which began between noon and 2:00 p.m. No subject had been exposed previously to the vection stimulus.

Visual and Computer Analysis of EGG Signals

Three cpm EGG waves (2.5-3.5 cpm) were considered normal; 4-9 cpm waves were considered evidence of tachygastria. Visual inspection of the EGG recording was used to determine the predominant gastric rhythm. Computer analysis representing approximately 45 minutes of EGG signals recorded from each subject were compared with the visual interpretation of the EGG signal in order to confirm the predominant frequency peaks and to ascertain shifts in EGG frequency which were not appreciated by visual inspection. Computer analyses of EGG records utilized analog to digital transformation, Fourier analysis and running spectral analyses. Methods of computer analysis of EGG signals have been reported (Stern et al, 1987).

Statistical Analysis

Within group comparisons for neuroendocrine measures were carried out with ANOVA and Dunnett's tests and between group comparisons were performed by two way ANOVA and unpaired t tests where expected differences were anticipated. P values < 0.05 were considered significant.

RESULTS

Gastric Myoelectrical Responses to Vection

Fifteen subjects were symptom-free during vection and served as asymptomatic controls. Each of these subjects remained in a 3 cpm EGG rhythm during vection as shown in Figure 1. Figure 1 shows the EGG tracings from the three active electrodes recorded from a subject who experienced no symptoms during vection. During baseline clear 3 cpm EGG signals are seen and during vection and recovery the 3 cpm pattern remains stable, although more respiratory artifact is noted at a frequency of 18-19 per minute.

In contrast, nineteen subjects, nine men and ten women, developed gastric dysrhythmias, nausea and other symptoms of motion sickness such as sweating, headache and dizziness during vection. The average nausea score for the nineteen subjects was 210 and ranged from 61 to 300 with zero indicating no nausea and 300 indicating severe nausea, almost vomiting. Figure 2 shows the EGG recordings from a subject who developed nausea and tachygastria during vection. During baseline the normal 3 cpm EGG pattern is seen (EKG artifact is present also). After six minutes of vection, the subject reported nausea and the EGG waves were narrow-based with increased amplitude and frequency of approximately 6 cpm, i.e. tachygastria. Ten minutes into the recovery period, 3 cpm signals are beginning to be re-established and nausea was resolving.

Computer analysis of the entire 45 min EGG recording from another subject who developed tachygastria and motion sickness is shown in Figure 3. The running spectral analysis (RSA) shows the predominate baseline EGG rhythm is 3 cpm,

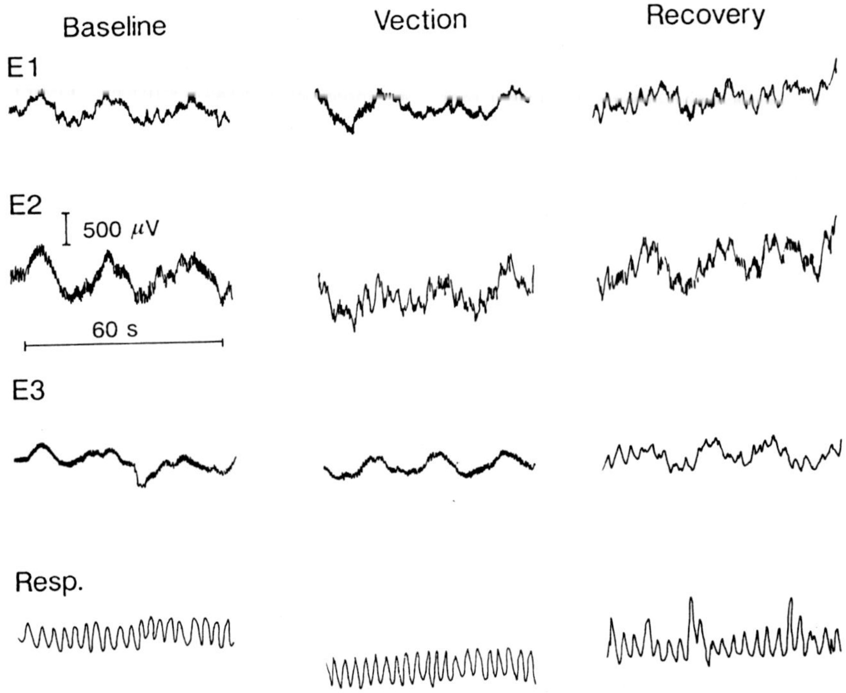

Fig. 1. Normal 3 cpm EGG signals recorded from subject who experienced no symptoms during vection.

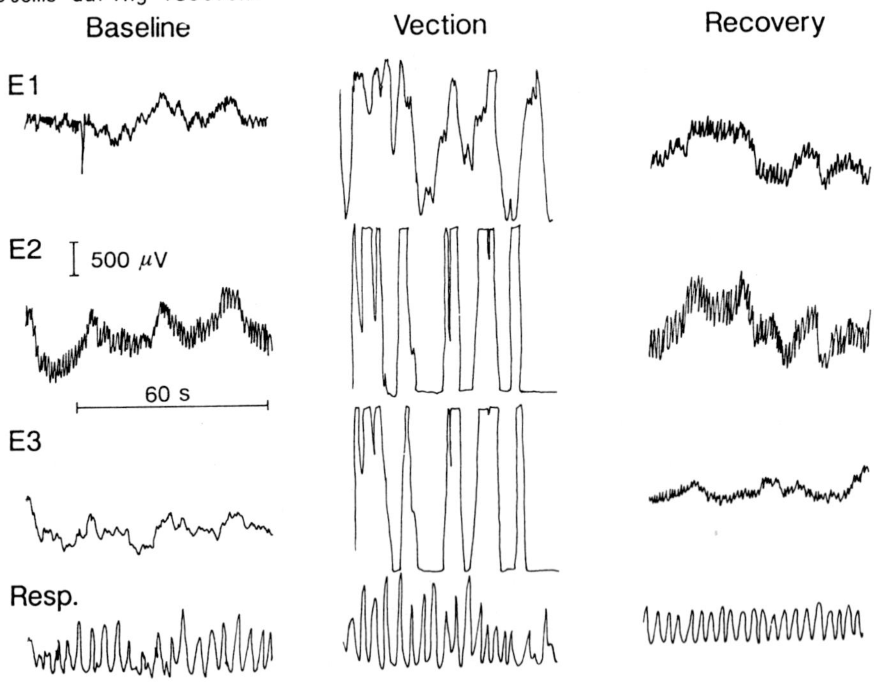

Fig. 2. Tachygastria in healthy subject with nausea during vection.

whereas after approximately five minutes of vection the 3 cpm peaks are lost abruptly and several peaks between 4 and 10 cpm appear in this subject who reported nausea. After the drum is turned off, the tachygastrias resolved, the nausea disappeared and by the end of the recovery period, 3 cpm peaks are re-established. The inserts show the actual EGG trace during these periods: the 3 cpm EGG signal at baseline; the 5-6 cpm tachygastria during vection-induced motion sickness and the re-establishment of 3 cpm rhythms at the end of recovery.

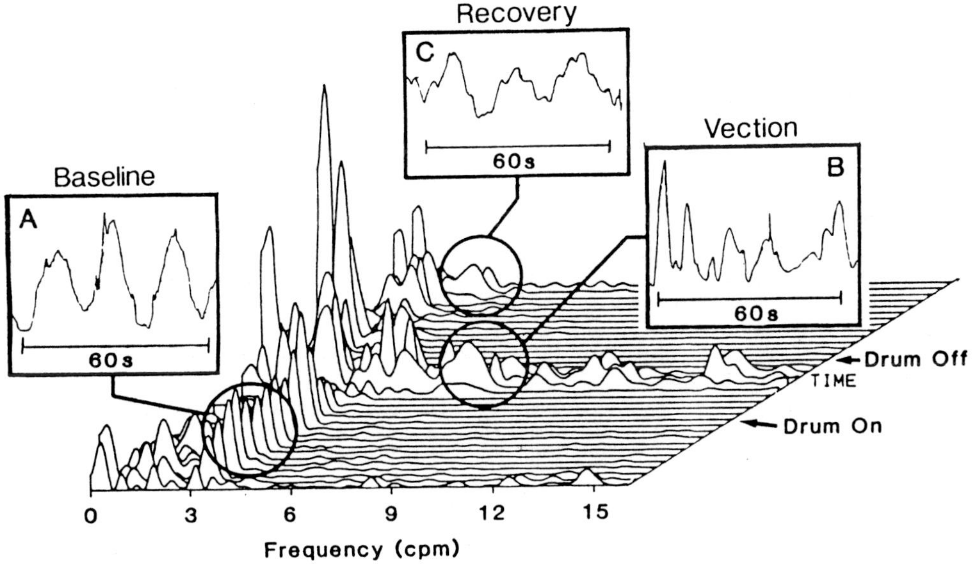

Fig. 3. Composite of computer analysis of EGG frequency and actual EGG recordings during baseline and vection-induced nausea and tachygastria in a healthy subject.

Neuroendocrine Responses to Vection

Cortisol levels at the -15 min baseline point were significantly greater in the subjects who developed tachygastrias and nausea compared with the subjects who remained symptom-free during vection (29.6 vs 14.9 mcg/dl, $P<0.01$). Cortisol responses in the two groups after vection were also significantly different at the +20 minute point in recovery (28.5 mcg/kg in the motion sickness group and 16.8 mcg/kg in asymptomatic subjects, $P<0.01$). Beta-endorphin levels also were significantly higher ($P<0.05$) in the subjects who would develop motion sickness at the -15 minute baseline and at the +10 and +20 minute points in the recovery period compared with the subjects who did not develop motion sickness.

There were no within or between group differences in the epinephrine, norepinephrine and dopamine levels obtained at the baseline periods before drum rotation. Norepinephrine increased significantly, however, in the subjects with nausea at +1 minute (a point when nausea and tachygastrias were present) compared with the subjects who remained in 3 cpm EGG rhythms and reported no motion sickness (354.6 pg/ml vs 223.1 pg/ml, P<0.01). Norepinephrine also rose transiently and significantly from baseline to +1 minute - (275.4 pg/ml to 354.6 pg/ml, P<0.05) in the motion sickness group.

Endogenous epinephrine levels increased significantly (P<0.05) throughout the recovery period in subjects with gastric dysrhythmias and motion sickness; in contrast, epinephrine levels in the subjects with no motion sickness were not elevated in the recovery period and did not differ significantly from baseline levels. Endogenous dopamine levels in subjects with nausea and without nausea did not change significantly in response to vection. Within group and between group comparisons revealed no differences in dopamine responses to vection.

Baseline vasopressin values prior to vection were similar and less than 6 pg/ml for all subjects. At +1 minute after vection stopped, however, vasopressin levels in subjects who became nauseated ranged from 5.9 pg/ml to 183.0 pg/ml and averaged 38.4 pg/ml, a significant increase (P<0.01) compared with baseline. The increase in plasma vasopressin at +1 minute occurred at a time when nausea and tachygastrias were present. Plasma vasopressin concentration decreased to baseline levels in the majority of nauseated subjects by 10 and 20 minutes after the drum stopped. In contrast, vasopressin levels were unchanged in the subjects who remained in 3 cpm gastric rhythms and who did not develop nausea. Finally, within group and between group comparisons showed no significant changes in oxytocin levels before or after vection.

DISCUSSION

Results of these studies reveal novel brain-gut interactions when healthy subjects are exposed to illusory self-motion, a central nervous system stimulus which produces neurosensory mismatch among visual-vestibular and proprioceptive systems. In subjects who find this stimulus stressful, as indicated by the development of sweating, epigastric distress and nausea, the normal 3 cpm baseline gastric myoelectrical rhythm is disrupted and gastric dysrhythmias develop. In contrast, subjects with no symptoms during vection maintain normal 3 cpm gastric rhythms. Thus, gastric dysrhythmias are objective physiological events which correlate with the presence of nausea and other upper gastrointestinal symptoms evoked during vection.

These studies also sought to investigate potential neuroendocrine systems which may play a role in the production of gastric dysrhythmias and symptoms of motion sickness. Results indicate that elevated baseline cortisol and beta-endorphin levels identified the subjects who would develop motion sickness and gastric dysrhythmias during vection. Since peripheral plasma cortisol levels reflect ACTH release and ACTH release is primarily controlled by CRF (Ney et al, 1963; Orth et al, 1983), these data suggest that the hypothalamic-pituitary-adrenal axis (HPA) is activated during baseline periods in those subjects who will become motion sick. The asymptomatic subjects, on the other hand, do not activate the HPA axis. Whether or not the increases in cortisol (and possibly ACTH and CRF) lower the gastric threshold for vection-induced gastric dysrhythmias requires further study.

One minute after drum rotation stopped, nausea and gastric dysrhythmias were present in those subjects who developed motion sickness during vection. Plasma samples drawn at this time point revealed elevations in epinephrine, norepinephrine and vasopressin in the symptomatic subjects. Increases in these neurohormones were significantly greater than levels in the asymptomatic subjects. Moreover, the increases in norepinephrine and vasopressin were transient, i.e. baseline levels were re-established by the 10 minute point after vection stopped. Thus, transient fluxes in norepinephrine and vasopressin may have had a role in the shift from normal 3 cpm rhythms to gastric dysrhythmias recorded during vection. These findings also indicate that vection affects hypothalamic vasopressinergic pathways in the symptomatic subjects. Vasopressin responses have been associated with nausea syndromes evoked by apomorphine (Feldman et al, 1988), chemotherapeutic agents (Fisher et al, 1982), and (paradoxically) ingestion of water (Rowe et al, 1979). Moreover, activation of hypothalamic-neurohyphophysis vasopressin responses were selective in that oxytocin release was not affected by the vection stimulus in either group of subjects.

Epinephrine remained elevated throughout the recovery period and cortisol and beta-endorphin levels increased significantly in the late recovery period. These findings may be interpreted as neuroendocrine responses to stresses which were experienced previously. We suggest that the stresses were the symptoms of motion sickness per se and not the experience of vection, because the asymptomatic subjects also experienced vection but did not activate vasopressinergic, sympathetic or HPA axis responses.

In summary, gastric dysrhythmias are evoked in healthy subjects who develop nausea during vection, but not in subjects who remain symptom free. The symptomatic group is also distinguished by anticipatory hypercortisolism, activation of the sympathomeduallary (epinephrine), sympatho-nonadrenal (norepinephrine) and hypothalmic-neurohyphophyseal (vasopressin) axes. Activation of these axes may have a role in the development of human gastric dysrhythmias and symptoms of nausea during vection.

REFERENCES

Abell T.L. & Malagelada, J-R. (1985): Glucagon-evoked gastric dysrhythmias in humans shown by an improved electrogastrographic technique. Gastroenterology 88, 1932-1940.

Abell, T.L., Malagelada, J-R., Lucasa, A.R. (1987): Gastric electromechanical and neurohormonal function in anorexia nervosa. Gastroenterology 93, 958-965.

Dichgans, J. & Brandt, T (1973): Optokinetic motion sickness and pseudocoriolis effects induced by moving visual stimuli. Acta Otolarying 76, 339-348.

Feldman, M., Samson, W.K., O'Dorisio, T.M. (1988): Apomorphine-induced nausea in humans: release of vasopressin and pancreatic polypeptide. Gastroenterology 95, 721-726.

Fisher, R.D., Rentschler, R.E., Nelson, J.C., Godfrey, T.E., Wilbur D.W. (1982): Elevation of plasma antidiuretic hormone (ADH) associated with chemotherapy-induced emesis in man. Can. Treat. Rep. 66, 25-29.

Geldof, H., van der Schee, E.J., van Blankenstein, M., Grashuis, J.L. (1986): Electrogastrographic study of gastric myoelectrical activity in patients with unexplained nausea and vomiting. Gut 27, 799-808.

Hamilton, J.W., Bellahsene, B.E., Reichelderfer, M., Webster, J.H., Bass, P. (1986): Human electrogastrograms. Comparison of surface and mucosal recordings. Dig. Dis. Sci. 31, 33-39.

Koch, K.L., Stern, R.M., Stewart, W.R., Dwyer, A.E. (1986): Effect of long-term domperidone therapy on gastric electromechanical activity in

symptomatic patients with diabetic gastroparesis. Gastroenterology 90 (Abstract), 1496.
Koch, K.L., Stern, R.M., Vasey, M.W., Dwyer, A. (1987): Gastric dysrhythmias and nausea of pregnancy. Dig. Dis. Sci. 32 (Abstract), 917.
Meyer, J.E. (1987): Motility of the stomach and gastroduodenal junction. In Physiology of the gastrointestinal tract, ed. L.R. Johnson, pp.393-410. New York: Raven Press.
Ney, R.L., Shimizu, N., Nicholson, W.E., Island, D.P., Liddle, G.W. (1963): Correlation of plasma ACTH concentration with adrenocortical response in normal human subjects, surgical patients and patients with Cushing's disease. J. Clin. Invest. 42, 1669-1677.
Orth, D.N., Jackson, R.V., DeCherney, G.S., DeBold, C.R., Alexander, A.N., Island, D.P., Rivier, J. (1983): Effect of synthetic ovine corticotrophin-releasing factor. Dose response of plasma adrenocorticotropin and cortisol. J. Clin. Invest. 71, 587-595.
Rowe, J.W., Shelton, R.L., Helderman, J.H., Vestal, R.E., Robertson, G.L. (1979): Influence of the emetic reflex on vasopressin release in man. Kidney Int. 16, 729-735.
Smout, A.J.P.M., van der Schee, E.J., Grashuis, J.L. (1980): What is measured in electrogastrography? Dig. Dis. Sci. 25, 170-187.
Stern, R.M., Koch, K.L., Leibowitz, H.W., Lindblad, M.S., Shupert, C.L., Stewart, W.R. (1985): Tachygastria and motion sickness. Aviat. Space Environ. Med. 56, 1074-1077.
Stern, R.M., Koch, K.L., Stewart, W.R., Lindblad, I.M. (1987): Spectral analysis of tachygastria recorded during motion sickness. Gastroenterology 92, 92-97.
Wolf, S. (1943): The relation of gastric function to nausea in man. J. Clin. Invest. 22, 877-882.
You, C.H., Lee, K.Y., Chey, W.Y. (1983): Gastric electromyography in normal and abnormal states in humans. In Functional disorders of the digestive tract, ed. W.Y. Chey, pp. 167-173. New York: Raven Press.
You, C.H., Lee, K.Y., Chey, W.Y., Menguy, R. (1980): Electrogastrographic study of patients with unexplained nausea, bloating and vomiting. Gastroenterology 79, 311-314.

The influence of psychological stress on esophageal motility

Ian J.S. Cook

Departments of Medicine and Gastroenterology, Royal Adelaide Hospital, North Terrace, Adelaide, South Australia

Behavioural factors and stress have been implicated in the expresion of symptoms arising from nearly every component of the gastrointestinal tract. In respect of the esophagus, an association between presumptive esophageal symptoms and behavioural abnormalities is clear. While psychogenic stimuli can elicit abnormal esophagal motor responses, it has not been established whether such responses are related causally to symptoms. The clinical impression that psychological factors are linked to esophageal dysmotility (Jacobsen, 1927) has only recently been examined rigorously using validated psychometric measures and well defined manometric criteria. Clouse and Lustman (1983) found, in patients referred for manometry, that 84 per cent of patients with dysmotility had psychiatric diagnoses compared to 31 per cent of those with normal motility. Richter et al (1986) found patients with non-cardiac chest pain and "nutcracker" esophagus to have a comparable psychological profile to patients with IBS. While these data establish an association between the potentially "stress-prone" individual and esophageal dysmotility, a causal link between psychogenic stress and esophageal symptoms remains speculative.

A critical analysis of the available evidence linking stress with symptoms must take into account the regional specialization within the esophagus based on functional differences. For the purpose of this review, the regions examined are the upper esophageal sphincter (UES), esophageal body and the lower esophageal sphincter (LES). The UES is a tonically contracted striated muscle under vagal control from the medulla. Tone within the UES is dependent on the level of arousal, being low during stable sleep or anaesthesia and rising sharply on waking. In healthy volunteers, a dichotic listening task markedly augments resting UES pressure and the magnitude of this response correlates with extraintestinal measures of the stress response (Cook et al, 1987). On the basis of earlier studies in patients with globus sensation, it was believed that these patients demonstrate increased basal UES tone (Watson & Sullivan, 1974). Recent studies, accommodating the radial asymetry and axial mobility of the UES with appropriate manometric techniques, found basal UES pressure in these patients to be comparable to healthy controls (Cook et al, 1989). That study found patients with globus sensation to be more anxious, neurotic and depressed than controls. However, the observed UES pressure augmentation in response to a dichotic listenting stressor, while significant, was comparable to that seen in healthy controls and did not precipitate globus sensation in these patients.

Within the striated and smooth muscle components of the esophageal body both primary and secondary peristalsis is dependent on vagal efferents. The esophagus is also generously supplied by vagal afferents which are responsible for modulation of peristaltic characteristics according to bolus volume and consistency. Only a small fraction of the vagal afferent information from the esophagus reaches the level of awareness by the individual. It is not surprising then that, in the majority of individuals with disturbed esophageal motor patterns, one cannot demonstrate a one to one relationship between dysmotility and symptoms. Hence, while certain psychogenic stimuli can induce measurable changes in esophageal body contractile activity, there is no available evidence that these changes are of functional significance. Rubin et al (1962), using non-perfused catheters, reported 3 of 5 healthy subjects developed significantly more non-propulsive, swallow-initiated, esophageal contractions during affectively charged interviews. However, this phenomenon has not been reproduced by other workers (Young et al, 1987; Soffer et al, 1988). Esophageal responses to exogenous stimuli vary according to the stimulus type. Stacher et al (1979) for example found that acoustic stimuli reproducibly invoke spontaneous synchronous esophageal contractions in healthy volunteers. While this study clearly demonstrates that the esophagus is sensitive to potent external stimuli, the contractions were of low amplitude and were unassociated with symptoms. Young et al (1987) reported a significant but modest (10-17 per cent) increase in peristaltic amplitude in response to stress in healthy controls. Soffer et al (1988), using a number of validated stressors, could not reproduce these findings. Similarly caloric labyrinthine stimulation designed to induce nausea has no effect on peristalsis unless vomiting ensues (Cook et al, 1987). Hence, the response of the esophageal body in the healthy individual to experimental stress is stimulus-specific, quantitatively small and unassociated with symptoms.

The function of the lower esophageal sphincter is to prevent inappropriate gastroesophageal reflux. The major mechanism facilitating reflux in healthy individuals and patients with reflux disease is the non-swallow associated, transient LES relaxation (Dent et al, 1980). The level of awareness appears to be an important determinant of these transient LES relaxations. For example, these events are absent during stable sleep and anaesthesia but are observed during arousal. These observations suggest that transient LES relaxations might be triggered from the brain. This notion is supported by the findings of Barone et al (1984) that direct stimulation of the cat dorsal motor nucleus of the vagus elicits LES relaxation. Anecdotally heartburn has been linked with stressful life events. However, in healthy individuals, psychogenic stress does not significantly influence the frequency or duration of post-prandial reflux episodes (Cook and Collins, 1987). Furthermore, caloric labyrinthine stimulation, while causing a modest reduction in basal LES pressues, does not significantly increase the frequency of transient LES relaxations nor reflux events (Cook et al, 1987). Although external stimuli do not appreciably influence LES motor function in healthy volunteers, these hypotheses have not been tested in patients with pathological gastroesophageal reflux disease.

From the above it can be concluded in healthy individuals that stress certainly induces motor changes in the UES; can evoke minor changes in esophageal contractions and appears to have little effect on LES function. Questions remaining are whether these motor changes can cause symptoms (the available data would suggest not) and whether stress induced dysmotility may influence symptoms in individuals with underlying, clearly defined manometric abnormalities such as diffuse esophageal spasm.

When considering potential therapies in patients presumed to have symptoms secondary to esophageal dysmotility, it must be borne in mind that the individual's inherent susceptibility to stress might not only render the esophagus more sensitive to external stimuli, but also determine the individual's perception of and responses to esophageal symptoms. Hence, non-specific behavioural or psychopharmacological therapies may provide symptomatic improvement without influencing motor patterns (Clouse et al, 1987). Further controlled trials in well defined patient populations are required before the role of such therapies is established.

REFERENCES

Barone, F.C., Lombardi, D.M., and Ormsbee, H.S. (1984): Effects of hindbrain stimulation on lower esophageal sphincter pressure in the cat. Am. J. Physiol. 247: G70-G78.

Clouse, R.E., and Lustman, P.J. (1983): Psychiatric illness and contraction abnormalities of the esophagus. N Eng. J. Med 22: 1337-1342.

Clouse, R.E., Lustman, P.J., Eckert, T.C., Ferney, D.M., and Griffith, L.S. (1987): Low does Trazodone for symptomatic patients with esophageal contraction abnormalities. Gastroenterology 92: 1027-1036.

Cook, I.J., Dent, J., Shannon, S., and Collins, S.M. (1987): Measurement of upper esophageal sphincter pressure. Effect of acute emotional stress. Gastroenterology 93: 526-532.

Cook, I.J., Dent, J., Shannon, S., and Collins, S.M. (1987): Evidence for central nervous system control of the lower esophageal sphincter from its response to vestibular stimulation. Gastroenterology 92: A1353.

Cook, I.J., Dent, J., and Collins, S.M. (1989); Upper esophageal sphincter tone and reactivity to stress in patients with a history of globus sensation. Dig. Dis. Sci (In press).

Cook, I.J. (1987): Influence of acute mental stress on the frequency and duration of gastroesophageal reflux in normal volunteers. Can. J. Gastroenterology 1: 7-10.

Dent, J., Dodds, W.J., Friedman, R.H., Sekiguchi, T., Hogan, W.J., Arndorfer, R.C., Petrie, D.J. (1980): Mechanism of gastroesophageal reflux in recumbent asymptomatic human subjects. J. Clin. Invest. 65: 256-267.

Jacobson, E. (1927): Spastic Esophagus and Mucous Colitis: Etiology and treatment by progressive relaxation. Arch. Int. Med. 39: 433-445.

Richter, J.E., Obrecht, W.F., Bradley, L.A., Young, L.D. and Anderson, K.O. (1986): Psychological comparison of patients with nutcracker esophagus and irritable bowel syndrome. Dig. Dis. Sci. 31: 131-138.

Rubin, J., Nagler, R., Spiro, H.M., and Pilot, M.L. (1962): Measuring the effection of emotions on esophageal motility. Psychosom. Med. 24: 170-176.

Soffer, E.E., Scalabrini, P., Pope, C.E., and Wingate, D.L. (1988): Effect of stress on oesophageal motor function in normal subjects and in patients with the irritable bowel syndrome. Gut 29: 1591-1594.

Stacher, G., Schmierer, G., and Landgraf, M. (1979): Tertiary esophageal contractions evoked by acoustical stimuli. Gastroenterology 77: 49-54.

Stacher, G. (1983): The responsiveness of the esophagus to environmental stimuli. In Psychophysiology of the Gastrointestinal Tract, eds R. Holzl and W.R. Whitehead, pp. 21-31. New York: Plenum.

Watson, W.C., and Sullivan, S.N. (1974): Hypertonicity of the cricopharyngeal sphincter: A cause of globus sensation. Lancet 1: 1417-1419.

Young, L.D., Richter, J.E., Anderson, K.O. et al. (1987): The effects of psychological and environmental stress on peristaltic esophageal contractions in healthy volunteers. Psychophysiology 24: 132-141.

Gastric emptying and intestinal transit in pain stress

D.G. Thompson, MD, MRCP

Department of Medicine, Hope Hospital (University of Manchester School of medicine), Eccles Old Road, Salford M6 8HD, United Kingdom

INTRODUCTION

The effects of stress induced by experimental means upon gastric and intestinal function have interested clinical gastrointestinal physiologists since the time of Beaumont.

Until recently, however, information obtained from studies has been fragmentary and occasionally contradictory.

In the last decade, improvements in knowledge of human upper gastrointestinal function now provide some explanation for previously inconclusive results. It is now well known, for example, that the fasted pattern of activity of the upper gut is cyclical, varying between total quiescence and intense activity. Unless these predictable alterations in activity are controlled for in experiments on stress, results are likely to be difficult to interpret. During feeding, a further change in pattern also occurs so that responses obtained to experimental stress during the fasting period are not necessarily relevant for those occurring after feeding.

This new physiological information has now provided an opportunity for a return to the subject to be made and a number of studies have recently been conducted to explore further the relationships between stress and upper intestinal function.

PAIN STRESS

The choice of pain for studies of the effects of experimental stress on upper gut function is both scientific and pragmatic. Much information has now accumulated on the autonomic and physiological effects of pain induced by immersion of the hand in cold water, upon the cardiovascular system (Hines & Brown, 1932; Wolff, 1951; Lovalls, 1975). It is recognised that the response to this stimulus is predominantly mediated via stimulation of sympathetic neural activity. This is, in turn, consequent upon the perception of discomfort induced by the hand cooling. Studies of responses in persons habituated to hand immersion in cold water and persons with disordered or hysterical loss of pain perception (Wolff, 1951) show no major autonomic responses. In normal individuals, however, the stimulus has a number of advantages over other techniques for inducing sympathetic arousal. It is inexpensive, simple, reproducible and control stimulation is easy to provide. With the possible exception of individuals with marked vasospastic responses to cold, the procedure is safe in healthy subjects and although necessarily unpleasant, is associated with no physical harm.

Physiologically measurable responses in the cardiovascular system include a marked pressor response, an increase in pulse rate, together with a consistent elevation of circulating noradrenaline and lesser elevation of plasma adrenaline (Atterhog et al., 1981; O'Brien et al., 1987). The stimulus thus provides extraintestinal markers of effect against which any physiological responses in the gut can be judged.

EFFECTS OF PAIN STRESS ON GASTRIC EMPTYING AND SECRETION

Information about the effects of pain stress on gastric emptying has been largely acquired from studies using repeated immersion of the hand in cold water during measurement of gastric efflux and gastric secretion by intubation methods (Thompson & Richelson, 1981).

Methods

In these studies healthy volunteers were stressed using repeated hand immersion in an ice-water mixture for 15 minutes. On a separate occasion they received control stimulation, repeated immersion of the same hand in warm water.

Gastric emptying and secretion was measured concurrently by an intubation technique which involved repeated sampling of the stomach and duodenum following ingestion of a standard liquid test meal containing ^{14}C polyethylene glycol.

The test or the control stimulus was applied ten minutes after meal ingestion, by repeatedly immersing the non-dominant hand in cold or warm water for one minute intervals. The hand was removed for 15 seconds between immersions, repeating these cycles for a period of 20 minutes. Measurements of blood pressure, pulse and skin temperature were measured throughout both test periods to provide an extra-intestinal index of the stress response.

Gastric emptying was markedly delayed by the test stimulus, the reduction in meal emptying being 32 $\pm$ 13 ml (mean$\pm$SE) during the 20 minute stimulation period. In addition to the delay in gastric emptying, gastric secretion and gastric acid output were also reduced.

Following the cessation of the stimulus, however, there was a consistently increased rate of secretion compared to the test stimulus suggestive of a post-stimulation rebound effect (Fig. 1).

The observed delay in gastric emptying appears to be an important and consistent effect of pain stress. This gastric stasis is best explained by an inhibition of gastric tone or by pyloric closure (Fone, 1988) since there was no accompanying increase in duodenal motor activity to indicate an increased breaking effect on gastric emptying and since the other major determinant of emptying, antral peristaltic activity, is not normally a major factor in the emptying of liquid meals.

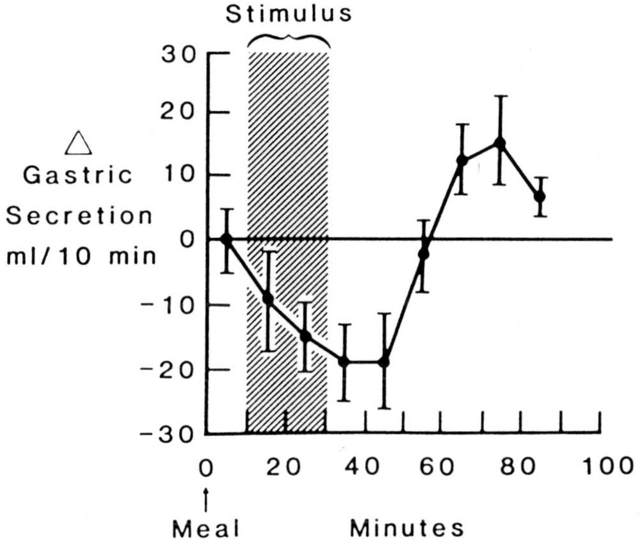

Figure 1 Differences in gastric secretion rates/10 min between the test and control stimulus are shown following the ingestion of a meal. The test stimulus (cold pain) induces an inhibition, followed by a rebound enhancement, in secretion. (reproduced by permission of GUT).

THE EFFECTS OF PAIN STRESS ON GASTROINTESTINAL TRANSIT

A number of studies on the effect of pain stress on the transit of nutrient through the upper intestinal tract have now been performed using exhaled breath hydrogen monitoring (Bond & Levitt, 1975). The choice of this model function being determined largely by its simplicity and non invasive nature which makes it suitable for repeated studies on normal individuals.

<u>Method</u>

The technique is based on the fact that poorly absorbed carbohydrate which passes through the stomach and small intestine becomes available for bacterial fermentation in the colon with the production of gaseous hydrogen as a metabolic by-product. This hydrogen passes rapidly through the colon wall, into the circulation and thence to the lungs where it is excreted, and is detectable, in exhaled breath using a simple electrochemical cell detector (Corbett et al., 1981). When simple precautions and carefully standardised conditions are employed (Thompson et al., 1985) the technique is highly reproducible within individuals, although wide variability between individuals is evident, (McIntyre, 1988).

THE EFFECTS OF PAIN STRESS ON UPPER INTESTINAL TRANSIT

Studies using a similar experimental stress protocol to that employed for gastric emptying studies above, indicate that a delay in transit can be induced by cold stress compared to control stimulation (O'Brien et al, 1987). It is evident that this delay varies with the intrinsic speed of transit of an individual, being greater in individuals with rapid than with slow transit.

The precise anatomical site of action of the mechanisms responsible for the transit delay is presently uncertain but is likely to include an effect on gastric emptying together with alteration in small intestinal propulsive activity together with an effect on intestinal secretion since pain stress is also known to inhibit intestinal fluid transport (Barclay & Turnberg, 1985).

STUDIES INTO THE PATHWAYS INVOLVED IN THE PAIN STRESS RESPONSE

Because the non-invasive nature of the transit model lends itself to repeated studies on individuals, multiple studies have now been conducted in normal volunteers and without adrenoreceptor blocking drugs during pain stress.

Repeated Studies in One Individual

The convenience of the technique can be seen from a series of 36 transit studies performed on one individual (Fig. 2). It was found that the administration of a beta-adrenoreceptor blocking agent prior to the administration of the pain stress significantly attenuated the effect of the stress on orocaecal transit.

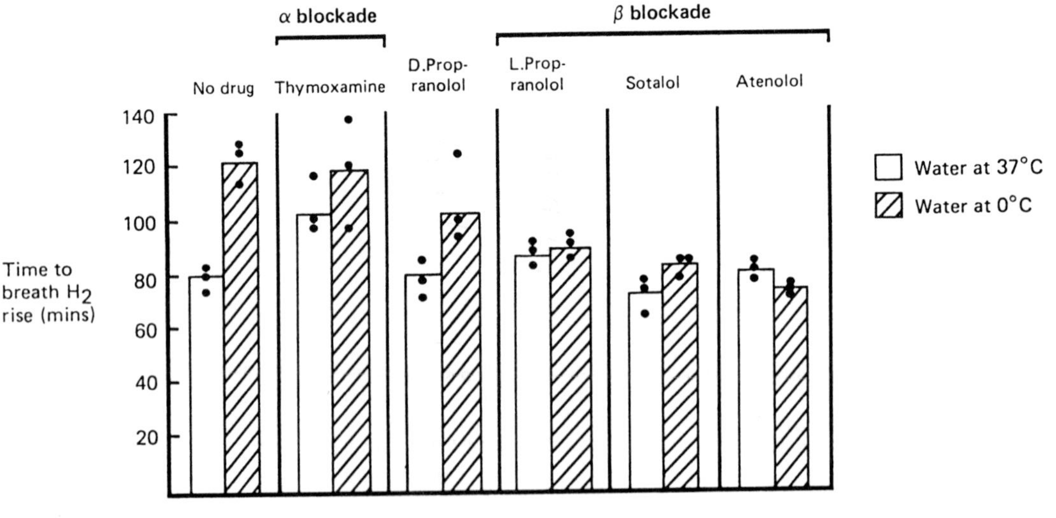

Figure 2: Orocaecal transit rates in one individual on 36 occasions are shown. Each point represents the transit rate for a single study. Vertical bars show the mean values for each group of three studies. (reproduced with permission of GUT).

The response appears moreover to have a major beta-1 adrenoreceptor mediated component since beta-1 specific blockers such as atenolol produce similar responses to propranolol (a non-specific beta-1 and beta-2 receptor antagonist). Furthermore the effects appear to be largely peripheral (outside the blood-brain barrier) since the attenuation was found to be equally effective with atenolol (a drug which does not cross the blood-brain barrier) as with sotolol, which is similarly beta-1 adrenoreceptor specific but which does cross the brain barrier. In addition, prior administration of D-propranolol, the stereo-isomer of L-propranolol which has similar membrane stabilising effects to L-propranolol but no beta blocking action, failed to attenuate the inhibitory effect.

Controlled Trial of Effect of Beta-Adrenoreceptor Blockade on the Stress Response

To explore this beta-1 receptor mediated effect further, a controlled trial was conducted in 9 individuals to evaluate the inhibitory action of Atenolol on the cold pain induced transit delay (O'Brien, 1989). As in the pilot study, transit was significantly delayed by pain stress after administration of placebo while the effect of pain stress was significantly attenuated by prior beta-1 adrenoreceptor blockade.

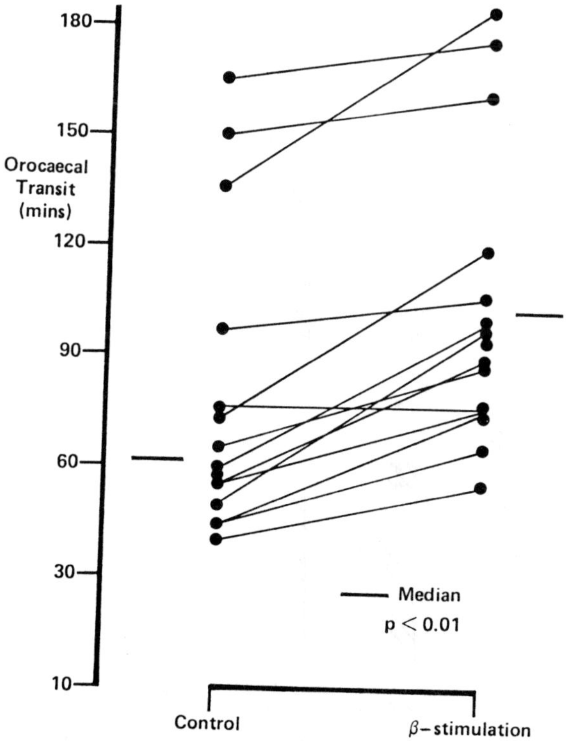

Figure 3 The delay in transit induced by the β -adrenoreceptor agonist isoprenaline is shown. The lines joint the test and control data for the fourteen individuals.

The Effect of Beta Adrenoreceptor Agonists on Intestinal Transit

In an attempt to explore further the mode of action of cold pain on transit, studies have been performed using isoprenaline (beta-1 and beta-2 adrenoreceptor agonist) and salbutamol (beta-2 adrenoreceptor specific agonist) on intestinal transit (McIntyre, 1988). As in the cold pain experiments, isoprenaline but not salbutamol was able to delay orocaecal transit (Fig. 3). This isoprenaline effect was inhibited by prior atenolol suggesting again a beta-1 adrenoreceptor specific effect.

Effect of Beta Adrenoreceptor Antagonists on Orocaecal Transit

In a further series of experiments, beta adrenoreceptor blockers were administered to unstimulated individuals prior to orocaecal transit (McIntyre, 1988). These experiments have shown that a significant acceleration of transit can be induced in individuals by beta blockade (Fig. 4). The magnitude of the acceleration depends, however, upon the individual's transit rate, being considerably greater in those individuals with slow intestinal transit than in those individuals with rapid intestinal transit, suggesting the presence of a resting beta-receptor mediated inhibitory tone on transit.

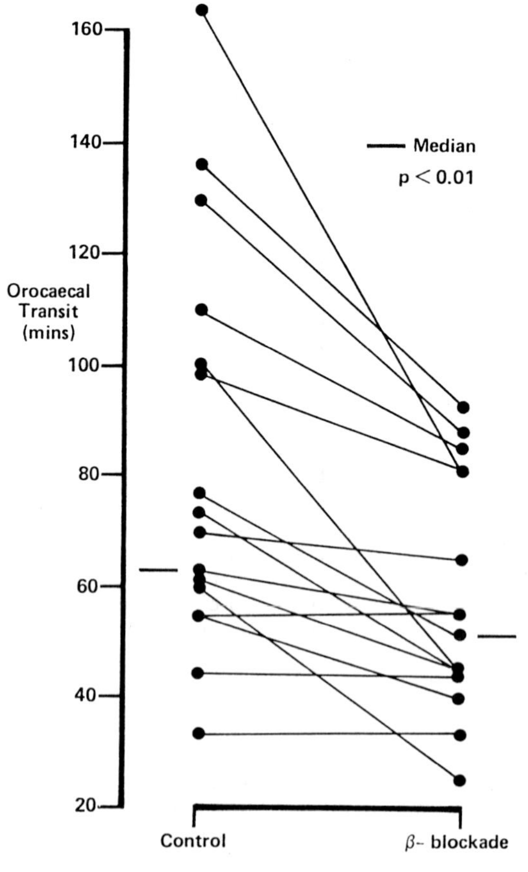

Figure 4: The transit acceleration associated with the administration of a beta blocker is shown in sixteen individuals.

Significance of the Findings

The presence of a beta-1 adrenoreceptor mediated pathway in the cold pain effect on transit, is evident from the above experiments. That a beta-1 adrenoreceptor pathway is involved strongly indicates that the effect is mediated via neural sympathetic pathways employing noradrenaline, since noradrenaline is known to act principally on alpha-1 and alpha-2 receptors whereas adrenaline is largely alpha-2 and beta-2 specific (Ariens & Simonis, 1983).

The precise anatomical location of the receptor involved cannot unfortunately be determined from the current experiments. It seems likely, however, that the principal site of action is gastrointestinal smooth muscle rather than enteric nervous system. Evidence for this supposition is based upon the current knowledge of adrenoreceptor subtype localisation in the gut. It is known that sympathetic fibres to the gut end almost exclusively upon the enteric nervous system ganglia rather than smooth muscle cells (Furness & Costa, 1974) and that these synaptic pathways to ganglia are largely alpha-specific (Gillespie & Hoyi, 1974). In contrast, the smooth muscle of the human intestine possess adrenoreceptors which are beta-specific (Hedges & Turner, 1969).

Beta adrenoreceptors differ from alpha receptors in their control of cellular function in that they largely modulate cellular function by influencing tissue cyclic AMP. The effects of beta adrenoreceptor stimulation on smooth muscle would therefore be expected to provide a more prolonged influence on smooth muscle tone rather than short term effects on contractile pattern of the gut.

RELEVANCE OF TRANSIT STUDIES TO INTESTINAL NUTRIENT PASSAGE

The relevance of the transit studies to the extraction of nutrients from the gut has been indicated by a further series of studies which have explored the extraction of fructose from the upper gastrointestinal tract (McIntyre, 1988).

Methods

The rationale for the design of these experiments is that fructose is not well extracted from the small intestinal lumen so that small intestinal capacity for fructose extraction can be saturated in all individuals if sufficient fructose is placed in a test meal. Overloading the intestine with fructose thus results in the appearance of fructose at the caecum with consequent fermentation and hydrogen production. A series of test meals containing progressively increasing doses of fructose can thus be given to an individual. The quantity of fructose in the meal at which a breath hydrogen rise is first noticed indicates that the functional absorptive capacity of the intestine has just been exceeded.

Using this technique in normal individuals it has been found that lactulose transit correlates closely with the dose of fructose required to produce a breath hydrogen rise, i.e. the longer the breath hydrogen transit, the greater the fructose threshold. Furthermore, the studies indicate that isoprenaline and beta blockade can influence the fructose absorptive capacity being increased by isoprenaline and decreased by beta blockers.

These studies therefore indicate that pain stress would influence nutrient extraction in a similar way.

Relevance of pain stress effects to other experimental stressor models

With the employment of an increasing number of experimental stressors in addition to cold pain such as dichotomous listening (O'Brien et al, 1987) and delayed auditory feedback (Valori et al, 1986), it is becoming increasingly difficult to conceive of stress responses in a unified way. In similar individuals, for example, the effects of cold pain and mental stimulation, while being qualitatively similar in the cardiovascular system, are quantitatively different in the gastrointestinal tract (O'Brien et al, 1987). It is thus difficult to extrapolate the results of experiments performed using one model to those performed using another.

CONCLUSION

The above studies indicate the role of sympathetic and in particular noradrenergic pathways in the perturbation of human upper gastrointestinal function by cold induced pain stress and provide a model for the exploration of central nervous system mediated effects on upper gut function.

REFERENCES

Ariens, E.J. & Simonis, A.M. (1983): Physiological and pharmacological aspects of adrenergic receptor classification. Biochem. Pharmacol. 32, 1539-1545.

Atterhog, J-H., Eliason, K. & Hjemdahl, P. (1981): Sympathoadrenal and cardiovascular responses to mental stress, isometric handgrip and cold pressor test. Brit. Heart J. 46, 311-319.

Barclay, G.R. & Turnberg, L.A. (1985): Influence of physical and psychological stress on fluid and electrolyte absorption in the human jejunum in vivo. Gut 26, A554-A555.

Bond, J.H. & Levitt, M.D. (1975): Investigation of small bowel transit time in man utilizing pulmonary hydrogen mea~urements. J. Lab. Clin. Med. 85, 546-555.

Corbett, C.L., Thomas, S., Read, N.W. et al (1981): Electrochemical detector for breath hydrogen determination: measurement of small bowel transit time in normal subjects and patients with irritable bowel syndrome. Gut 22, 836-840.

Fore, D., Horowitz, M., Maddox, A. et al (1988): Cold stress induces isolated pyloric pressure waves in healthy volunteers. Gastroenterology 94, A133.

Furness, J.B. & Costa, M. (1974): The adrenergic innervation of the gastrointestinal tract. Ergeb der Physiol. 69, 1-52.

Gillespie, J.S. & Khoyi, M.A. (1974): The site and receptors responsible for the inhibition of sympathetic nerves of intestinal smooth muscle and its parasympathetic motor nerves.

J. Physiol. 267, 767-789.

Hedges, A. & Turner, P. (1969) Beta receptors in human isolated smooth muscle. Br. J. Pharm. 37, 547-548.

Hines, E.A. & Brown, C.E. (1932): A standard stimulus for measuring vasomotor reactions: Its application in the study of hypertension. Proc. Staff Meeting Mayo Clin. 7, 332-335.

Lovallo, W. (1975): The cold pressor test and autonomic function: a review and integration. Psychophysiology 12, 268-282.

McIntyre, A.S., Thompson, D.G., Burnham, W.R. & Walker, E. (1988): The mode of action and functional consequence of beta-adrenergic tone in the human gut. Gastroenterology 94, A296.

O'Brien, J.D., Thompson, D.G., Burnham, W.R., Holly, J. & Walker, E. (1987): Action of centrally mediated autonomic stimulation on human gastrointestinal transit: a comparative study of two stimuli. Gut 28, 960--969.

O'Brien, J.D., Thompson, D.G., Day, S.J., Burnham, W.R. & Walker, E. (1989): Perturbation of upper gastrointestinal transit and antroduodenal motility by experimentally applied stress: the role of beta adrenoreceptor mediated pathways. Gut 1989 (in press).

Stanghellini, V., Malagelada, J.R., Zinsmeister, A.R., Go, V.L.W. & Kao, P.C. (1983): Stress mediated gastroduodenal motor disturbance in humans: Possible humoral mechanisms. Gastroenterology 85, 83-91.

Thompson, D.G., Richelson, E. & Malagelada, J-R. (1981): Perturbation of upper gastrointestinal function by cold stress. Gut 24, 277-283.

Thompson, D.G., Binfield, P., DeBelder, A., O'Brien, J., Warren, S. & Wilson, M. (1985): Extraintestinal influences on exhaled breath hydrogen measurements during the investigation of gastrointestinal disease. Gut 26, 1349-1352.

Valori, R.M., Kumar, D. & Wingate, D.L. (1986) Effects of different types of stress and of prokinetic drugs on the control of the fasting motor complex in humans. Gastroenterology 90, 1890-1900.

Wolff, H.H. (1951): The mechanism and significance of the cold pressor response. Q. J. Med. 20, 261-273.

The influence of psychological stress on intestinal motility

D.L. Wingate, R.M. Valori and D. Kumar

Gastrointestinal Science Research Unit, London Hospital Medical College, 26 Ashfield Street, London E1 2AJ, England

Although 'psychological stress' may be difficult to define with precision, it is surely common ground that it implies the conscious perception of stress. The comparatively few reports on the effects of stress on small bowel function that exist in the literature almost certainly reflect a consensus that small bowel function is not susceptible to stress, and this in turn reflects the fact that individuals cannot readily identify symptoms of small bowel dysfunction. The digestive symptomatology of stress is referred - rightly or wrongly - to other regions of the digestive tract; for example, dyspepsia and epigastric fullness to the stomach and diarrhoea to the colon.

The small intestine is a long, featureless and almost uniform tube; there are no structural features that offer clues to its motor function. Until the last two decades, knowledge of small bowel motor physiology was largely deduced on 'black box' principles; comparison of small bowel input and output led to the conclusion that the small bowel is the principal site of fluid and nutrient absorption, and the progress of markers between one end and the other show an average transit time, in man, of about 3 hours (Davis et al, 1985). The discovery (Szurszewski, 1969) or rediscovery (Wingate, 1981) of the migrating motor complex (MMC) has led to the realisation that the motor activity of the small intestine is highly organised and that, moreover, this organisation takes place at the level of the intrinsic enteric system (ENS). Paradoxically, it is the homogeneity of the small intestine along its length that confers the great variation in motor activity of which the small bowel is capable; peristalsis (which is the primary motor pattern of the small bowel) can be organised into an infinity of patterns of transient contractions, propagating contractions, segmentation and motor quiescence. This functional plasticity, unrestrained by anatomical specialisation, offers the clearest expression of ENS control that is available for study, and consequently it is a valuable test-bed for studying the interaction between the ENS and the central nervous system (CNS). Equally, psychological stress is an unequivocal CNS input, independent of peripheral receptors.

The stimulus for the study of stress on the small intestine arose from the observations by Thompson et al (1980) of the variability of the inter-MMC interval in the proximal small bowel in untrained human subjects, compared with the findings in trained laboratory dogs by Code and Marlett (1975), who laid great stress on the regularity of the fasting MMC in their animals. Since human

MMCs were shown to be more regular during sleep, it seemed possible that the irregularity might be due to stress experienced by the human subjects when awake; experimental psychological stress offered a means of testing the hypothesis. Accordingly, a stress protocol, utilising the dichotomous listening test as a stressor, was devised and tested in human volunteers. The results showed that over 2 hours, the stressor induced an inhibition of MMC activity, but this inhibition faded when exposure to the stressor continued for a further 2 hours (McRae et al 1982). A similar, but not identical, protocol utilised by Cann et al (1983), showed that small bowel transit of a standard meal appeared to be accelerated by this stressor; thus, it would appear that both fasting and postprandial motility may be modulated by psychological stress.

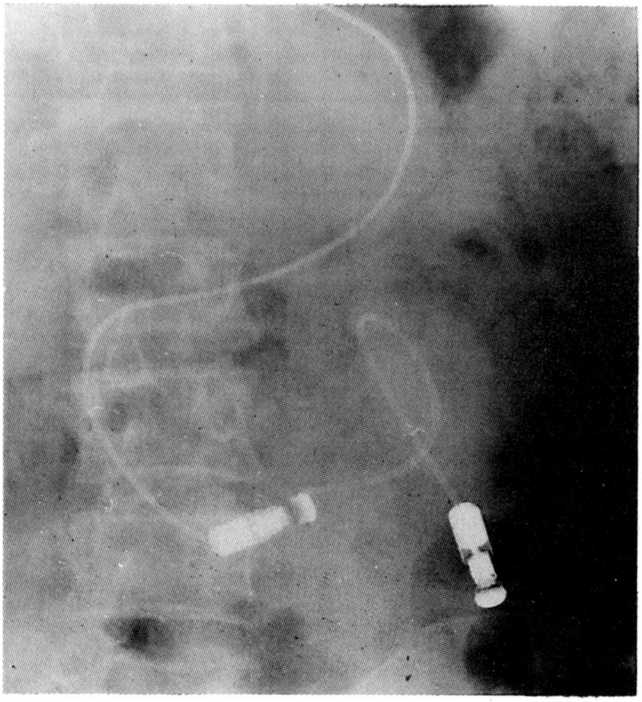

Figure 1: Plain film of the abdomen showing two radiotelemetric pressure sensors (RTCs) stationed in the proximal small bowel of a healthy volunteer.

Improved methodology, utilising two radiotelemetric pressure capsules (RTCs) stationed in the proximal small bowel (Figure 1) was used in a further study (Valori et al, 1986) that was designed to study the effect of prolonged exposure to stressors while avoiding the phenomenon of adaptation that had been previously reported by McRae and co-workers. Subjects were studied continuously for 48 hours, including two 8-hour days under fasting conditions (Figure 2).

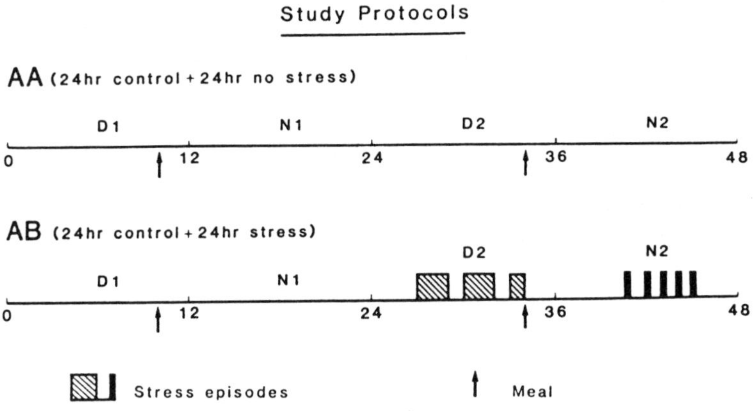

Figure 2: Schematic representation of the study protocol for the control (AA) and test (AB) groups.

For a control group, no stressors were applied on either day. The test group had one day without stress but, on the second day, were subjected to 3 different psychological stressors, each for 2-hour periods separated by a one-hour rest period. During the second night, the test group were also woken at one-hour intervals between midnight and 5.00 am by bright lights and loud music, which were extinguished when the subjects had keyed the correct answers to five simple mental arithmetic problems into the keyboard of the computer controlling the sound and light.

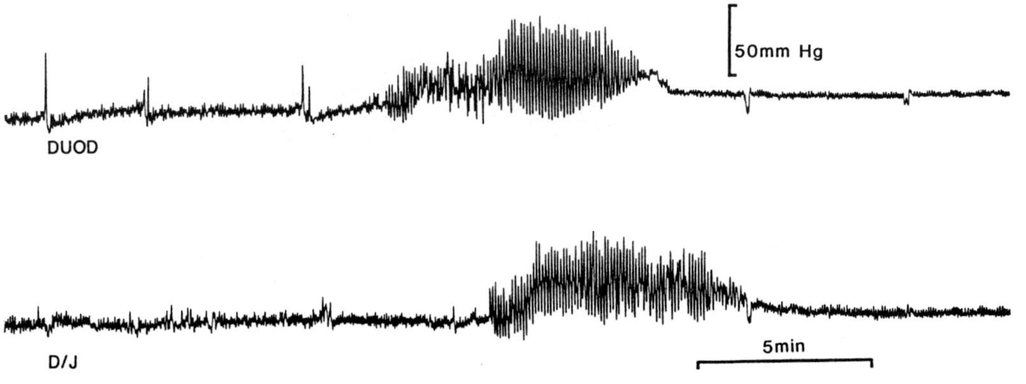

Figure 3: Phase III episodes of an MMC recorded from RTCs stationed as illustrated in Figure 1.

During the entire study, small bowel pressure activity was continuously recorded from the two RTCs (Figure 3) and the incidence of Phase III episodes identified from the recording during different phases of the study was compared. Simple tests to measure overall stress response were used to assess the efficacy of the stressors.

The results in the test group showed a consistent reduction (Figure 4) in the number of MMCs recorded in the test group during the 8-hour stress period, compared with the same period on the previous day when no stressors were administered; this difference was statistically significant ($p<0.02$). There was no difference in MMC incidence between the study days in the control group who were not exposed to stressors.

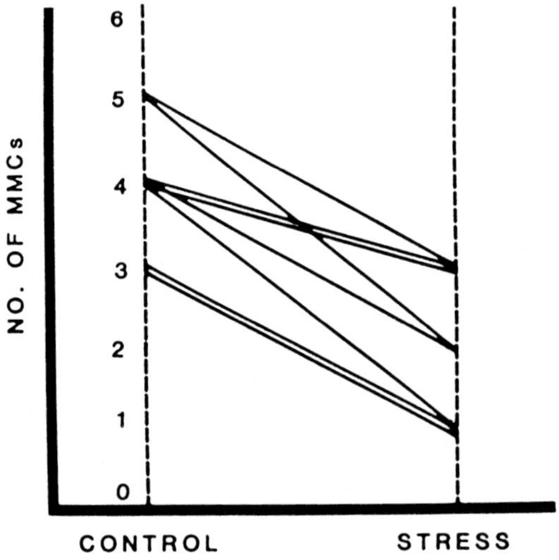

Figure 4: Incidence of MMCs in the test group during the 8 hours of stress (right) compared with the equivalent 8 hours of rest (left).

The nocturnal stress, however, had only a slight effect on MMC incidence. This was surprising, as all the subjects considered that the repetitive awakening was extremely unpleasant; one subject described it as "the most unpleasant night that I can remember". The difference between the diurnal and nocturnal stressors was in their duration; diurnal stressors were applied continuously for 2-hour periods, whereas the nocturnal stress was brief, averaging no more than 5 minutes. This difference suggests that the effect of stress on small bowel motility is not sustained after the stressor is removed; this would explain why the nocturnal stressor, which on aggregate amounted to no more than 25 minutes during the whole night, failed to significantly perturb the MMC biorhythm.

We have tested the hypothesis that the inhibitory effect of stressors on MMCs is short-lived by evaluating the incidence of MMCs during the stressor day. For this evaluation, we have not only used the data from healthy volunteers, but also from a series of 22 patients suffering from irritable bowel syndrome (IBS) and a disease control group of 5 patients with inflammatory bowel disease (IBD) who were submitted to the same protocol (Kumar and Wingate, 1985).

Figure 5 illustrates the temporal distribution of MMCs in the healthy test group and the inflammatory bowel group during the rest and stress days. It will be noted that on the stress day, there is a tendency for MMCs to occur in the inter-stress rest periods. Figure 6 shows the equivalent data for the IBS group, showing a similar distribution of MMCs. The figure also shows that some IBS patients (7/22 = 32%) appear to be much more susceptible to the effects of stress in that MMCs were completely abolished during the stressor day; such total abolition of MMCs was not seen in healthy volunteers or in the IBD group.

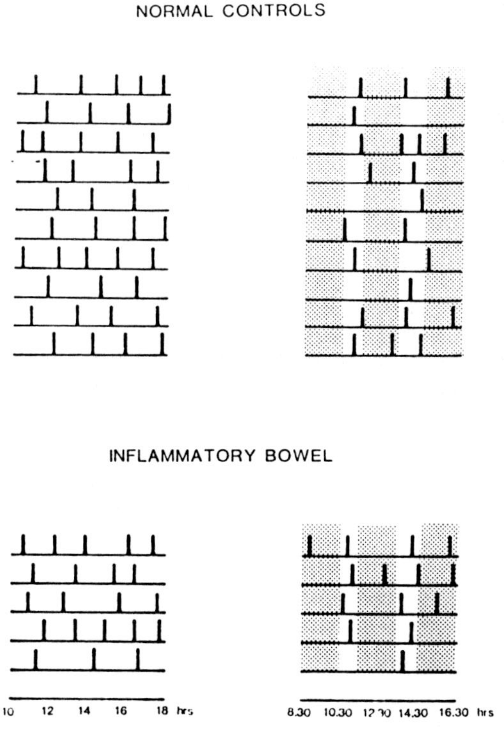

Figure 5: Temporal distribution of MMCs in healthy volunteers (above) and IBD patients (below) during rest (left) and stress (right) days. Vertical bars indicate Phase III episodes and shaded areas indicate stressor periods.

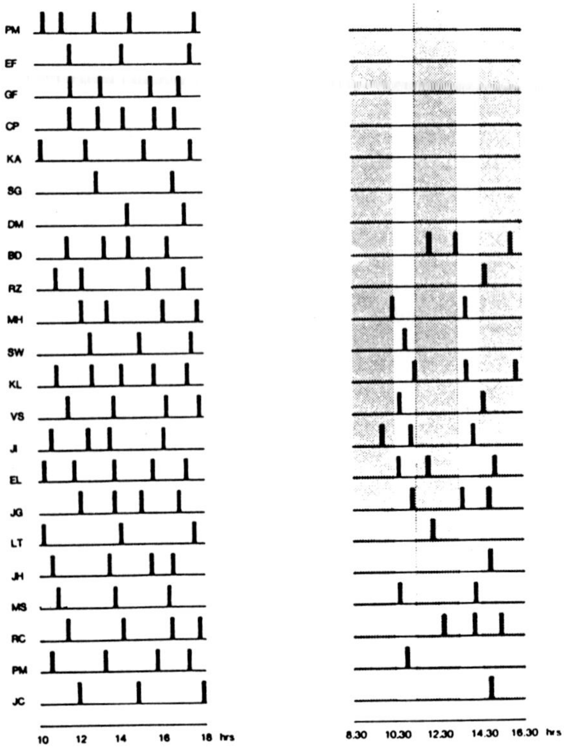

Figure 6: Temporal distribution of MMCs in IBS patients; for explanation, see caption of Figure 5.

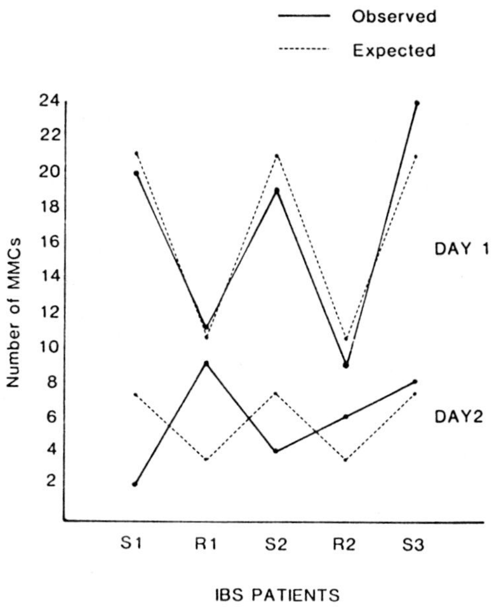

Figure 7: Temporal distribution of MMCs in IBS patients. See explanation, see text.

Further analysis of the data indicates that the effect is not merely a suppression of MMCs during a period of stress. Figure 7 illustrates this analysis for the IBS patients (the analysis of data from the volunteer group is not illustrated here but shows identical trends). The explanation of the figure is as follows. For each of the 2 days, the total number of MMCs in the study group has been aggregated for each of the three 2-hour periods used for stressor exposure on the second day of the study and for the two intervening hours corresponding to the inter-stress rest periods on the second day. This distribution is shown for the first (rest) day in the upper solid line. The upper broken line shows the incidence calculated for each period if it is assumed that MMC incidence is random; the coincidence of the 2 lines shows that under rest conditions, MMC incidence occurs at an average frequency during the day. The lower part of the figure shows the same calculation for the second (stress) day. There is a marked deviation between the solid and broken lines. This shows that not only were there less MMCs during stress than predicted on the basis of a random distribution, but there were more during the inter-stress rest periods than were predicted. The deviation between the predicted and actual incidence on the stress day diminishes with the passage of time, suggesting that individuals are more susceptible to stress at the beginning of the day; this is consistent with the observation that symptoms of IBS - a stress-related disorder - are common in patients shortly after waking but often pass off by mid-morning.

Thus, it appears that not only is the inhibitory effect of stress on small bowel motility not prolonged on the cessation of stress, but that there is also a 'rebound' effect, almost as though the gut was trying to 'catch up'. An identical phenomenon has been reported by Thompson et al (1983) who studied the effect of cold pain stress on gastric emptying and acid secretion, suggesting that while psychological and pain stress involve different neural inputs, they may evoke an identical mechanism of response affecting the gut.

In summary, our data show that:

1 Psychological stressors inhibit the incidence of MMCs in the human proximal small bowel;

2 The inhibition is much more profound in some patients with irritable bowel syndrome;

3 The inhibitory effect is confined to the duration of the stressor;

4 Inhibition of MMCs appears to be followed by a 'rebound' phase of stimulation.

REFERENCES

Cann PA, Read NW, Cammack J, Childs H, Holden S, Kashman R, Longmore J, Nix S, Simms N, Swallow K & Weller J. (1983): Psychological stress and the passage of a standard meal through the stomach and small intestine in man. Gut 24:236-240

Code CF & Marlett JA. (1975): The interdigestive myoelectric complex of the stomach and small bowel of dogs. J Physiol (Lond) 246:289-309

Davis SS, Hardy JD & Fara JW. (1985): Transit of pharmaceutical dosage forms through the small intestine. Gut 27:886-892

Kumar D & Wingate DL. (1985): The irritable bowel syndrome: a paroxysmal motor disorder. Lancet ii:973-977

McRae S, Younger K, Thompson DG & Wingate DL. (1982): Sustained mental stress alters human jejunal motor activity. Gut 23:404-409

Szurszewski JH. (1969): A migrating electric complex of the canine small intestine. A J Physiol 217:1757-1763

Valori RM, Kumar D & Wingate DL. (1986): Effects of different types of stress and of 'prokinetic' drugs on the control of the fasting motor complex in humans. Gastroenterology 90:1890-1900

Wingate DL. (1981): Backwards and forwards with the migrating complex. Dig Dis Sci 26:641-666

Noise and intestinal motor alterations

J.F. Erckenbrecht

Department of Gastroenterology, Heinrich-Heine-University of Duesseldorf, Moorenstrasse 5, D-4000 Duesseldorf 1, Federal Republic of Germany

Noise above a threshold so far undefined induces changes of the function of various internal organs. These include the blood vessels, the heart, the skin, and the eye pupilla. In addition, changes of gastrointestinal motor activity during noise exposure are well recognized since more than 50 years (1). Diseases to which disturbances of gastrointestinal motility are said to contribute seem to be more frequent in professions with high noise load and seem to lead to higher rates of morbidity in this population (2). We, therefore, studied the effects of short and long term noise exposure on various functions of the gastrointestinal tract.

1. Effect of noise on bowel habits in normal healthy volunteers

In a controlled study 16 healthy male volunteers were exposed to a 90 dB broad frequency noise which was applied by headphones for 24 hours. To avoid adaptation the headphones were removed for 2 minutes after each 8 minute period of noise application. The 24 h stress period was interrupted by a 12 h night rest. Stool weight and stool frequency were recorded throughout the entire 36 h test period. In addition, oro-cecal transit time of a standardised carbohydrate rich meal (1000 kcal) was measured by the H_2-breath test. The results of the stress period were compared to a control period in the same individuums without noise application. As shown in figure 1, longterm noise exposure resulted in a 50 % increase of stool frequency and a 100 % increase of stool weight. In addition, oro-cecal transit time, which mainly represents small bowel transit time, was accelerated from about 5 hours to about 4 hours (3).

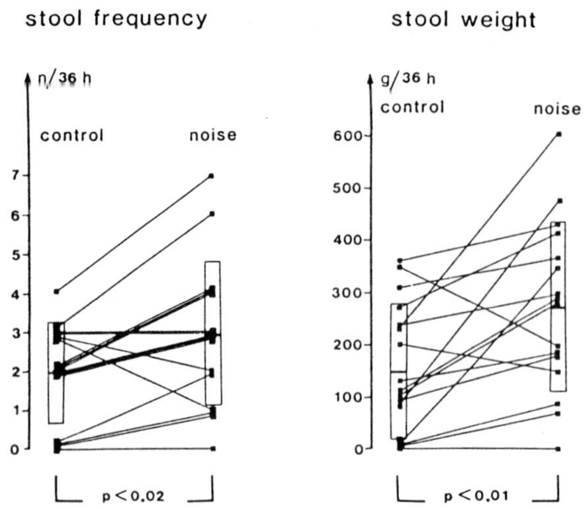

Figure 1

2. Effect of noise on postprandial colonic motility in normal healthy volunteers

To further elucidate the underlying pathomechanism by which the above cited gross changes of intestinal motility during noise exposure were brought about, postprandial colonic motility was evaluated in a seperate study. Eleven healthy volunteers were exposed to a 105 dB broad frequency noise for 50 min and to control situation without noise application. Intraluminal pressures of the rectum and the sigmoid colon were recorded

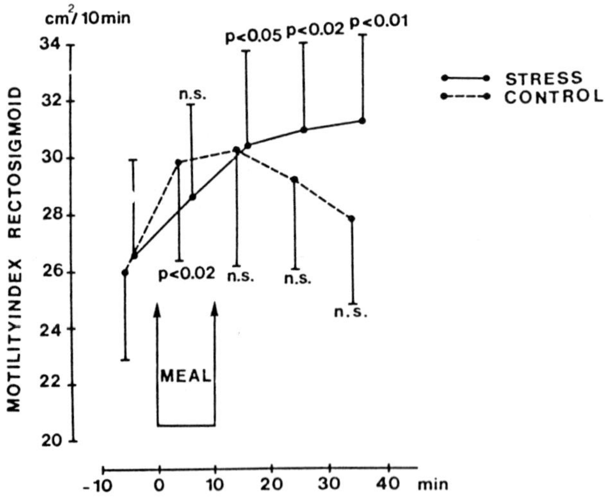

Figure 2

continuously from 10 minutes before to 40 minutes after oral uptake of a standardized 1000 kcal meal containing 50 % fat. As shown in figure 2, a significantly delayed but prolonged increase of postprandial sigmoid colon motility following noise exposure could be observed as compared to the control situation without noise (4).

3. Effect of noise on fasted gastrointestinal motility and fluid absorption

The aim of this study was to clarify the question whether in addition to postprandial small bowel transit acceleration fasting intestinal motility and transmural fluid and electrolyte transport are influenced by noise exposure. In a controlled cross-over trial 16 male healthy volunteers were subjected to a 100 dB broad frequency noise applied intermittently for 5 hours. Motility and transmural fluid transport in the duodenum and jejunum were measured by means of a perfused 5-lumen catheter. Compared to a control situation in the same volunteers, noise application did not alter the number, duration, and propagation velocity of phase III activity, or the cycle length of the interdigestive migrating motor complex (MMC). Furthermore, transmural transport of water and electrolytes was unaffected by noise application (5).

4. Stress effects on colonic sensitivity

Since we became interested whether stress may not only interfere with efferent gastrointestinal control mechanisms but also efferent information processing from the gut, we studied the effects of 2 different stressors, mental and physical stress, on gastrointestinal sensitivity. Mental stress (dichotomous listening test, colour word conflict test, and a mental arithmetic test) and physical stress (cold pressor test) were applied to 10 and 11 male healthy volunteers, respectively. Gastrointestinal sensitivity was determined by the ability to perceive gastrointestinal distension by repetively inflating an intrarectal balloon until the volunteers perceived the balloon, an urge to defecate, and lower abdominal pain. Heart rate and blood pressure were significantly increased both during mental and physical stress. As shown in figure 3 perception of gastrointestinal distension was differentially affected by mental and physical stress. Intrarectal volumes to induce an urge for defecation were increased during physical stress but were unaffected by mental stress. The opposite was true for the induction of lower abdominal pain by gastrointestinal distension. Intrarectal volumes to induce pain were decreased by mental stress but were unaffected by physical stress. The observed effects of mental and physical stress in the gastrointestinal system were unrelated to the stress induced changes in the cardiovascular system as measured by heart rate and blood pressure (6).

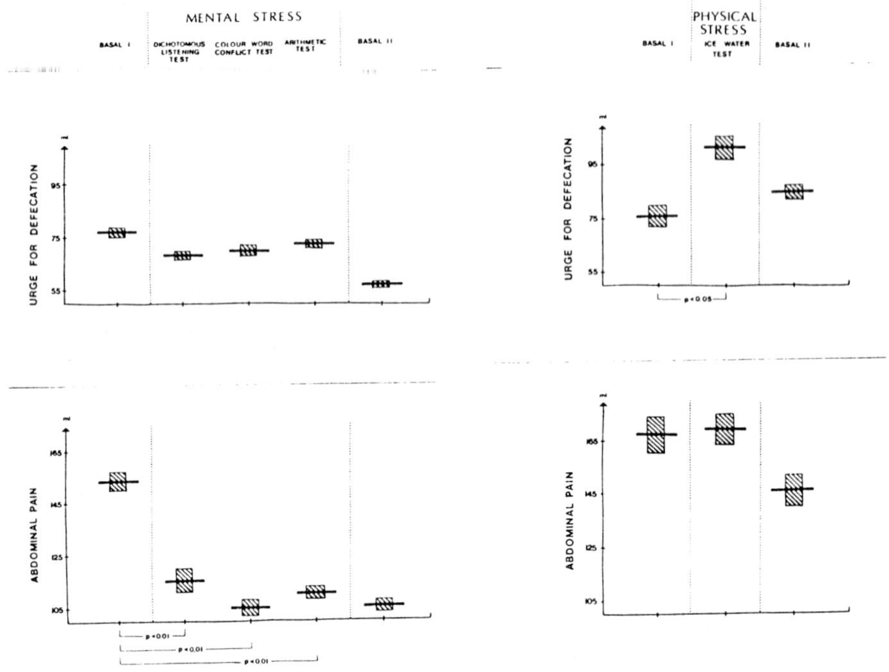

Figure 3

LITERATUR

1. Smith EL, Laird DA. The loudness of auditory stimuli which affect the stomach contractions in healthy human beings. J Acous Soc Am 1930; 2: 94 - 98

2. Jansen G: Einfluß hoher Lärmintensitäten auf den menschlichen Organismus. Wehrmed Monatschr 1981; 25: 371 - 379

3. Erckenbrecht JF, Ziemer B, Lesch B, Rehm S, Kothe E, Berges W, Wienbeck M. The effect of longterm mental stress by noise on transit of a meal through the small and large bowel. Gut 1984; 25: A 1311

4. Erckenbrecht JF, Lesch M, Ziemer B, Schwarze S, Jansen G, Wienbeck M. Wirkungen von Lärm auf die postprandiale Dickdarmmotilität. Z Lärmbekämpfung 1988; 35, 74 - 77

5. Erckenbrecht, Borgos J, Schöpe-Stiller A, Schwarze S, Wienbeck M, Jansen G. Wirkungen von Lärm auf die Motilität und Flüssigkeitsresorption im menschlichen Dünndarm. Z Lärmbekämpfung 1988; 35: 42 - 46

6. Erckenbrecht JF, Hoeren C, Skoda G, Enck P, Berges W, Wienbeck M. Differential effects of mental and physical stress on perception of gastrointestinal distension. Gastroenterology 1988; 94: 115

Correlations of cardiovascular and gastroduodenal motility responses to acute mental stress

Gerald Holtmann, Reinholde Kriebel and Manfred V. Singer

Division of Medicine, Department of Gastroenterology and Institute of Medical Psychology, University of Essen, Hufeland Str. 55, D-4300 Essen 1, FRG.

Since the uncontrolled single case observations of Beaumont (1833) and Wolff & Wolf (1947), there is no doubt that centrally acting stimuli may alter gastroduodenal motility in humans. In a controlled study McRae et al. (1982) demonstrated that acute mental stress induced by noise or mental arithmetics increased the length of the migrating motility complex in healthy humans. Dichotomous listening did not change gastric emptying but decreased the time interval of the oral-coecal-passage of a test meal (Cann et al., 1983). Vertigo induced by labyrinthine stimulation significantly inhibited gastric emptying (Thompson et al., 1982). Additionally, Stanghellini et al. (1983) demonstrated that cold pressure test and labyrinthine stimulation decreased the antral phasic pressure response to a meal (Stanghellini et al., 1983). It is widely assumed that mental stress induces a sympathetic activation with release of catecholamines and cardiovascular responses (Dimsdale and Moss, 1980). This sympathetic activation might be related with the motility changes.

However, up to now nothing is known about the correlations between autonomic stress responses and changes of gastrointestinal motility. The aim of the present study was therefore to evaluate the correlations between cardiovascular and motility changes in humans. In healthy volunteers we studied the effects of a sympathetic activating situation (mental stress) on cardiovascular system and upper gastrointestinal motility responses and correlated the changes of cardiovascular stress response with the changes of gastroduodenal motility.

This study was supported by a grant from the Deutsche Forschungsgemeinschaft (Si 228/6-2).

METHODS

Subjects

Eleven adult male volunteers gave written informed consent to participate in this study. All subjects had previously participated in studies with similar techniques. Thus they were habituated to the discomfort induced by the nasogastric tubes. The age ranged from 20 to 39 years. None of the volunteers had a history of any relevant acute or chronic gastrointestinal illness. All were in good health. After an overnight fast the subjects were intubated with a nasogastric and nasoduodenal multilumen tube. The tip of the 5-lumen nasoduodenal tube was placed just distal the Ligament Treitz. Pressure recording ports were placed in the region of the antrum, near the papilla vateri and 15 cm distal in the duodenum. The pressure recording catheters (polyvinyl tubes with sideholes, obtained from Dural Plastics, New South Wales, Australia) were perfused with deionized water at 0.1 ml/min. A 4-lumen gastric tube was positioned fluoroscopically with the tip in the antrum and the aspiration ports at the most dependent part of the stomach. To determine the emptying of the stomach, a gastric recovery marker (phenolsulphonphthalein) was perfused through the proximal port at a rate of 0.1 ml/min. Gastroduodenal motility was measured by perfusing the catheters with deionized water, tubes were connected with a low compliance perfusion system (Arndorfer et al., 1977). After ensuring an optimal position of the tubes, the subjects were transferred to a separated single room where they were positioned on a table with the head raised to about 30°. After the subjects was seated, the cuff of a Dinamap 845 automated oscillometric blood pressure device was attached to the arm. Data on the reliability of this automated blood pressure device have been published and indicate very high correlations between its measurements and intraarterial measurements of blood pressure (Yelderman and Ream, 1979; Ramsey, 1979). The study was started with a period of at least 40 min to allow subjects to adjust to the setting.

Experimental design

After the first or second duodenal phase III of the migrating motility complex (MMC), acute mental stress was induced in randomized order. During the 60-min stress period the subjects had to solve anagrams and to do mental arithmetics (up to 20 mathematical operations per minute) against a financial reward. The mental stress period of 60 min consisted of four 8 min segments of problem solving phases and four feedback periods of 7 min each during which the subject was informed about the results in the preceeding problem solving phase (Figure 1). This feedback was randomized and standardized (3 x positive, 1 x negative) and was independent from

the correctness of the answers given. Emptying of the interdigestive secreted gastric juice was measured by marker recovery (Phenolsulphonphthalein). The duration of the duodenal MMC (time interval between two consecutive phases III) with and without mental stress was measured.
Differences between means were tested for statistical significance by one-way analysis of variance. The influence of cardiovascular changes on alterations of interdigestive motility was studied by means of stepwise regression analysis and Spearman correlations.

Fig. 1: Schematic representation of the experimental design

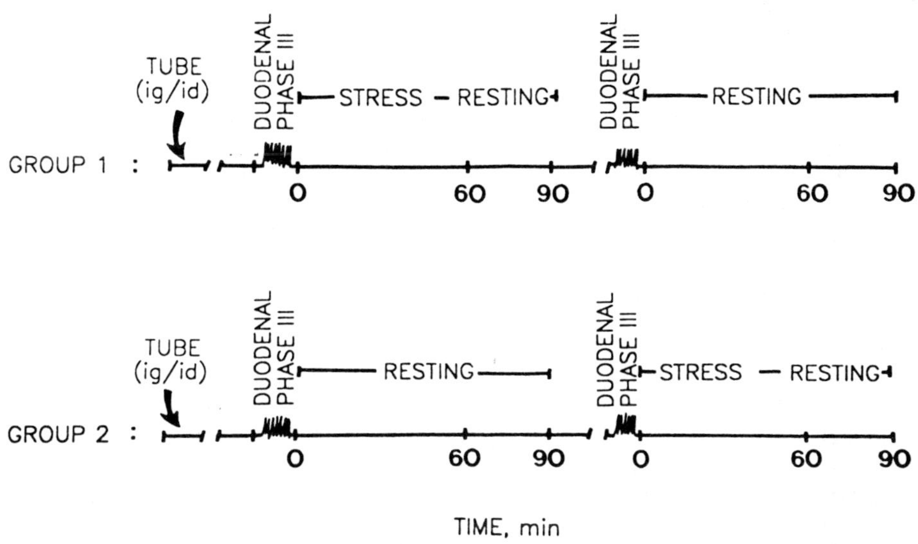

RESULTS

Gastroduodenal motility

The mean duration of the MMC was 117.6 ± 8.2 min (x ± SEM, N=11). There was no significant difference between the first and the second MMC observed. In 10 of the subjects studied, mental stress increased the duration of the MMC. Therefore, during the stress period the duration of the MMC was significantly increased by 60 per cent (143.4 ± 14.1 min vs. 91.4 ± 9.9 min). A significant effect of the experimental sequence was not found, although in subjects exposed to the stressor after the first duodenal phase III complex MMC's tended to be longer than in the group stressed after the second phase III complex. The difference, however, was not significantly different.

Gastric emptying

Mean gastric emptying with and without mental stress of all 15-min collecting periods was 21.1 ml ± 9. During acute mental stress periods emptying was not significantly altered as compared to the corresponding control periods (Table 1).

Cardiovascular stress responses

Acute mental stress significantly increased heart rate and blood pressure as compared to control (resting) values. The individual increase of heart rate during the actual stress period ranged from 0.9 to 17.3 bpm. Mean increases of heart rate and blood pressure are given in table 1.

Tab. 1 : Cardiovascular and gastroduodenal motility responses to mental stress (x±SEM, N=11, *p<0.05 vs control)

		Stress		Post-Stress
Time periods (min)		0 - 30	30 - 60	60 - 90
heart rate (beats/ min)	control	64 ±2	64 ±3	65 ±3
	stress	69 ±3*	71 ±3*	66 ±3
syst. blood press. (mmHg)	control	128 ±3	129 ±3	127 ±3
	stress	136 ±2*	135 ±2*	133 ±3
diast. blood press. (mmHg)	control	75 ±2	75 ±2	77 ±3
	stress	82 ±2*	79 ±2*	79 ±3
gastric emptying (ml/30 min)	control	25 ±8	18 ±6	20 ±8
	stress	24 ±24	22 ±10	18 ±8

Correlations between cardiovascular and motility changes

Mental stress increased the cycle length of the MMC and increased blood pressure and heart rate. However, analysis by means of multiple correlations and stepwise regressions did not yield any significant influence of the cardiovascular responses on the increase of the MMC. The same seems to be true for changes of gastric emptying (Tab. 2).

Table 2: Correlations of cardiovascular responses (increase of arterial blood pressure and heart rate) with motility responses (changes in the duration of the MMC and changes of gastric emptying) in response to acute mental stress. Spearman correlation coefficients of 11 subjects are given for the three distinct experimental periods (0-30, 30-60 and 60-90 min). SAP=systolic arterial pressure, DAP=diastolic arterial pressure, MAP=mean arterial pressure, HR=heart rate.

	correlation (r)			
	increase in the duration of the MMC	changes of transpyloric fluid movements 0 - 30	30 - 60	60 - 90 min
changes during				
0 - 30 min				
HR (/min)	-0.11	0.56	0.11	0.10
SAP (mmHg)	-0.16	0.23	0.15	0.02
DAP (mmHg)	0.00	0.01	-0.35	0.06
MAP (mmHg)	-0.11	0.28	0.09	-0.18
30 - 60 min				
HR (/min)	0.26	0.37	-0.05	0.15
SAP (mmHg)	0.01	0.05	-0.05	0.17
DAP (mmHg)	-0.21	0.11	-0.27	-0.16
MAP (mmHg)	-0.15	-0.03	-0.14	-0.08
60 - 90 min				
HR (/min)	-0.11	0.26	0.52	0.07
SAP (mmHg)	0.06	-0.44	-0.14	-0.30
DAP (mmHg)	0.23	0.60	0.34	0.07
MAP (mmHg)	0.05	0.12	0.04	0.08

DISCUSSION

The results of the present investigation can be summarized as follows: 1. acute mental stress increases the cycle length of the migrating motor complex; 2. acute mental stress does not alter basal gastric emptying; 3. there are only slight but insignificant correlations between cardiovascular and motility changes.

There is now considerable evidence that centrally activating stimuli such as mental stress influence gastro-duodenal motility. Data from the present investigation demonstrate, that the occurrence of duodenal phase III complexes is significantly inhibited. In contrast, acute mental stress did not alter gastric emptying of basally secreted gastric juice. With respect to the stress induced changes of the gastrointestinal motility similar findings have been made by MacRae et al. (1982), Cann et al. (1983) and Valori et al. (1986) although in these studies no pure mental (psychological) stressors had been used. It can be concluded, that stimuli increasing central nervous system activity decrease the frequency of duodenal phase III complexes. In contrast gastric emptying (basal and postprandial) is not altered by mental stress and stimuli increasing central nervous activity. Recently Camilleri et al. (1984) demonstrated that painful dermatomal stimulation by a transcutaneous electrical nerve stimulator impaired the antral

phasic pressure response to a meal. Interestingly this painful stimulus did not induce any cardiovascular changes or changes of circulating plasma catecholamines. However, plasma ß-endorphin levels increased. Although it is known that intravenous infusion of ß-endorphins inhibits antral phasic pressure activity in healthy individuals, this effect was only observed at doses associated with plasma levels higher than those obtained in Camillieri's study (Camilleri et al. 1984). This plasma level cannot be induced by any external physiological stimulus.
It is known, that cardiovascular responses to acute stress are mediated by catecholamines and sympathetic activation. Therefore, the release of catecholamines such as epinephrine which are responsible for cardiovascular responses might mediate changes of motility. However, a close "dose-response" relation between stress induced cardiovascular changes and alteration of gastroduodenal motility is not found. This finding suggests, that changes of upper gastrointestinal motility induced by acute mental stress are not mediated by direct sympathetic actions. Other mediators e.g. release of gastrointestinal hormons (Graeffner et al., 1987) have to be taken in account. Previous studies have shown, that the release of human pancreatic polypeptide (PP) is influenced by the adrenergic tone (Sive et al., 1980). On the other hand PP levels reflect cholinergic (vagal) tone (Schwartz et al., 1979). Therefore, sympathetic activation might influence cholinergic activity and changes of cholinergic activity and alterations of the cholinergic activity have to be considered as the mediators of motility changes. On the other hand the study of Camillieri et al. (1984) indicates that ß-endorphins might be involved in stress responses of the gastrointestinal motility. Further studies are needed to elucidate mechanisms mediating stress responses of the gastroduodenal motility.

REFERENCES

Arndorfer, R.C.; Steff, J.J.; Dodds, W.J.; Linehan, J.H. Hogan, W.J. (1977) Improved infusion system for intraluminal esophagal manometry. Gastroenterology, 73, 23-27

Axelrod, J. Reisine, T.D. (1984). Stress hormones: their interactions and regulation. Science, 224, 452-459

Beaumont, W. (1833) Experiments and observations on the gastric juice and the physiology of digestion. Platsburg: F.P. Allen

Camillieri, M.; Stanghellini, P.C.; Kao, C.H.; Li A.R., Zinsmeister and J.R. Malagelada (1984). Effects of synthetic ß-endorphin on upper gut motility (Abstract) Gastroenterology 86, 1039

Cann, P.A.; Read, N.W.; Cammack, N.W.; Childs, H. Holden, S.; Kashman, R.; Longmore, I.; Nix, S.; Simms, N. Swallow, K. Weller, J. (1983) Physiological stress and the passage of a standard test meal through the stomach and small intestine in man. GUT 24, 236-242

Dimsdale, J.E. & Moss, J. (1980) Plasma catecholamine in stress and exercise. J. Am. Med. Assoc. 243, 340-342
Graeffner, H., Bloom, S.R. Farnebo, L.O. Järhult, J. (1987) Effects of pysiological increases of plasma noradrenaline on gastric acid secretion and gastrointestinal hormons. Digestive Disease and Sciences, 3, 715-719.
McRrae, S. Younger, K. Thompson, D.L. (1982). Sustained mental stress alters human jejunal motor activity. GUT 23, 404-409
Thompson, D.G., Richelson, E.; Malagelada, J.R. (1982). Pertubation of gastric emptying and duodenal motility through central nervous system. Gastroenterology 83, 1200-1206
Schwartz, T.W.; Stenquist, B.; Olbe, L.; Stadil, F. (1979) Synchronous oscillation in the basal secretion of pancreatic polypeptide and gastric acid. Depression by cholinergic blockade of pancreatic polypeptide concentrations in plasma. Gastroenterology, 76, 14-19
Stadil and Rehfeld (1973) release of gastrin by epinephrine in man. Gastroenterology, 65, 210-215
Stanghellini, V.; Malagelada, J.-R.; Zinsmeister, A.R. Go, V.L.W.; Kao, P.C. (1983) Stress-induced gastroduodenal motor disturbances in humans: possible humoral mechanisms. Gastroenterology, 85, 83-91
Ramsey, M (1979) Noninvasive automatic determination of mean arterial blood pressure. Med. Biol. Eng. Comput. 17, 11-18
Thompson, D.G., Richelson, E.; Malagelada, J.R. (1983). Pertubation of upper gastrointestinal function by cold stress. GUT 24, 277-283
Thompson, D.G., Richelson, E.; Malagelada, J.R. (1983). Pertubation of upper gastrointestinal function by cold stress. GUT 24, 277-283
Valori, R.M.; Kumar, D.; Wingate, D.L.; (1986) Effects of different types of stress and the "prokinetic drugs" on the control of the fasting motor complex in humans. Gastroenterology, 90, 1890-1900
Wolf, S. & Wolff, H.G. (1947) An experimental study of a man and his stomach. New York: Oxford University Press
Yelderman, M.; Ream, A.D. (1979) Indirect measurement of mean blood pressure in the anesthetized patient. Anesthesiology 50, 253-256

Effect of cold pressure test on gallbladder contraction induced by a standardized meal in normal human subjects

Leonardo Marzio, Franca DiFelice, Velia Celiberti, Maria Grazia Laico

Istituto di Fisiopatologia Medica, Universita' «G. D'Annunzio», Ospedale SS. Annunziata, 66100 Chieti, Italy

INTRODUCTION

Recent studies (Stanghellini et al. 1983, 1984) have shown that stressful, centrally acting simuli modify fed gastrointestinal motility in humans with reversion of the motor pattern from fed to fasting. No data are at present available if gallbladder contraction induced by food may be modified by stress as well. The aim of this study has been therefore to evaluate the effect of acute stress on gallbladder contraction induced by a standard meal in a group of normal human subjects.

MATERIALS AND METHODS

Seven normal subjects (4 M, 3 F) of mean age 28 years (range 22-35) free from any gastrointestinal disturbances were studied. Each subject gave a written informed consent to the study which was approved by the ethic committee of our University. After 12 hours fasting each subject ate a meal composed by dried egg yolk (4 g), sorbitol (10 g), malt (3 g), cacao (2.5 g), ethilic alcohol 95° (3 g) used conventionally to test gallbladder contraction in radiology departments.

Gallbladder volume was assessed before the meal and subsequently every 10 min up to 120 min by real-time ultrasonography , using the formula $\pi/6 * a * b * c$ (Dodds et al. 1985) where a,b and c are the maximum antero-posterior, transverse and longitudinal gallbladder measurements respectively. In a preliminary study on a control group in our laboratory we showed that the test meal used for this study induced a maximal gallbladder contraction between 35 to 45 min from its administration. Each subject received the test meal twice with a 48 hours interval in between. Thirtyfive min after the meal a cold pressure test was performed for 10 min in one occasion and a placebo test with water 37°C was used in the second occasion as control. The test was performed introducing the non dominant hand in water at 4°C for 1 min with 15 sec interval between each immersion for a total period of 10 min or less if the subject felt that the pain was intolerable. The test was randomly assigned to each subject in a double blind manner. Gallbladder volume during the test was observed every 5 min. In order to make a statistical comparison a percent gallbladder volume (%GBV) was computed as follows: %GBV= RV/FV * 100 where FV is the volume after 12 hours fasting, RV is the residual volume calculated at each observation after the meal. The ANOVA test for repeated measurements and the Student's t test for paired data were used to test differences. Values are expressed as mean±SD.

RESULTS

Fasting gallbladder volume was similar in the two studies (cold pressure test: 28±4 cm^3;control: 31±5 cm^3). In the control study the standard meal induced a gallbladder contraction which reached a maximum after 35-40 min. Gallbladder volume returned to 80% initial volume 105 min after the meal (fig.1). When the cold pressure test was applied maximum gallbladder volume after meal was significantly less than the one reached in the control study (fig.1). Gallbladder refilling after maximum contraction was also accelerated with return to 80% fasting values 90 min after the meal.

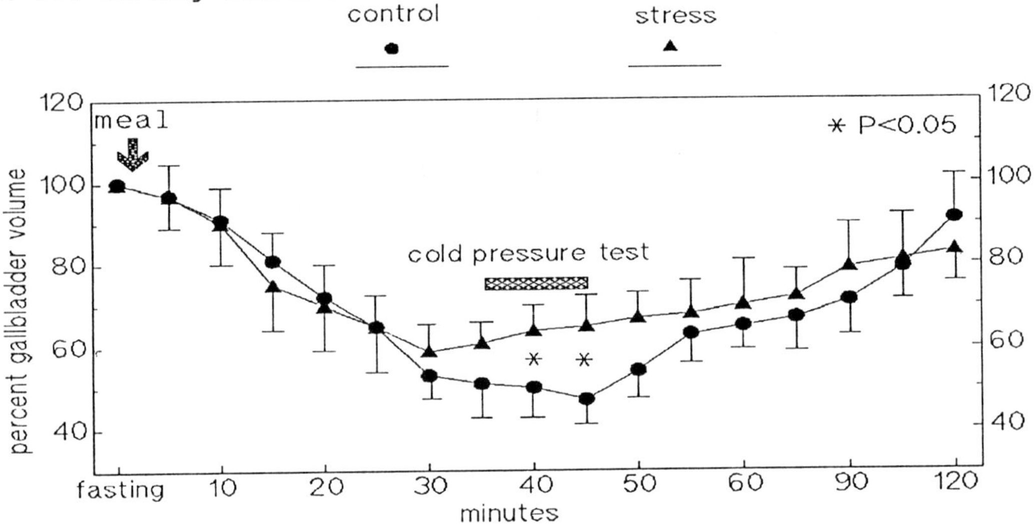

Fig.1. Line bar of percent gallbladder volume (mean±SD) observed after 12 hours fasting and after a standard meal in seven normal subjects. Thirty min after the meal a cold pressure test with water 4°C, was applied to each subject for 10 min (black triangles). Water at 37°C was used as control (black circles).

DISCUSSION

This study shows that maximum gallbladder contraction induced by a standard meal is significantly inhibited by cold pressure test in normal human subjects.

Gallbladder contraction after a meal is under the influence of various components, that is the vagus nerve, the rate of delivery of food from the stomach into the proximal duodenum, and the amount of substances liberated from the duodenal mucosa, mainly cholecystokinin, which are known to contract the gallbladder. The vagal component seems to influence the first part of gallbladder response to the meal that is the first 5 to 10 min of the meal before the beginning of gastric emptying, the gastric and duodenal component determine amount and duration of gallbladder contraction after the beginning of gastric emptying. In the present study cold pressure test was applied 35 min after the meal presumably after the cessation of the vagal component, therefore an inhibition of gastric emptying of the meal with a reduction in cholecystokinin release may be suggested. Cold pressure test has been in fact shown in humans to inhibit the high antral waves seen postprandially and to reverse the fed motility pattern into a fasting one. Furthermore cold pressure test has been shown to release endogenous substances such as catecholamines and endorphins which are known to have an inhibitory effect on gastric emptying (Sullivan et al. 1981). If these substances antagonize gallbladder contraction induced by a meal remains to be shown.

REFERENCES

Dodds, W.J., Groh, W.J., Darweesh, R.M.A., Lawson, T.L., Kishk, S.M.A., Kern, M.K.(1985). Sonographic measurements of gallbladder volume. AJR 145:1003-1011.

Stanghellini, V., Malagelada, J-R., Zinsmeister, A.R., Go, V.L.W., Kao, P.C. (1983): Stress-induced gastroduodenal motor disturbances in humans: possible humoral mechanisms. Gastroenterology 85: 83-91.

Stanghellini, V., Malagelada, J-R., Zinsmeister, A.R., Go, V.L.W., Kao, P.C. 1984) Effect of opiate and adrenergic blockers on the gut motor response to centrally acting stimuli. Gastroenterology 87:1104-1113.

Sullivan, S.N., Lamki, L., Corcoran, P. (1981):Inhibition of gastric emptying by enkefalin analogue. Lancet 2: 86-87.

Influence of cold water stress on colonic myoelectrical spiking activity in irritable bowel syndrome patients

Jacques Frexinos, Ghislain Staumont, Michel Delvaux, Jean Fioramonti and Lionel Buéno

Department of Nutrition and Gastroenterology, Centre Hospitalier Universitaire, 31054 Toulouse and Department of Pharmacology, INRA, 180 chemin de Tournefeuille, 31300 Toulouse, France

SUMMARY. *The influence of cold water stress (CWS) on colonic myoelectrical spiking activity was investigated in 12 IBS patients complaining of painful sensations without disturbance of bowel habits. The periods of stress were compared to periods of vigilance in the same patients. No significant effect was observed after CWS test on different kinds of spike burst activities (LSB,SSB and MLSB) on the whole colon or at any colonic level investigated (transverse, left and sigmoid colon).*

Emotional tensions influence abdominal symptoms and bowel function in irritable bowel syndrome (IBS) patients (Mendeloff et al.,1970). Recent studies on colonic motor recordings obtained in humans after periods of stress reported either a stimulation (Welgan et al.,1988; Narducci et al.,1985) or no effect on colonic motility (Schang et al.,1988; Sarna et al.,1982). But observations have been obtained in different experimental conditions. Moreover, the great variety of stressful conditions used limits the comparisons between different studies. The present study investigated in IBS patients the influence of a standartized stress by hand immersion in cold water (CWS) on the myoelectrical spiking activity recorded on the transverse, left and sigmoid colon.

SUBJECTS AND METHODS..

Subjects.
Twelve IBS patients, 4 men and 8 women aged 27-63 yr, were studied. They had one or two bowel movements per day, but painful sensations. They have never taken laxatives and any other medication for at least 3 weeks before investigations. The absence of organic disease was confirmed by clinical examination, gastroscopy and colonoscopy. The probe was positionned in the right colon during colonoscopy. Informed consent was obtained from each patient.

Recording system.
The probe, made of a polyvinyl tube 0.5 cm in diameter and 150 cm in length supported eight groups of three electrodes placed at 4 mm intervals. A full description of the probe was published elsewhere (Frexinos et al.,1985). Bipolar recordings were made with an eight-channel electroencephalograph (minihuit Alvar, Paris, France) using a short time constant (0.03 sec) and a paper speed of 7.2 cm/min.

Recording session.
All subjects were fasted for at least 14 hrs before introduction of the probe. A careful bowel cleansing was performed 24, 12 and-6 hrs before placing the probe. A thread attached to the tip of the probe was introduced into the operator channel of the colonoscope, permitting us to pull the probe to the right colon. Usually it was placed at 9:00 am, and recording session began at 5:00 pm, after a radiographic control of the position of the probe.

CWS was applied during 20 minutes the second day of recording at 10:00 am. It consisted of alternatively immersing one hand in ice cold water (4°C) for two minutes and removing the hand for two minutes , and so on for 20 minutes. During the two hours preceding CWS, the patients were in bed, but kept busy with neutral conversations and administrative questionnaires. This two hours period was considered as control and called period of vigilance. Blood arterial pressure and heart rate were continuously monitored during the session from 8:00 to11:00.

Analysis of the signal.

Long (LSB) and short (SSB) spike burst activities were analysed by visual inspection of the records from 8:00 to 11:00 on the second day of recording. Each kind of spiking activity was expressed as percentage of time. Propagated spike bursts (MLSB) were measured over at least 6 of the 8 channel records and expressed as number per hour. This visual analysis was done by the same observer who was unware of the period studied. Results were expressed as mean ± sem. Then the duration of the total spike burst activity was analysed on two consecutive electrode sites in each part of colon considered (transverse, left and sigmoid colon) and on the eight channels plotted together. This cumulative spiking acticity (total activity) was expressed as percentage of time. Values obtained for two hours before the test (period of vigilance) were compared to values obtained for one hour after the beginning of CWS (period of stress) using a paired T Wilcoxon test.

RESULTS.

The tip of the probe was placed into the right colon in five cases, reached the right flexure in five and only the left flexure in two. Two kinds of spike bursts have been previously observed with this technique (Frexinos et al.,1985). The first consisted of short spike bursts (SSB) lasting 3-3.5 sec and recurred at regular rate of 10-11/min. These bursts always appeared to be localized at one electrode site without any propagation to an adjacent group of electrodes. The second consisted of long spike bursts (LSB) lasting 10-11 sec and are either localized at one to three electrodes, either rapidly propagated in the aboral direction over the whole length of the colon investigated (MLSB) (Fig.1).

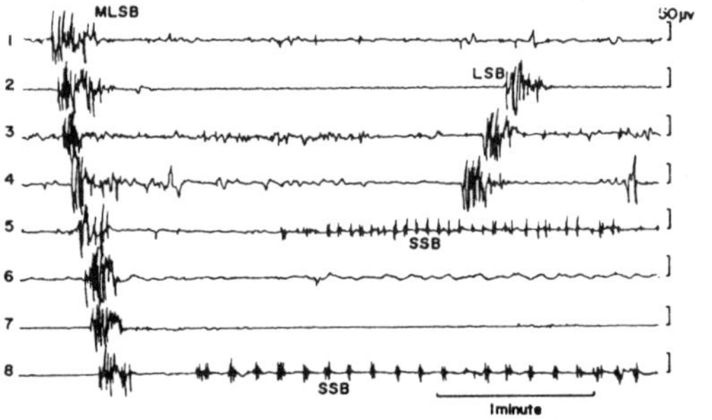

Fig.1 A representative electromyogramm obtained in a patient from the right colon (1) to the rectosigmoid junction (2) showing the different kinds of spike bursts: short spike bursts (SSB) at the 5th and 8th electrode sites, long spike bursts (LSB) orally propagated over 3 electrode sites or rapidly propagated over the whole colon (migrating long spike burst, MLSB). (from Frexinos et al.,1987.b).

CWS produced a significant ($P<0.01$) rise on systolic pressure and in pulse rate (mean rise of 16.1 ± 4.2 mmHg and of 8.9 ± 3.7 beats/min).

Table 1. Myoelectrical spiking activity (percentage of time or number per hour (MLSB), mean ± sem, n=12) recorded on the whole colon investigated during the periods of vigilance and CWS.

	LSB	SSB	MLSB	Total activity
Vigilance	7.3 ± 2.5	2.5 ± 2.0	0.3 ± 0.4	11.7 ± 6.2
CWS	9.1 ± 2.9	2.1 ± 1.8	0.7 ± 0.6	15.0 ± 5.9

No significant difference ($P>0.05$) between the two groups.

Table 2. Total myoelectrical spiking activity (percentage of time, mean ± sem, n=12) recorded on different colonic segments during the periods of vigilance and CWS.

	transverse (n=10)	left	sigmoid	whole colon
Vigilance	9.7 ± 4.9	12.3 ± 6.4	13.8 ± 8.1	11.7 ± 6.2
CWS	12.2 ± 5.1	14.8 ± 7.0	17.3 ± 8.6	15.0 ± 5.9

No significant difference ($P>0.05$) between the two groups.

The comparison of values of spiking activity expressed as percentage of time for LSB and SSB activities and as number per hour for MLSB activity indicated no significant difference (P>0.05) between control (period of vigilance from 8:00 to 10:00) and the period of CWS (from 10:00 to 11:00) (table.1).
The comparison of mean values of cumulative spiking activity expressed as total activity indicated no significant difference (P>0.05) between the period of vigilance (control) and the period of CWS at any colonic level investigated (table.2).

DISCUSSION.

This study shows that cold pain had no effect on colonic myoelectrical activity analysed on the whole colon (LSB,SSB and MLSB) or on diferent colonic segment (transverse,left and sigmoid). These results confirm previous data obtained in IBS patients (Narducci et al.,1985) as in healthy humans with CWS (Schang et al.,1988) or stressful interviews (Sarna et al.,1982). However our study disagree with other results reported after psychological stress in IBS patients (Welgan et al.,1988) or CWS in healthy subjects (Narducci et al.,1985). These discrepancies probably involve the choice both of subjects studied and of experimental stressors used. A considerable variability of colonic motility is observed in humans (Frexinos et al.,1985), leading us to use a non parametric paired test for statistical analysis. Moreover colonic motor pattern of IBS patients depends upon bowel symptoms and subgroups can be defined (Frexinos et al.,1987.b). Recently an increase of LSB and MLSB activities was reported after CWS in a painless diarrhea group whereas no significant difference was observed in isolated painful sensation groups (Frexinos et al.,1987.a).
Furthermore CWS was choosen as a standardized and classical stress test according to the well established effects on gastrointestinal functions. A significant reduction of antral phasic contractions (Stanghellini et al.,1983) was reported as a delay of gastric emptying (Thompson et al.,1983), an increase of oro-cecal transit time (O'brien et al.,1987) or a reduction of jejunal absorption (Barclay & Turnberg,1988). But even if cold pain is associated with significant rise in blood pressure and in pulse rate as in our study, the question arises to know if such a stressful model can be considered as available for life events or social relationships. But other stressful situations as anger, interview or mental stimulation appeared less standardized and so less reproducible.
In conclusion, hand immersion in cold water had no effect on colonic myoelectrical activity in a group of patients complaining of painful sensations without disturbances of bowel habits. However we cannot extrapolate that stress does not affect the colonic motility in other stressful situations and/or experimental conditions as well as in other subgroups of IBS patients.

REFERENCES.

Barclay,G.R., Turnberg,L.A. (1988): Effect of cold-induced pain on salt and water transport in the human jejunum. *Gastroenterology.* 94, 994-998.

Frexinos,J., Fioramonti,J., Buéno,L. (1985): Diurnal changes in myoelectric spiking activity of the human colon. *Gastroenterology.* 88, 1104-1110.

Frexinos,J., Buéno,L. (1987.a): Influence of stress on colonic myoelectrical activity in IBS patients. *Gastroenterology.* 92, 1396 (abstract).

Frexinos,J., Fioramonti,J., Buéno,L. (1987.b): Colonic myoelectrical activity in IBS painless diarrhoea. Gut.28,1613-1618.

Mendeloff,A.I., Monk,M., Singh,C.I., Lilienfeld,A. (1970): Illness experience and life stresses in patients with irritable colon and ulcerative colitis. *N.Engl.J.Med.* 282, 14-17.

Narducci,F., Snape,W.J., Battle,W.M., London,R.L., Cohen,S. (1985): Increased colonic motility during exposure to a stressful situation. *Dig.Dis.Sci.* 30, 40-44.

O'Brien,J.D., Thompson,D.G., Burnham,W.R.,Holly,J. Walker,E. (1988): Action of centrally mediated autonomic stimulation on human upper gastrointestinal transit: a comparative study of two stimuli. *Gut.* 28, 960)-969.

Sarna,S., Latimer,P., Campbell,D., Waterfall,W.E. (1982): Effect of stress, meal and neostigmine on rectosigmoid electrical control activity (ECA) in normals and in irritable bowel syndrome patients. *Dig.Dis.Sci.* 27, 582-591.

Schang,J.C., Devroede,G., Hebert,M., Hemond,M., Pilote,M., Devroede,L. (1988): Effects of rest, stress,and food on myoelectrical spiking activity of left and sigmoid colon in humans. *Dig.Dis.Sci.* 33, 614- 618.

Stanghellini,V., Malagelada,J.R., Zinsmeister,A.R., Go,V.L.W., Kao,P.C. (1983): Stress-induced gastroduodenal motor disturbances in humans: possible humoral mechanisms. *Gastroenterology.* 85, 83-91.

Thompson,D.G., Richelson E., Malagelada J.R. (1983): Perturbation of upper gastrointestinal function by cold stress. *Gut.* 24, 277-283.

Welgan,P., Meshkinpour,H.,Beeler,M. (1988): Effect of anger on colon motor and myoelectrical activity in irritable bowel syndrome. *Gastroenterology.* 94, 1150-1156.

3rd SESSION :

Animals models and mechanisms

Moderators : *T. Burk, J. Fioramonti*

Restraint stress and intestinal transit in rats

Thomas F. Burks, Julie M. Peterson, Cynthia L. Williams and Thomas H. Kramer

Department of Pharmacology, College of Medicine, The Univeristy of Arizona, Tucson, Arizona, U.S.A. 85724

Physical and psychological stress can produce profound alterations in gastrointestinal motility and propulsion. In humans, experimental stress has been shown in a number of studies to alter specific aspects of gastrointesinal motility. Several types of experimental stress have been used in clinical studies of gastrointestinal motility. For example, labyrinthine stimulation and vertigo produced by instilling cold water into the external auditory canal of one ear was found to decrease gastric emptying in healthy volunteers and to decrease contractions of the antrum of the stomach (Thompson et al., 1982). Painful immersion of one hand in ice water delayed gastric emptying (Thompson et al., 1983). Labyrinthine stimulation with cold water and painful immersion of one hand in cold water were also found in other studies to decrease antral contractions (Stanghellini et al., 1983). Dichotomous listening to recordings inhibited the development of the migrating motility complexes of the jejunum that is characteristic of the fasting motility pattern in humans (McRae et al., 1982). Electronic video games, driving in traffic and other psychological stressors also decreased the incidence of fasting migrating motor complexes in normal subjects (Valori et al., 1986). However, another study with fed subjects found that labyrinthine stimulation tended to convert random duodenal postprandial contractions to migrating motor complexes characteristic of fasting (Thompson et al., 1982). Experimental stress can produce changes in gastrointestinal propulsion as well as changes in patterns of motility. Two preliminary studies indicated that painful immersion of one hand in cold water reduced orocecal transit of intestinal contents in humans (O'Brien et al., 1985a, 1985b).

Experimental stress has usually been found to increase the incidence and amplitudes of contractions of the colon in humans. Immersion of one hand in ice water increased colonic contractions (Almy and Tulin, 1947; Narducci et al., 1985). Card-sorting and ball-sorting psychological stress was also found to increase the number of colonic contractions (Narducci et al., 1985). But exposure of normal subjects to a stressful interview was not found to induce consistent changes in colonic motility (Latimer et al., 1981). Overall, however, most studies in human subjects indicate that experimental pschological and painful stressors decrease gastric emptying, affect small intestinal patterns of motility, and usually increase the incidence or amplitudes of colonic contractions.

Increased colinic contractions in response to stress also occur in patients with irritable bowel syndrome (IBS). Patients with IBS displayed higher rates of colonic contractions than normal subjects (Latimer et al., 1981) and the contractile response of the colon to stress may also be exaggerated in comparison with normal subjects (Narducci et al., 1985). Studies in humans suggest that the most consistent motility alteration associated with stress is an increase in colonic contractions. Small bowel motility and transit in humans may be increased or decreased, depending on the stressor to which they are exposed (Cann et al., 1983a, 1983b).

<u>Animl Models of Stress</u>

We have carried out studies in rats to develop a suitable model for stress-induced alterations in gastrointestinal motility and transit (Williams and Burks, 1989). The effects of several potential stressors on small intestinal transit are summarized in Table 1.

Table 1. Effects of stressors on small intestinal transit in unanesthetized rats.

Decreased small intestinal transit	No change in small intestinal transit
Wrap restraint	Electroconvulsive shock
Cold water swim	Footshock
Cold restraint	Warm water swim
Ether vapors	Cold exposure

As expected, different stressors produced different effects. Partial restraint of unanesthetized rats produced by wrapping the foresholders and thorax with paper tape ("wrap restraint") was found consistently to decrease small intestinal transit. In a cold water swimming test, rats were required to swim intermittently for 10 sec periods in water maintained at 4°C. Other animals were required to swim similarly in water maintained at 20° C. The cold water swimming test resulted in decreased small intestinal transit, whereas the warm water swimming test did not alter small intestinal transit. Electroconvulsive shock (Galligan et al., 1983a) and electrical foot shock (Galligan et al., 1983b) induced analgesia, but had no effect on small intestinal transit. The effects of cold were assessed by maintaining animals for 1 hour at an ambient temperature of 4°C (Williams and Burks, 1989). Other rats were restrained in wire mesh restraints for 1 hour at an ambient temperature of 4° C. Cold exposure alone did not alter small intestinal transit. However, cold restraint produced significant inhibition of small intestinal transit. Exposure of rats to vapors of diethyl ether for 5 min decreased small intestinal transit. Thus, different stressors had different effects on small intestinal transit, wrap restraint was selected as the most appropriate model for further studies.

Release of Adrenocorticotropic Hormone and β-Endorphin

To ascertain that the changes in transit induced by wrap restraint were associated with accepted markers of stress, plasma levels of ACTH and β-endorphin were measured by radioimmunoassay (Williams et al., 1988). Wrap restraint resulted in a rapid, 8-fold increase in plasma ACTH levels (from 95 ± 5 to 822 ± 38 pg/ml) within 20 min, levels remained elevated for 30 min, and returned to control values by 60 min. The pattern of release of β-endorphin was similar. Wrap restraint stress resulted in a rapid increase in plasma β-endorphin concentrations that peaked 20 min after application of stress, and remained elevated (60-75 pM) for 60 min. The increases in plasma levels of ACTH and β-endorphin indicated that wrap restraint is a true stress stimulus.

Effect of Time of Day

The effect of stress on small intestinal transit was strongly dependent on the time of day at which the experiment was performed. The greatest changes in intestinal transit and plasma ACTH concentrations occurred in late afternoon hours. Animals tested at 5:00 PM, immediately before the beginning of the dark phase, showed the greatest response in both stress-induced inhibition of intestinal transit and release of ACTH. The similarity of the two responses to wrap restraint stress was striking and there was a pronounced correlation ($r = 0.95$) between the inhibition of small intestinal transit and stimulation of ACTH release over the entire 24 hour period. The degree of intestinal dysfunction produced by stress was dependent on the time of day that the animals were stressed, suggesting a circadian influence on stress-induced changes in intestinal propulsion. It has been reported that symptoms are most severe for patients with IBS in the early morning, the equivalent of late afternoon in rats and other nocturnal species, possibly suggesting a circadian influence on the sensitivity of the human bowel to stress (Kumar and Wingate, 1985; Kumar et al., 1986).

Functional Effects of Wrap Restraint Stress

Studies were carried out in female Sprague-Dawley rats to determine effects of wrap restraint stress on gastric emptying, small intestinal transit, and colonic transit (Williams et al., 1988). Small intestinal and colonic transit were measured by the geometric center method (Miller et al., 1981). Wrap restraint stress did not affect the rate of gastric emptying in rats. As observed in other studies, wrap restraint stress inhibited small intestinal transit, reducing the geometric center of transit from 5.4 to 4.1 (a geometric center of 1 indicates no transit, a geometric center of 10 indicates complete transit through the small intestine). Interestingly, wrap restraint stress greatly increased colonic transit. In addition, restraint stress resulted in an increase in fecal excretion.

Motility Effects of Stress

Wrap restraint stress in rats was found to produce changes in transit in the small intestine and colon that mimic in some respects stress-induced changes of transit in humans. To determine the effects of stress on intestinal motility, we measured intraluminal pressure in the small intestine, cecum and colon of rats before and after wrap restraint. Wrap restraint stress consistently caused increased incidence and amplitude of contractions in the small intestine, cecum and colon. In the small intestine, wrap restraint stress was associated with reduction or abolition of migrating motor complexes and increased regular or irregular contractions. In the cecum and colon, wrap restraint stress caused an increase in the frequency of contractions and often in the amplitude of contractions.

Mediators of Stress Responses

The observation that stress-induced changes in ACTH levels and intestinal transit in rats occur in parallel suggests that endocrine messengers may play a role in mediating the effects of stress on the gastrointestinal tract. The hypothalamic-pituitary-adrenal axis is the endocrine system most central to the stress response (Rivier and Plotsky, 1986). Corticotropin-releasing factor (CRF) acts on the pituitary to cause release of ACTH and β-endorphin concomitantly in response to stress (Guillemin et al., 1977). CRF also acts at extrapituitary sites to alter motor outflow in the autonomic nervous system. Thus, CRF-mediated stress effects could result either from pituitary-adrenal or extrapituitary actions of CRF. Surgical ablation of the adrenal glands and pituitary did not alter wrap restraint stress-induced inhibition of small intestinal transit in rats (Williams et al., 1988). Moreover, intravenously administered ACTH or β-endorphin did not affect small intestinal transit, even when the doses administered were much greater than the doses required to reach plasma concentrations of the hormones under stress conditions. Therefore, stress-induced changes in gastrointestinal transit in rats seem not to be mediated by pituitary or adrenally derived factors.

Evidence for a direct mediator role of CRF in stress-induced changes in gastrointestinal motility in rats has recently been presented (Williams et al., 1987). CRF, administered intravenously (i.v.) or intracerebroventricularly (i.c.v.), produced significant changes in the propulsive activity of the gastrointestinal tract. Gastric emptying was inhibited in a dose-dependent manner, at doses of 1.0 to 10.0 μg i.v. or i.c.v. In addition, CRF, in doses of 0.3 to 10.0 μg, inhibited small intestinal transit and increased colonic transit, resulting in increased fecal output. Thus, there was a striking parallelism between gastrointestinal effects of stress and exogenously administered CRF, especially when CRF was administered at an i.c.v. dosage of 0.3 μg (Table 2). Low doses of CRF, like

Table 2. Similarities of effects of wrap restraint stress and corticotropin-releasing factor (CRF, 0.3 μg, i.c.v.) on gastrointestinal functions.

Function	Wrap restraint stress	CRF (0.3 μg, i.c.v.)
Gastric emptying	0	0
Small intestinal transit	↓	↓
Colonic transit	↑	↑
Fecal excretion	↑	↑

0 = no effect, ↓ = decrease, ↑ = increase

stress, decreased small intestinal transit, increased colonic transit, and increased fecal excretion, without affecting gastric emptying. To determine whether endogenously released CRF might mediate gastrointestinal motility responses to stress in vivo, a CRF antagonist, alpha-helical CRF-(9-41) (Rivier et al., 1985), was employed. The CRF antagonist, given i.v. or i.c.v. in a dose of 50 μg, had no effect alone on small intestinal transit or colonic transit. However, it effectively antagonized the effects of exogenous CRF on small intestinal and colonic transit when CRF and the antagonist were administered via the same route. Administration of the CRF antagonist i.c.v. or i.v. immediately before wrap restraint stress completely blocked the stress-induced increase in colonic transit and significantly diminished the stress-induced increase in fecal excretion. However, the CRF antagonist did not antagonize stress-induced inhibition of small intestinal transit. The results of these studies suggest that endogenous CRF may mediate the effects of stress on intestinal motility and transit, particularly in the cecum and colon. Blockade of endogenous CRF can prevent the response of the colon to stress, suggesting that CRF may be directly responsible for mediating the effects of stress on colonic function. Recent studies in our laboratory have provided preliminary evidence that exogenously administered CRF produces striking increases in contractions of the cecum. CRF released by stress may act in the brain to alter autonomic nervous system outflow or may act directly within the enteric nervous system of the gastrointestinal tract to alter propulsive activity.

A CRF link in stress-induced changes in gastrointestinal motility is supported by other reports. Application of partial restraint in rats, like CRF administered i.c.v. (Lenz et al., 1988), was found to decrease gastric emptying, inhibit small intestinal transit, and increase colonic transit. In mice fed a milk powder meal containing fat, acoustic stress and cold stress were found to increase gastric emptying (Bueno and Gué, 1988). Administration of CRF antiserum given intraperitoneally (i.p.) blocked the effects of acoustic and cold stress on gastric emptying. Interestingly, administration of CRF antiserum by i.p. injection also blocked the effects of i.c.v. CRF on gastric emptying. These important experiments suggest that the stress-induced alterations of gastric emptying were abolished by immunoneutralization of circulating CRF. It is not certain whether the CRF released by stress that affects gastrointestinal motility arises from the brain or from a peripheral site.

Conclusions

Many stress models have been tested in rats to determine effects of stress on gastrointestinal motility. In several respects, acute wrap restraint stress mimics the effects of experimental and pathological stress in humans: there is inhibition of small intestinal transit, stimulation of colonic transit, stimulation of small intestinal and colonic motility, and increase in fecal excretion, but no change in gastric emptying. Acute wrap restraint stress fulfills the criteria of a true stress response in that plasma levels of ACTH and β-endorphin are increased. Other restraint models and acoustic stress in animals also affect gastrointestinal motility.

Evidence has been put forward that some components of the gastrointestinal response to stress may be mediated by extrapituitary actions of CRF. The CRF link may be in the central nervous system or in the periphery. Additional experimentation will be required to determine the precise site of CRF action. Identification of CRF as a critical link in the effect of stress on gastrointestinal motility and transit provides new opportunities to understand one of the most typical responses of the body to stress.

ACKNOWLEDGEMENTS

This work was supported by USPHS grants DA02163 and DK32547.

REFERENCES

Almy, T.P., and Tulin, M. (1947): Alterations in colonic function in man under stress: experimental production of changes simulating the "irritable colon." Gastroenterology 8, 616-626.

Bueno, L., and Gué, M. (1988): Evidence for the involvement of corticotropin-releasing factor in the gastrointestinal disturbances induced by acoustic and cold stress in mice. Brain Res. 444, 1-4.

Cann, P.A., Read, N.W., Brown, C., Hobson, N., and Holdsworth, C.D. (1983a): Irritable bowel syndrome: relationship of disorders in the transit of a single solid meal to symptom patterns. Gut 24, 405-411.

Cann, P.A., Read, N.W., Cammack, J., Childs, H., Holden, S., Kashman, R., Longmore, J., Nix, S., Simms, N., Swallow, K., and Weller, J. (1983b): Psychological stress and the passage of a standard meal through the stomach and small intestine in man. Gut 24, 236-240.

Galligan, J.J., Porreca, F., and Burks, T.F. (1983a): Dissociation of analgesic and gastrointestinal effects of electroconvulsive shock-released opioids. Brain Res. 271, 354-357.

Galligan, J.J., Porreca, F., and Burks, T.F. (1983b): Footshock produces analgesia but no gastrointestinal motility effects in the rat. Life Sci. 33 (Suppl. 1), 473-475.

Guillemin, R., Vargo, T., Rossier, J., Minick, S., Ling, N., Rivier, C., Vale, W. and Bloom, F. (1977): β-Endorphin and adrenocorticotropin are secreted concomitantly by the pituitary gland. Science 197, 1367-1369.

Kumar, D., and Wingate, D.L. (1985): IBS: a paroxysmal disorder. Lancet 2, 973-977.

Kumar, D., Wingate, D.L., and Ruckebusch, Y. (1986): Circadian variation in the propagation velocity of the migrating motor complex. Gastroenterology 91, 926-930.

Latimer, P., Sarna, S., Campbell, D., Latimer, M., Waterfall, W., and Daniel, E.E. (1981): Colonic motor and myoelectrical activity: a comparative study of normal subjects, psychoneurotic patients, and patients with irritable bowel syndrome. Gastroenterology 80, 893-901.

Lenz, H.J., Burlage, M., Raedler, A., and Greten, H. (1988): Central nervous system effects of corticotropin-releasing factor on gastrointestinal transit in the rat. Gastroenterology 94, 598-602.

McRae, S., Younger, K., Thompson, D.G., and Wingate, D.L. (1982): Sustained mental stress alters human jejunal motor activity. Gut 23, 404-409.

Miller, M.S., Galligan, J.J., and Burks, T.F. (1981): Accurate measurement of intestinal transit. J. Pharmacol. Methods 6, 211-217.

Narducci, F., Snape, W.J., Battle, W.M., London, R.L., and Cohen, S. (1985): Increased colonic motility during exposure to a stressful situation. Dig. Dis. Sci. 30, 40-44.

O'Brien, J.D., Thompson, D.G., Holly, J., Burnham, W.R., and Walker, E. (1985a): Stress disturbs human gastrointestinal transit viá a beta-1 adrenoreceptor mediated pathway. Gastroenterology 88, 1520.

O'Brien, J., Thompson, D.G., Holly, J., Burnham, W., and Walker, E. (1985b): Beta-blockers can protect human upper gastrointestinal function from disturbance by stress. Gut 26, A559.

Rivier, C.L., and Plotsky, P.M. (1986): Mediation by corticotropin releasing factor (CRF) of adrenohypophysial hormone secretion. Ann. Rev. Physiol. 48, 475-494.

Rivier, J., Rivier, C., and Vale, W. (1985): Synthetic competitive antagonists of corticotropin-releasing factor-induced ACTH secretion in the rat. Science 224, 889-891.

Stanghellini, V., Malagelada, J.-R., Zinsmeister, A.R., Go, V.L.W., and Kao, P.C. (1983): Stress-induced gastroduodenal motor disturbances in humans: possible humoral mechanisms. Gastroenterology 85, 83-91.

Thompson, D.G., Richelson, E., and Malagelada, J.-R. (1982): Perturbation of gastric emptying and duodenal motility through the central nervous system. Gastroenterology 83, 1200-1206.

Thompson, D.G., Richelson, E., and Malagelada, J.-R. (1983): Perturbation of upper gastrointestinal function by cold stress. Gut 24, 277-283.

Valori, R.M., Kumar, D., and Wingate, D.L. (1986): Effects of different types of stress and of "prokinetic" drugs on the control of the fasting motor complex in humans. Gastroenterology 90, 1890-1900.

Williams, C.L., and Burks, T.F. (1989): Stress, opioids, and gastrointestinal transit. In Neuropeptides and Stress. ed. Y. Tache', J.E. Morley and M.R. Brown, pp. 175-187, New York: Springer-Verlag.

Williams, C.L., Peterson, J.M., Villar, R.G., and Burks, T.F. (1987): Corticotropin-releasing factor directly mediates colonic responses to stress. Am. J. Physiol. 253, G582-G586.

Williams, C.L., Villar, R.G., Peterson, J.M., and Burks, T.F. (1988): Stress-induced changes in intestinal transit in the rat: a model for irritable bowel syndrome. Gastroenterology 94, 611-621.

Stress-induced alterations of gastric emptying

Yvette Taché

Center for Ulcer Research and Education, Veterans Administration Medical Center and Department of Medicine and Brain Research Institute, University of California, Los Angeles, California 90073, U.S.A.

The influence of stressful events on gastric emptying has been recognized since the beginning of the 19th century. Among the pioneer investigators who have revealed such an interaction is the French physiologist, Jean Charles Cabanis (Cabanis, 1981), who described in 1802 the perturbing effect of emotions on gastric motor function as following: "A vigorous and healthy man has just eaten a good meal; ...the digestive juices dissolve them easily and quickly. Should this man receive bad news, or should sad and baneful passions suddenly arise in his soul, his stomach will immediately cease to act on the foods contained in them. The very juices in which the foods are already almost entirely dissolved will remain as though struck by a moral stupor, and... digestion ceases entirely". Thirty years later, Beaumont's observations performed in his fistulous subject brought objective clinical evidence that "... fear, anger or whatever depresses or disturbs the nervous system ..." was accompanied by delay in gastric digestion and emptying (Beaumont, 1833). In 1936, Selye (Selye, 1936) formulated the concept of biological stress and established in laboratory animals that the stomach is an important target organ adversely affected by various stressors. These early clinical and experimental observations opened up a new field of investigation related to the influence of stress on gastric function.

This chapter will review knowledge on the effects of stress on gastric emptying and mechanisms through which stress-related alteration of gastric emptying occurred, particularly the possible role of selected brain neuropeptides.

ALTERATIONS OF GASTRIC EMPTYING BY VARIOUS STRESSORS

Various physical, psychological or chemical acute stimuli have been used to study the influence of stress on gastric emptying of a liquid or solid nutritive meal or non caloric solution in animals and human. As summarized in Table 1, delayed gastric emptying is induced by labyrinthine stimulation (Thompson et al. 1982), painful stimuli (cold) applied on one hand (Thompson et al. 1983) and preoperative anxiety (Simpson, and Stakes, 1987) in man, ionizing radiations and acquisition of free operant avoidance in monkeys (Dorval et al. 1985; Dubois, and Natelson, 1978), loud noise in the dog (Peeters et al. 1989), handling combined with noise in guinea pig (Costall et al. 1983), passive avoidance (Enck et al. 1988), hemorrhage (Limlomwongse et al. 1988), restraint by trunk clamping (Lenz et al. 1988b), ether anesthesia, abdominal surgery, trephination (Taché et al. 1989b), unpredictable, unavoidable tail shock (Taché and Garrick, unpublished observations) or cold exposure for 2-3 h in rats (Koo et al. 1985). By contrast, an increase in the rate of gastric emptying has been reported in subjects viewing stressful films (Rosman et al. 1987) or in mice exposed to loud music (Buéno, and Gué, 1988; Gué et al. 1987) or in rats or mice exposed for 30 to 60 min to cold (Buéno, and Gué, 1988; Taché et al. 1988b). No change in gastric emptying has also been observed in monkey following first exposure to unavoidable, unpredictable shock (Natelson, and Dubois, 1980) or in man exposed to psychological stress of task performance under dichotomous listening and interruption (Cann et al. 1983; OBrien et al. 1987).

Taken together these studies indicate that delayed gastric emptying appears the most common and consistent effect resulting from exposure to various stressors, particularly in human, monkey, dog or rats. However variability in the pattern of response does exist since no change or an increase in gastric transit has also been observed following exposure to some stressors. Such variability may be related to differences in the nature, intensity and duration of the stressors employed, previous stress experience, species under study as well as the composition of the meal (caloric or non caloric, solid or liquid). Which of these factors are the key variables determining the pattern of the gastric response needs to be further documented under similar conditions.

Table 1. Effects of various stressors on gastric emptying

Stressors	Species	Meal	Gastric Emptying	References
Fear, anger	Man	Cal.	Delay	(Beaumont, 1833)
Labyrinthine stimulation	Man	Liq.Cal.	Delay	(Thompson et al. 1982)
Painful stimuli	Man	Liq.Cal.	Delay	(Thompson et al. 1983)
Preoperative anxiety	Man	Non Cal.	Delay	(Simpson, and Stakes, 1987)
Stressful films	Man	Egg	Increase	(Rosman et al. 1987)
Dichotomous listening	Man	Cal.	No change	(Cann et al. 1983; OBrien et al. 1987)
Operant avoidance	Monkey	Water	Delay	(Dubois, and Natelson, 1978)
Radiation	Monkey	Water	Delay	(Dorval et al. 1985)
Handling, noise	Guinea pig	Non Cal.	Delay	(Costall et al. 1983)
Acoustic	Dog	Cal.	Delay	(Peeters et al. 1989)
Passive avoidance	Rat	1:1 Food-water	Delay	(Enck et al. 1988)
Hemorrhage	Rat	Liq. non cal.	Delay	(Limlomwongse et al. 1988)
Cold, 2-3 h	Rat	Liq. non cal.	Delay	(Koo et al. 1985)
Tail shocks	Rat	Liq. non cal.	Delay	(Taché et al. 1989b)
Surgery	Rat	Liq. non cal.	Delay	(Taché et al. 1989b)
Trunk clamping	Rat	Liq. non cal.	Delay	(Lenz et al. 1988b)
Wrap restraint	Rat	Liq. non cal.	No change	(Taché et al. 1988b; Williams et al. 1987; 1988)
Cold, 30-80 min	Rat	Liq. non cal.	Increase	(Koo et al. 1985; Taché et al. 1988b)
Cold, 20 min	Mice	Milk	Increase	(Buéno, and Gué, 1988)
Music ($\leq$ 190 dB)	Mice	Milk	Increase	(Buéno, and Gué, 1988)

Liq.:liquid; cal.: caloric.

CENTRAL NERVOUS SYSTEM ACTION OF SELECTIVE BRAIN PEPTIDES TO INFLUENC GASTRIC EMPTYING

The mechanisms through which various stressors influence gastric transit remain poorly understood. Several studies indicate that it represents a centrally mediated effect which is probably initiated by stressor specific neurochemical pathways and modulated by the internal biochemical status of animals (OBrien et al. 1987; Simpson, and Stakes, 1987; Thompson et al. 1982; Williams, and Burks, 1988).

Growing evidence indicates that several peptides delivered into the cerebrospinal fluid act into the brain to influence gastric emptying in the rat (Taché, 1988a) (Table 2). TRH injected into the cisterna magna increases gastric emptying independently from the activation of pituitary-thyroid axis (Maeda-Hagiwara, and Taché, 1987). Other peptides injected into the cerebrospinal fluid including calcitonin (Lenz, 1988a; Taché et al. 1987a), calcitonin-gene related peptide, CGRP, (Lenz, 1988a; Raybould et al. 1988), corticotropin-releasing factor, CRF, (Lenz et al. 1988c; Taché et al. 1987b; Williams et al. 1987), and bombesin (Porreca, and Burks, 1983) inhibit gastric emptying of a non nutrient meal in the rat through autonomic dependent pathways. In the dog, injection of bombesin, CRF and neurotensin have been reported to delay gastric emptying of a peptone meal (Lenz, 1987b). Specific brain nuclei on which these peptides act to influence gastric transit have not yet been investigated.

Table 2. Central nervous system action of peptides to influence gastric emptying in experimental animals

Peptides	**Dose nmol/animal**	**Species**	**Meal**	**Gastric Emptying**	**References**
TRH	0.03-0.3	Rat	Non cal.	Increase	(Maeda-Hagiwara and Taché, 1987)
Bombesin	0.06-0.6	Rat	Non cal.	Decrease	(Porreca and Burks, 1983)
	12	Dog	Cal.	Decrease	(Lenz, 1987b)
Calcitonin	0.003-0.03	Rat	Non cal.	Decrease	(Lenz 1988a; Taché et al. 1987a)
	12	Dog	Cal.	No change	(Lenz, 1987b)
CGRP	0.02-0.2	Rat	Non cal.	Decrease	(Lenz 1988a; Raybould et al. 1988)
	12	Dog	Cal.	No change	(Lenz, 1987b)
CRF	0.06-1	Rat	Non cal.	Decrease	(Lenz et al. 1988c; Taché et al. 1987b; Williams et al. 1987)
	12	Dog	Cal.	Decrease	(Lenz, 1987b)
	0.03	Mice	Cal.	Increase	(Buéno, and Gué, 1988; Gué et al. 1987)
Neurotensin	12	Dog	Cal.	Decrease	(Lenz, 1987b)
ß-Endorphin	12	Dog	Cal.	No change	(Lenz, 1987b)
GRF	0.2	Rat	Non cal.	No change	(Taché et al. 1987b)

Cal.: Liquid caloric meal; non cal.: Liquid non caloric meal.

The understanding of the physiological role of these peptides in relation with brain regulation of gastric emptying under basal or stress conditions is still rudimentary. This is due in part to the lack of specific chemical approach for altering selectively endogenous neuropeptidergic systems. However recent neuroanatomical, neuropharmacological and physiological evidence suggests a likely involvement of brain CRF and TRH in mediating alteration of gastric emptying in response to stressors.

ROLE OF BRAIN CRF IN MEDIATING STRESS-INDUCED INHIBITION OF GASTRIC EMPTYING IN THE RAT

Brain CRF has been demonstrated to play a role in the endocrine, behavioral, cardiovascular and gastrointestinal responses to stress (Berridge, and Dunn, 1987; Brown et al. 1986; Krahn et al. 1986; Lenz et al. 1987a; 1988b; Rivier, and Plotsky, 1986; Rivier et al. 1986; Stephens et al. 1988; Tazi et al. 1987; Williams et al. 1987). Convergent information suggests that central CRF may be involved in the gastric stasis elicited by various stressors in the rat.

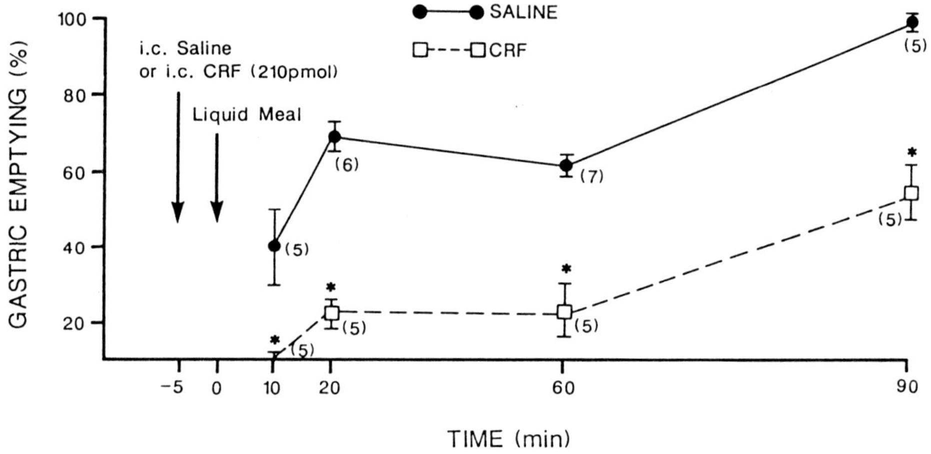

Fig. 1. Time course of intracisternal injection of rat CRF induced inhibition of gastric emptying of a methylcellulose phenol red solution in conscious rats. Number in parenthesis are number of rats per group. * P<0.05 compared to saline-treated group.

First, CRF-immunoreactivity and receptors have been localized in hypothalamic and medullary nuclei regulating visceral function (De Souza, 1987; Merchenthaler, 1984; Swanson et al. 1983) and various stressors activate CRF release in the brain (Haas, and George, 1988; Plotsky, and Vale, 1984). Second, injection of CRF into the cerebrospinal fluid inhibits gastric emptying of a non nutrient meal in the rat (Lenz et al. 1988c; Taché et al. 1987b; Williams et al. 1987) (Fig. 1) and of a peptone meal in the dog (Lenz, 1987b). CRF action is receptor mediated since it was blocked by the CRF antagonist, α-helical CRF19-41, injected into the cerebrospinal fluid (Griffiths et al. 1982; Kubek et al. 1983; Taché et al. 1989b). Finally, the CRF antagonist injected into the cerebrospinal fluid blocks restraint (Lenz et al. 1988b), ether, abdominal surgery, trephination (Taché et al. 1989b) and unescapable tail shock (Taché and Garrick, unpublished observation) induced delay in gastric emptying of non nutrient meal in the rat. Taken together these findings substantiate a possible role of endogenous brain CRF in mediating the inhibition of gastric emptying elicited by exposure to various stressful stimuli in the rat.

ROLE OF BRAIN TRH IN MEDIATING COLD STRESS-INDUCED STIMULATION OF GASTRIC EMPTYING IN THE RAT

Unlike most other stressors, short exposure to cold (4°C) induced stimulation of gastric emptying in rats (Koo et al. 1985; Taché et al. 1988b). Although cold exposure was combined with restraint, the restraint procedure in itself at room temperature does not alter gastric emptying (Taché et al. 1988b; Williams et al. 1987; 1988). The cold-related increase in emptying may represent a stressor specific effect related to activation of brain TRH. In support of such a role of TRH is the fact that cold exposure is a well established specific stimuli activating brain TRH release (Arancibia et al. 1983; Arancibia, and Assenmacher, 1987). Secondly, in rats, injection into the cisterna magna of small amount of TRH, unlike other peptides (Table 2), markedly stimulated gastric emptying through vagal-cholinergic dependent pathways (Maeda-Hagiwara, and Taché, 1987) (Fig. 2). Moreover, neuroanatomical studies have localized abundant distribution of TRH-like immunoreactive fibers and receptors in sites of origin of vagal preganglionic neurons regulating gastric motor function, namely the dorsal motor nucleus of the vagus (Kubek et al. 1983; Mantyh, and Hunt, 1985; Palkovits et al. 1986). These findings provide neuropharmacologic, neuroanatomic and physiologic evidence in support of a possible role of medullary TRH in mediating cold-induced increases in gastric emptying in the rat. Peptide specific antagonist when available will be an important tool to establish further such a TRH involvement. Central injection of CRF prevents the stimulatory effects of TRH on gastric function (Garrick et al. 1988; Taché et al. 1983). The fact that longer exposure to cold leads to an inhibition of gastric emptying (Koo et al. 1985) may be related to the interactions between brain CRF and TRH. The longer exposure to cold may trigger more CRF release which blocks the effect of TRH as previously demonstrated.

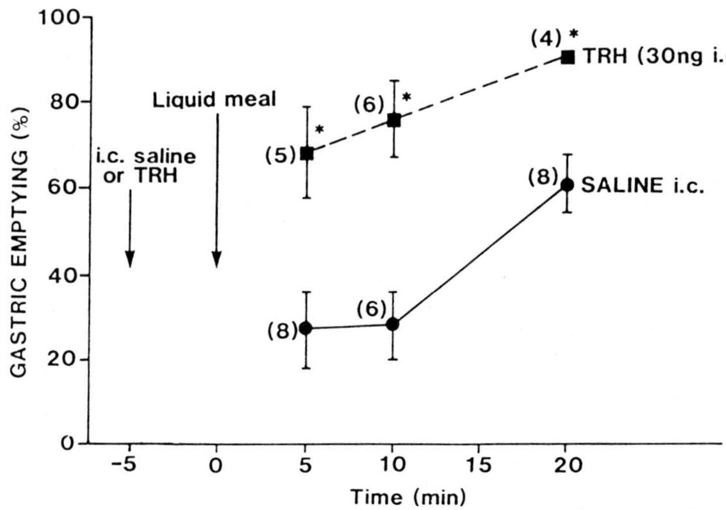

Fig. 2. Time course of intracisternal TRH-induced stimulation of gastric emptying of a methylcellulose phenol red solution in conscious rats. For other details see legend of Figure 1. From Maeda-Hagiwara, and Taché, 1987.

PERIPHERAL MECHANISMS INVOLVED IN STRESS-INDUCED ALTERATIONS OF GASTRIC EMPTYING

Among possible peripheral mechanisms suggested to participate in stress-induced disturbance of gastric emptying are the alteration of parasympathetic nervous system, activation of sympathetic nervous system activity, stimulation of the pituitary-adrenal axis and/or release of opioid peptides and enhanced release of pancreatic polypeptide and gastrin (Peeters et al. 1989; Stanghellini et al. 1983). However, most studies which have evaluated the effects of stress on gastric emptying have not further investigated and defined the underlying peripheral mechanisms under their experimental conditions. The increase in ACTH, corticosteroid and ß-endorphin secretion in response to stress does not appear to play an important role in mediating the alteration of gastric emptying since elevated levels of ACTH, ß-endorphin and corticosterone can be produced by exogenous injection of these compound or certain stimuli without concomitant alteration of gastric emptying in the rat or mice (Buéno, and Gué, 1988; Williams et al. 1988). The rapid onset of change in gastric emptying induced by stress favors a direct neurally mediated mechanism rather than a secondary event to alterations of hormone secretion.

Further work needs to be done to reveal the mechanisms through which stress alters gastric emptying particularly in relation with caloric content of the meal and different types of stressors. It is well established that emptying of non-nutrient, osmotically neutral physiological saline is emptying from the stomach rapidly at an exponential rate related to the volume (McHugh, 1983). By contrast, emptying of a caloric meal is characterized by a lag and linear phase of solid emptying which is influenced by duodenal reflexes inhibitory mechanisms (McHugh, 1983). To what extent stress influences these inhibitory mechanisms is still unknown.

CONCLUSIONS

Delayed gastric emptying appears the most common pattern of response induced by exposure to various stressors in rats, monkeys and human, although stimuli specific patterns of response have also been observed, in particular, increased gastric emptying following cold exposure. Despite the early recognition of stress influence on gastric transit, still very little is known regarding the exact central and peripheral neurohumoral mechanisms by which stress exerts its influence. Recently, growing experimental evidence in the rat indicates that brain CRF may play a role in mediating the inhibition of gastric emptying elicited by various stressors whereas the increase in gastric emptying induced by cold exposure may represent a specific effect related to specific increase release of brain TRH.

ACKNOWLEDGMENTS

The author thanks Ms. Anita Starlight for helping in the preparation of the manuscript. The author's work cited in the text was supported by the National Institute of Mental Health, Grant MH-00663 and the National Institute of Arthritis Metabolism and Digestive Disease, grants DK-33061, 30110 and AM 17238.

REFERENCES

Arancibia, S., Tapia-Arancibia, L., Assenmacher, I., and Astier, H. (1983): Direct evidence of short-term cold-induced TRH release in the median eminence of unanesthetized rats.

Neuroendocrinology 37, 225-228.

Arancibia, S., and Assenmacher, I. (1987): Sécrétion de TRH dans le troisième ventricle cérébral lors de l'exposition aigue au froid chez le rat non anesthésié. Effect des drogues ∝-adrénergiques. C. R. Soc. Biol. (Paris) 181, 323-331.

Beaumont, W. (1833). In Experiments and observations on the gastric juice and the physiology of digestion, ed W. Osler, pp. 1-280. New York: Dover Publications Inc.

Berridge, C.W., and Dunn, A.J. (1987): A corticotropin-releasing factor antagonist reverses the stress-induced changes of exploratory behavior in mice. Horm. Behav. 21, 393-401.

Brown, M.R., Gray, T.S., and Fisher, L.A. (1986): Corticotropin-releasing factor receptor antagonist: effects on the autonomic nervous system and cardiovascular function. Regul. Pept. 16 321-329.

Buéno, L., and Gué, M. (1988): Evidence for the involvement of corticotropin-releasing factor in the gastrointestinal disturbances induced by acoustic and cold stress in mice. Brain Res. 441, 1-4.

Cabanis, P.J.G. (1981). Introduction: On the relations between the physical and moral aspects of man. eds G. Mora, and M.D. Saidi, pp. 650. Baltimore: Johns Hopkins University Press.

Cann, P.A., Read, N.W., Cammack, J., Childs, H., Holden, S., Kashman, R., Longmore, J., Nix, S., Simms, N., Swallow, K., and Weller, J. (1983): Psychological stress and the passage of a standard meal through the stomach and small intestine in man. Gut 24, 236-240.

Costall, B., Gunning, S.J., Naylor, R.J., and Simpson, K.H. (1983): A central site of action for benzamide facilitation of gastric emptying. Eur. J. Pharmacol. 91, 197-205.

De Souza, E.B. (1987): Corticotropin-releasing factor receptors in the rat central nervous system: characterization and regional distribution. J. Neurosci. 7, 88-100.

Dorval, E.D., Meuller, G.P., Eng, R.R., Durakovic, A., Conklin, J.J., and Dubois, A. (1985): Effect of ionizing radiation on gastric secretion and gastric motility in monkeys. Gastroenterology 89, 374-380.

Dubois, A., and Natelson, B.H. (1978): Habituation of gastric function suppression in monkeys after repeated free-operant avoidance sessions. Physiol. Psych. 6, 524-528.

Enck, P., Wienbeck, M., Merlin, V., Erckenbrecht, J.F., and Berges, W. (1988): Panic induced changes of gastrointestinal transit in the rat. Gastroenterology 94, A115.(Abstract)

Garrick, T., Veiseh, A., Sierra, A., Weiner, H., and Taché, Y. (1988): Corticotropin-releasing factor acts centrally to suppress stimulated gastric contractility in the rat. Regul. Pept. 21, 173-181.

Griffiths, E.C., McDermott, J.R., and Smith, A.I. (1982): Mechanisms of brain inactivation of centrally-acting thyrotrophin-releasing hormone (TRH) analogues: a high performance liquid chromatography study. Regul. Pept. 5, 1-11.

Gué, M., Fioramonti, J., and Buéno, L. (1987): Comparative influences of acoustic and cold stress on gastrointestinal transit in mice. Am. J. Physiol. 253, G124-G128.

Haas, D.A., and George, S.R. (1988): Single or repeated mild stress increasess synthesis and release of hypothalamic corticotropin-releasing factor. Brain Res. 461, 230-237.

Koo, M.W.L., Ogle, C.W., and Cho, C.H. (1985): The effect of cold-restraint stress on gastric emptying in rats. Pharmacol. Biochem. Behav. 23, 969-972.

Krahn, D.D., Gosnell, B.A., Grace, M., and Levine, A.S. (1986): CRF antagonist partially reverses CRF- and stress-induced effects on feeding. Brain Res. Bull. 17, 285-289.

Kubek, M.J., Rea, M.A., Hodes, Z.I., and Aprison, M.H. (1983): Quantitation and characterization of thyrotropin-releasing hormone in vagal nuclei and other regions of the medulla oblongata of the rat. J. Neurochem. 40, 1307-1313.

Lenz, H.J., Raedler, A., Greten, H., and Brown, M.R. (1987a): CRF initiates biological actions within the brain that are observed in response to stress. Am. J. Physiol. 252, R34-R39.

Lenz, H.J. (1987b): Brain regulation of gastric secretion, emptying and blood flow by neuropeptides in conscious dogs. Gastroenterology 92, 1500. (Abstract)

Lenz, H.J. (1988a): Calcitonin and CGRP inhibit gastroinestinal transit via distinct neuronal pathways. Am. J. Physiol. 254, G920-G924.

Lenz, H.J., Raedler, A., Greten, H., Vale, W.W., and Rivier, J.E. (1988b): Stress-induced gastrointestinal secretory and motor responses in rats are mediated by endogenous corticotropin-releasing factor. Gastroenterology 95, 1510-1517.

Lenz, H.J., Burlace, M., Raedler, A., and Greten, H. (1988c): Central nervous system effects of corticotropin-releasing factor on gastrointestinal transit in the rat. Gastroenterology 94, 598-602.

Limlomwongse, L., Suanarunsawat, T., and Krishnamra, N. (1988): Hemorrhage with blood reinfusion and the relationship between gastroduodenal motility and bile reflux in rats. Can. J. Physiol. Pharmacol. 66, 608-612.

Maeda-Hagiwara, M., and Taché, Y. (1987): Central nervous system action of TRH to stimulate gastric emptying in rats. Regul. Pept. 17, 199-207.

Mantyh, P.W., and Hunt, S.P. (1985): Thyrotropin-releasing hormone (TRH) receptors. Localization by light microscopic autoradiography in rat brain using [$_3$H][3-Me-His$_2$]TRH as the radioligand. J. Neurosci. 5, 551-561.

McHugh, P.R. (1983): The control of gastric emptying. J. Auton. Nerv. Syst. 9, 221-231.

Merchenthaler, I. (1984): Corticotropin releasing factor (CRF)-like immunoreactivity in the rat central nervous system: extrahypothalamic distribution. Peptides 5(Suppl 1), 53-69.

Natelson, B.H., and Dubois, A. (1980): Gastric emptying and secretion in monkeys during unavoidable shock. Brain Res. Bull. 5, 63-66.

OBrien, J.D., Thompson, D.G., Burnham, W.R., Holly, J., and Walker, E. (1987): Action of centrally mediated autonomic stimulation on human upper gastrointestinal transit: a comparative study of two stimuli. Gut 28, 960-969.

Palkovits, M., Mezey, E., Eskay, R.L., and Brownstein, M.J. (1986): Innervation of the nucleus of the solitary tract and the dorsal vagal nucleus by thyrotropin-releasing hormone-containing raphe neurons. Brain Res. 373, 246-251.

Peeters, T.L., Gué, M., Depoortere, I., Vantrappen, G., and Buéno, L. (1989): Postprandial hormonal status and gastric emptying in stressed dogs. Dig. Dis. Sci. 33, 485.(Abstract)

Plotsky, P.M., and Vale, W. (1984): Hemorrhage-induced secretion of corticotropin-releasing factor-like immunoreactivity into the rat hypohysial portal circulation and its inhibition by glucocorticoids. Endocrinology 114, 164-169.

Porreca, F., and Burks, T.F. (1983): Centrally administered bombesin affects gastric emptying and small and large bowel transit in the rat. Gastroenterology 85, 313-317.

Raybould, H.E., Kolve, E., and Taché, Y. (1988): Central nervous sytem action of calcitonin-gene related peptide to inhibit gastric emptying in the conscious rat. Peptides 9, 735-737.

Rivier, C., Rivier, J., and Vale, W. (1986): Stress-induced inhibition of reproductive functions: role of endogenous corticotropin-releasing factor. Science 231, 607-609.

Rivier, C.L., and Plotsky, P.M. (1986): Mediation by corticotropin releasing factor (CRF) of adenohypophysial hormone secretion. Ann. Rev. Physiol. 48, 475-494.

Rosman, G., Roemer, R., Mauer, A., Siegel, J., Perri, J., Urbain, J., Malmud, L., and Krevsky, (1987): Differential effects of acutely induced stress on upper gastrointestinal motility. Gastroenterology 92, 1601.(Abstract)

Selye, H. (1936): Syndrome produced by diverse nocuous agents. Nature 138, 32.

Simpson, K.H., and Stakes, A.F. (1987): Effect of anxiety on gastric emptying in preoperative patients. Br. J. Anaesth. 59, 540-544.

Stanghellini, V., Malagelada, J.-R., Zinsmeister, A.R., Go, W.L.W., and Kao, P.C. (1983): Stress-induced gastroduodenal motor disturbances in humans: possible humoral mechanisms. Gastroenterology 85, 83-91.

Stephens, R.L., Yang, H., Rivier, J., and Taché, Y. (1988): Intracisternal injection of CRF antagonist blocks surgical stress-induced inhibition of gastric secretion in the rat. Peptides 9, 1067-1070.

Swanson, L.W., Sawchenko, P.E., Rivier, J., and Vale, W.W. (1983): Organization of ovine corticotropin-releasing factor immunoreactive cells and fibers in the rat brain: an immunohistochemical study. Neuroendocrinology 36, 165-186.

Taché, Y., Goto, Y., Gunion, M.W., Vale, W., Rivier, J., and Brown, M. (1983): Inhibition of gastric acid secretion in rats by intracerebral injection of corticotropin-releasing factor. Science 222, 935-937.

Taché, Y., Kolve, E., Maeda-Hagiwara, M., and Kauffman, G. (1987a): CNS action of calctioni to alter experimental gastric ulcers in rats. Gastroenterology 41, 651-655.

Taché, Y., Maeda-Hagiwara, M., and Turkelson, C.M. (1987b): Central nervous system action of corticotropin-releasing factor to inhibit gastric emptying in rats. Am. J. Physiol. 253, G241-G245.

Taché, Y. (1988a). Central control of gastrointestinal transit and motility by brain-gut peptides. In Pathogenesis of Functional Bowel Disease, ed W.J. Snape, pp. (In Press). New York: Plenum Press.

Taché, Y., Ishikawa, T., Stephens, R., and Hagiwara, M. (1988b): Stressor specific alterations of gastric function in rats: role of brain TRH and CRF. Gastroenterology 94, 452-Abstract.

Taché, Y., Stephens, R.L., and Ishikawa, T. (1989a). Stress-induced alterations of gastrointestinal function: involvment of brain CRF and TRH. In IV. New Frontiers of Stress Research, eds H. Weiner, I. Florin, D. Hellhammer, and M. Murison, pp. 1-11. : Hans Huber.

Taché, Y., Kolve, E., Stephens, R.L., and Rivier, J.E. (1989b): Role of corticotropin-releasing factor in mediating gastric ileus. Gastroenterology in press,

Tazi, A., Dantzer, R., Le Moal, M., Rivier, J., Vale, W., and Koob, G.F. (1987): Corticotropin-releasing factor antagonist blocks stress-induced fighting in rats. Regul. Pept. 18, 37-42.

Thompson, D.G., Richelson, E., and Malagelada, J.-R. (1982): Perturbation of gastric emptying and duodenal motility through the central nervous system. Gastroenterology 83, 1200-1206.

Thompson, D.G., Richelson, E., and Malagelada, J.-R. (1983): Perturbation of upper gastrointestinal function by cold stress. Gut 24, 277-283.

Williams, C.L., and Burks, T.F. (1988). Stress, opioids, and gastrointestinal transit. In Symposia Hans Selye: Neuropeptides and Stress, eds Y. Taché, J. Morley, and M.R. Brown, New York: Springer-Verlag.

Williams, C.L., Peterson, J.M., Villar, R.G., and Burks, T.F. (1987): Corticotropin-releasing fact directly mediates colonic responses to stress. Am. J. Physiol. 253, G582-G586.

Williams, C.L., Villar, R.G., Peterson, J.M., and Burks, T.F. (1988): Stress-induced changes in intestinal transit in the rat: a model for irritable bowel syndrome. Gastroenterology 94, 611-621.

Influence of different stressors on gastric emptying in mice and rats

Michèle Gué, Jean Fioramonti and Lionel Buéno

Department of Pharmacology INRA, 180 chemin de Tournefeuille 31300 Toulouse, France

BACKGROUND

Stress was defined as a specific morphological, biochemical, physiological and/or behavioral change experienced by an organism in response to a stressful event or stressor. The typical behavioral stress responses are fear, tension, apprehension and anxiety. Physiological stress responses include changes in gastric secretion and motility, and increases in heart rate and blood pressure. Biochemical changes include large increases in the levels of plasma corticosterone, cortisol and catecholamines as well as marked changes in brain neurotransmitter concentration, particularly in brain area involved in the regulation of gut motility.

It is now well established that stress exert a significant effect on the gastrointestinal system in animals as well as in humans : stressful stimuli have been reported to affect gastric emptying in both rats (KOO et al., 1985 ; LENZ et al., 1987 ; WILLIAMS et al., 1987), mice (BUENO & GUE, 1988 ; GUE et al., 1987), dogs (GUE et al., 1989) and humans (ERCKENBRECHT et al., 1985 ; THOMPSON et al., 1982). Whereas it is accepted that stressors induced changes in gastric emptying, little is known about the discrepancies obtained in different studies and the true response of gastric emptying induced by stress : enhancement or slowing down ?

More specifically we need to know the nature and range of the gut response to stress and its relationship to perception of general stress. In fact, data from literature involve too many different experimental conditions to compare results and any study would performed to probe the three major factors involved in experiments : the species, the nature of the meal (nutritive *vs* non-nutritive) and the stressor used. For example while cold exposure stress reduces gastric emptuing of a non nutritive used in rats (KOO et al., 1985) it increases that of a nutritive meal in mice (GUE et al., 1987).

Similar discrepancies are found when considering the effects of central administration of hypothalamic factors considered to play a major role in the initiation of stress-induced gastrointestinal motor disturbances. For example, few studies have demonstrated that central injection of thyrotropin-releasing hormone (TRH) stimulates in rats (CARINO & HORITA, 1987 ; MAEDA-HAGIWARA & TACHE, 1987) or inhibits in mice (BHARGAVA & PILLAI, 1984) the gastric emptying of non-nutritive meal. Furthermore, recent studies have shown that gastric emptying of a non-nutritive liquid meal was delayed in rats by central administration of corticotropin-releasing faction (CRF) (LENZ et al., 1987; TACHE et al., 1987 ; WILLIAMS et al., 1987) while central injection of CRF increased gastric emptying of milk in mice (BUENO & GUE,1988).

The purpose of this study was to examine comparatively factors (thought to be stressful), that might influence the gastric emptying of four different meals in rats and mice ; three different types of stimuli were used : a) acoustic stress (AS) produced by continuous playing of music delivered from a magnetic tape, at room temperature (20 ± 2°C) designed to initiate a moderate stressful event ; b) cold stress (CS) obtained by adjustment of the box temperature to 10 ± 1°C and c) immobilization stress (IS) produced by enclosing animals in flexible wire mesh designed to mimic a severe physical stress.

MATERIALS AND METHODS

- *Animals*

Sixteen groups of 8 males NMRI mice wheighing 25-30 g and sixteen groups of 8 males WISTAR rats weighing 150-200 g were maintained *ad libitum* on Purine laboratory chow and tap water. They were housed under conditions of controlled temperature (20 ± 1°C), humidity (40-50 %) and lighting (08 : 00 - 20 : 00 h). All experiments were performed in animals deprived of food for 24 h but given free access to water up to the beginning of the experiments.

- *Gastric emptying*

The oral test meal (0.5 ml. in mice, 2 ml. in rats) containing 1 µCi/ml of ^{51}Cr sodium chromate (CIS, Gif sur Yvette) was administered by gavage in animals fasted for 24 hours. Except the volume of the test meal similar procedure and regimen were used in the two species. Thirty minutes later mice and rats were killed by cervical dislocation. The stomach, the small intestine and the colon were excised and placed into individual tubes. The radioactivity was determined by placing the tubes in a gamma counter (MR 252 C, Kontron, Basel, Switzerland) for 2 min. Gastric emptying (GE) was calculated as the percent of total counts found in the small intestine and the colon as previously described (GUE et al., 1987). Values are given as means ± SD, and comparisons between controls and corresponding values in stressed animals were analyzed statistically using Student's t test ; the effects of treatments were determined by two-way analysis of variance in mice an rats respectively.

- *Tests - Meals*

The reference test meal (diet A) was reconstitute milk (1g of milk powder in 3 ml of water containing 1 µCi/ml of ^{51}Cr sodium chromate) as previously used (GUE et al., 1987). Two other nutritive synthetic meals containing proteins (casein), glucose, arabic gum (diet B) and peanut oil (diet C) were prepared and previously tested in groups of six mice and six rats in order to obtain comparative values of gastric emptying at t = 30 min (Table 1).

The last meal was a non-nutritive meal wich contained water and methyl cellulose (diet D). The methylcellulose test meal has a viscosity of ≅ 400 centipoises and a rate of gastric emptying similar to the others diets containing food constituents.

Table 1 : Composition of test meals. A-B-C were considered as nutritive meal and D as a non-nutritive meal.

DIET	A	B	C	D
Milk powder (g)	1.66			
Arabic gum (g)		1.00	1.00	
Glucose (g)		1.25	1.25	
Peanut oil (ml)			0.6	
Casein (g)		1.8	1.8	
Methyl cellulose				2.5

All diets were prepared in equal volumes adjusted to 5 ml with NaCl (9 ‰) ; diet C was added with 1 drop/5 ml of Tween 80 to emulsify arachis oil.

- *Stressors and experimental design*

Acoustic stress (AS) was obtained by placing the animals (rats and mice) in a closed box equiped with loudspeakers playing broad frequency taped music (< 90 dB) at room temperature (20 ± 2°C). Cold exposure stress (CS) was produced by lowering to 10 ± 1°C the box temperature in which the animals were placed and immobilisation stress (IS) was produced by enclosing animals in a flexible wire mesh (3 x 3 mm) initially formed into a cone and then bent to conform to the size of the individual animals.

The experiments were conducted in groups of 8 mice or 8 rats as follows : ten minutes after receiving one of the test meal (diet A, B, C, or D) the animals were submitted or not (control) during 20 min to one of the three stressors : AS, CS or IS and then immediately killed, i.e. 30 min after the test meal.

RESULTS

- *Incidence of diet on gastric emptying in both mice and rats*

The percentage of gastric emptying at 30 min after the administration of the diet A, B, C, or D was, respectively, 42.5 ± 5.9, 47.2 ± 2.7, 41.4 ± 4.4 and 59.9 ± 12.5 % in the no-stressed groups of mice.

In no-stressed rats, the stomachs showed, respectively, 54.6 ± 6.6, 48.1 ± 4.1, 49.9 ± 3.9 and 48.8 ± 9.0 % emptying over these different given meals. (Table 2).

Table 2 : Comparative influence of acoustic (AS), cold (CS) and immobilization (IS) stress on gastric emptying of four different test meals in mice and rats (mean ± S.D., n = 8).

	MICE				RATS			
	CONTROL	A.S	C.S.	I.S.	CONTROL	A.S.	C.S.	I.S.
Diet A [(a)]	42.5 ± 5.9	62.8 ± 15.5*	73.4 ± 7.6*	46.4 ± 7.6	54.6 ± 6.6	64.9 ± 4.2*	66.6 ± 6.9*	53.7 ± 6.7
Diet B	47.2 ± 2.7	51.7 ± 8.1	53.7 ± 5.1*	46.0 ± 7.2	48.1 ± 4.1	39.8 ± 10.0	48.5 ± 7.0	41.9 ± 8.1
Diet C	41.4 ± 4.4	41.5 ± 5.9	50.8 ± 14.2*	45.0 ± 9.2	49.9 ± 3.9	43.2 ± 9.2	48.6 ± 6.6	51.8 ± 17.0
Diet D	59.9 ± 12.5	51.6 ± 7.3	61.6 ± 5.3	61.5 ± 9.0	48.8 ± 9.0	59.3 ± 7.9	71.1 ± 14.6*	58.7±10.6

(a) see composition of diets in table 1
* significantly different from corresponding control values at $P \leq 0.05$
Gastric emptying was measured at t = 30 min after the test-meal and was expressed in percent of test meal emptied.

- *Effect of AS, CS and IS on gastric emptying*

Both AS and CS, applied 10 min after the meal, significantly increased the gastric emptying of the diet A in mice. The percentage of enhancement was, respectively, 47.8 and 72.2 %.

A similar increase in gastric emptying was observed in rats fed with milk and submitted to AS or CS (Fig. 1).

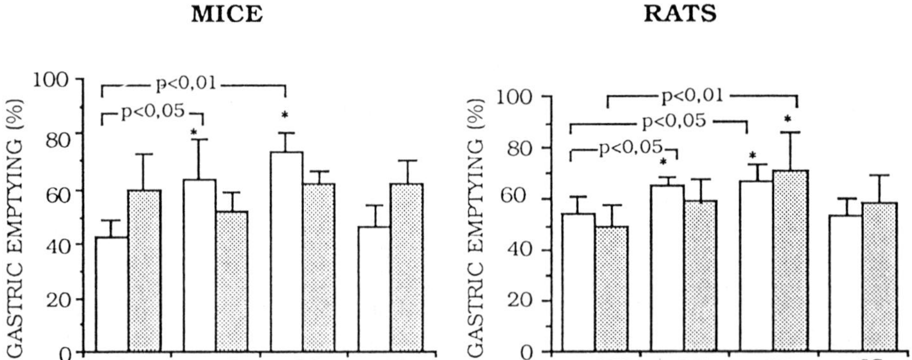

Fig. 1. Comparative influence of acoustic (AS) cold (CS) and immobilization (IS) stress on gastric emptying of nutritive (milk) vs non-nutritive (methyl-cellulose solution) meal in mice and rats (mean ± SD, n = 8, significantly different from control values).

In contrast, the gastric emptying of diet A was not altered by IS neither in mice (46.4 ± 7.6 vs 42.5 ± 5.9 %), nor in rats (53.7 ± 6.7 vs 54.6 ± 6.6 %).

The gastric emptying of synthetic nutritive meals with (diet C) or without fat (diet B) was significantly ($p < 0.05$) increased by CS in mice, while AS and IS were unable to affect it. These results differed from those obtained in rats in which none of the three stressors were able to alter the gastric emptying of diet B and C.

In contrast, the gastric emptying of the non-nutritive meal (diet D) was not affected by any stressors (CS, AS or IS) in mice. However, the percentage of gastric emptying that was 48.8 ± 9.0 in control group was increased to 71.1 = 14.6 % in rats submitted to CS, whereas the other stressors had no effect.

DISCUSSION

These results demonstrate that gastric emptying in mice as well as in rats was affected differently by various stressors. This work also extends to rats the previous data obtained in mice (GUE et al., 1987) showing that both acoustic and cold stress increase gastric emptying of milk.

Cold restraint-stress associating both cold exposure and immobilisation, was known to delay gastric emptying of a non-nutritive meal in rats (KOO et al., 1985, WILLIAMS et al., 1987). In fact, the previous study of KOO et al. (1985) shown that the effects of cold-restraint stress on gastric emptying is triphasic with an increase in the first hours of experiment which return to normal then slow down in the third hour of stress. Nevertheless, it appears in our experiments that response of gastric emptying is stressor specific as suggested by previous studies showing that cold stress stimulate gastric emptying of a non-nutritive meal (TACHE et al., 1987), while wrapping restraint stress does not affect it in rats. This observation is in accord with experiments performed in humans showing that cold water stress delays gastric emptying (THOMPSON et al., 1982), while psychologic stress does not (CANN et al., 1983).

It is classically admitted that the rate of gastric emptying of a liquid meal is linearly correlated with intragastric pressure (MINAMI & Mc CALLUM, 1984) and to the slow sustained contractions of the proximal stomach, while the emptying of solids depends on the distal stomach motility and opening of the pylorus (BECKER & KELLY, 1983).

Recently, we have shown that in dogs the influence of acoustic stress on gastric and intestinal motility were different between fed and fasted state (GUE et al., 1989). Furthermore, only meals containing nutrients are able to modify the gastrointestinal motor profile from fasted to fed patthern (SINAR et al., 1983). Consequently, the lack of effects of the three kinds of stressor (AS, CS and IS) on gastric emptying of the non-nutritive meal in mice let us to speculate that the influence of stress on gastric emptying depend particularly on the neural and hormonal mechanisms involved during the post prandial state.

On a other hand, IS was unable to affect gastric emptying of any diet neither in rats nor in mice. These results may be explained by the ineffectiveness of IS to induce ACTH release suggesting a lack of CRF release (NAKANE et al, 1985). Indeed, various model of stress influence differently the levels of circulating ACTH, suggesting that CRF release is related to the nature of the stressful event.

Although CS is able to increase gastric emptying of the three kinds of nutritive meals, its effects were attenuated on diet B and C containing arabic gum. Such difference may be related to the viscosity of diet B and C which is an important physical factor regulating the rate of gastric emptying overriding the effects of motor stimulants (WULSCHKE et al., 1986). Actually, we are unable to conclude about the influence of fat in the regulation of gastric emptying according to the lack of difference between gastric emptying of diet B and C. On a other hand, the absence of effects of acoustic stress on such diets may be related to the damping effect of arabic gum. Whereas in rats, CS does not altered significantly the gastric emptying of both diet B and C (as in mice), it increases the gastric emptying of a non-nutritive meal, while this effect was not observed in mice. This difference may be related to the species differences. Furthermore, it is known that central administration of TRH stimulates in rats (CARINO & HORITA, 1987 ; MAEDA-HAGIWARA & TACHE, 1987) and inhibits in mice (BHARGAVA & PILLAI, 1984) gastric emptying and intestinal transit suggesting that the CNS regulation of gut function may be different in the two species. Consequently, the lack of effects of CS on gastric emptying of diets B and C in rats would be related first to species difference in the time course of gastric emptying of viscous meal and secondly to the volume of test meal used.

In conclusion, we have shown in this study that the effects of stressors on gastric emptying depends more upon the stressors than the species (at least in rodents) used ; on a other hand, the nature of the test-meal used in such experiments is important and the composition of the meal, even for nutritive diet, should be consider as a major factor.

REFERENCES

Bécker, J.M., and Kelly, K.A. (1983) : Antral control of canine gastric emptying of solids. *Am. J. Physiol*. 245 (Gastrointest. Liver. Physiol. 6): G334-G338.

Bhargava, H.N. and Pillai, P. (1984) : Studies on the mechanism of thyrotropin releasing hormone-induced inhibition of gastrointestinal transit. *Peptides* 6: 185-187.

Buéno, L., and Gué, M. (1988) : Evidence for the involvement of corticotropin-releasing factor in the gastrointestinal disturbances induced by acoustic and cold stress in mice. *Brain Res*. 441: 1-4.

Cann, P.A., Read, N.W., Cammack, J., Childs, H., Holden, S., Kashman, R., Longmore, J., Nix, S., Simms, N., Swallow, K., and Weller, J. (1983) : Psychological stress and passage of a standard meal through the stomach and small intestine in man. *Gut* 24: 236-240.

Carino, M.A., and Horita, A. (1987) : Localization of THR-sensitive sites in rat brain mediating intestinal transit. *Life Sci*. 41: 2663-2667.

Erckenbrecht, J.F., Schoepe-Stillel, A., Borgos, J., Rehm, S., and Weinbeck, M. (1985) : The effects of mental stress by noise on motility and fluid absorption in the human upper small bowel. *Dig. Dis. Sci*. 30: 768 A.

Gué, M., Fioramonti, J., and Buéno, L. (1987) : Comparative influences of acoustic and cold stress on gastrointestinal transit in mice. *Am. J. Physiol*. 253 (Gastrointest. Liver. Physiol. 16): G124-G128.

Gué, M., Peeters, T., Vantrappen, G., and Buéno, L. (1989) : Stress-induced changes in gastric emptying and post prandial motility in dogs : hormonal correlates. *Gastroenterology* in press.

Koo, M. W.L., Ogle, C.W., and Cho, C.H. (1985) : The effect of cold-restraint stress on gastric emptying in rats. *Pharmacol. Biochem. Behav*. 23: 969-972.

Lenz, H.J., Burlage, M., Raedler, A., and Greten, H. (1987) : Central nervous system effects of corticotropin-releasing factor on gastric emptying and intestinal transit in rats (Abstract). *Gastroenterology* 92: 1500.

Maeda-Hagiwara, M., and Tache, Y. (1987) : Central nervous system action of TRH to stimulate gastric emptying in rats. *Regul. Pept*. 17: 199-207.

Minami, H., and McCallum, R.W. (1984) : The physiology and pathophysiology of gastric emptying in humans. *Gastroenterology* 86: 1592-1610.

Nakane, T., Audhya, T., Kanie, N., and Hollander, C.S. (1985) : Evidence for a role of endogenous corticotropin-releasing factor in cold, ether, immobilization, and traumatic stress. *Proc. Natl. Acad. Sci*. 82: 1247-1251.

Sinar, D.R., and Charles, L.G. (1983) : Glucose is the major component controling irregular spike activity after feeding in primates. *Gastroenterology* 85: 1319-1325.

Tache, Y., Maeda-Hagiwara, M. and Turkerlson, C.M. (1987) : Central nervous system action of corticotropin-releasing factor to inhibit gastric emptying in rats. *Am. J. Physiol* 253: G241-G245 .

Thompson, D.G., Richelson, E., and Malagelada, J.-R. (1982) : Perturbation of gastric emptying and duodenal motility through the central nervous system. *Gastroenterology* 83: 1200-1206.

Wilbur, B.G., and Kelly, K.A. (1973) : Effect of proximal gastric, complete gastric and truncal vagotomy on canine gastric electric activity, motility and emptying. *Ann. Surg*. 178: 295-303.

Williams, C.L., Peterson, J.M., Villar. R.G., and Burks, T.F. (1987) : Corticotropin-releasing factor directly mediates colonic responses to stress. *Am. J. Physiol*. 253 (Gastrointest. Liver. Physiol. 16): G582-G586.

Williams, C.L., Villar, R.G., Peterson, J.M., and Burks, T.F. (1988) : Stress-induced changes in intestinal transit in the rat : a model for irritable bowel syndrome. *Gastroenterology* 94: 611-621.

Wulschke, S., Ehrlein, H.J., and Tsiamitas, C. (1986) : The control mechanisms of gastric emptying are not overriden by motor stimulants. *Am. J. Physiol*. 251: (Gastrointest. Liver. Physiol. 14): G744-G751.

Role of corticotropin-releasing factor in the genesis of gastrointestinal motor disturbances induced by stress : an overview

Lionel Buéno

Department of Pharmacology INRA, 180 chemin de Tournefeuille 31300 Toulouse, France

BACKGROUND

In 1936, Selye discovered that toxic doses of drugs and other noxious treatments (stressful stimuli) produced hypertrophy of the adrenal cortex in intact but not in hypophysectomised rats suggesting that these effects are related to enhanced ACTH secretion. This result had given an enormous interest in the mechanisms controlling the ACTH secretion particularly to confirm the hypothesis of HARRIS (1937) that the secretory activity of the adenohypophysis may be controlled by a chemical transmitter substance from the hypothalamus. This substance was later named the corticotropin releasing factor (CRF) by SAFFRAN et al. (1955) and the existence of a hypothalamic CRF was convincingly demonstrated by PORTER et al. showing that extract of plasma from the *Sella turcica* of stressed hypophysectomized dogs caused adrenal ascorbic acid depletion (an indication of increased circulating ACTH) in cortisol-treated rats. However in the same time it was convincingly demonstrated that hypothalamic extracts evoke release of ACTH from pituitary tissue in vitro (GUILLEMIN et al., 1955) providing firm evidence for the existence of a hypothalamic CRF.

Twenty six years later CRF was structurally characterized as a 41 amino-acid peptide in sheep (VALE et al., 1981) and then in other species including humans and rats (RIVIER et al., 1983), pigs (PATTHY et al., 1985) and cows (ESCH et al., 1984). This peptide was shown to act primary as a physiologic regulator of pituitary ACTH secretion (RIVIER et al., 1982). However the widespread distribution of CRF and CRF receptors throughout the central nervous system (CNS) supports the concept that this peptide may subserve functions apart from its hypophysiotropic role (SWANSON et al. 1983, DE SOUZA, 1987). Indeed, intracerebroventricular (ICV) administration of CRF produces multiple antonomic, behavioral and visceral effects that are characteristic of stress reactions (BROWN et al. 1985 ; LENZ et al., 1987). Furthermore, stress-induced elevations of plasma ACTH and epinephrine levels are greatly attenuated by prior blockade of CRF receptors in the CNS (RIVIER et al., 1984 ; BROWN et al., 1985).

Consequently CRF was hypothesized to be an important mediator of the coordinated and integrated endocrine and antonomic responses to stress suggering interest for its role in the genesis of gastrointestinal secretory and motor alterations. Furthermore CRF is present in hypothalamic and medullary nuclei regulating visceral functions and particularly gastrointestinal motility (SWANSON et al., 1983 ; DE SOUZA, 1987).

1. EFFECTS OF CRF ON GASTROINTESTINAL MOTILITY

- Motility studies

In 1984, TACHE et al. showed that CRF injected centrally in rats affects gastric acid secretion in rats suggesting a role in the CNS control of gastric acid secretion. Several oligopeptides present in the brain and affecting gastric acid secretion are also able to affect the muscular activity of the gut when administered centrally in rats at picomolar doses (BUENO et FERRE, 1982). These results have suggested that CRF may also play a role in the control of digestive motility.

The first evidence that CRF injected centrally affects gastrointestinal motility was obtained in dogs (BUENO et al., 1986). In fasted dogs as in other species including humans, the motility of the gastric corpus and antrum is characterized by cyclic phases of grouped high amplitude contractions also called "activity front" or gastric migrating motor complex (MMC). These phases which last about 20 min, occur at 90-120 min intervals are propagated to the duodenum and then, migrate to the terminal ileum. In this species, intracerebroventricular (ICV) administration of ovine CRF (20 to 100 ng/kg) suppress these gastric cyclic MMCs which are replaced by small amplitude irregular contractions during several hours without affecting the cyclic motility of the jejunum (fig. 1). The lack of effects of ICV or IV infusion of ACTH as well as cortisol have suggested that, in dogs, CRF may be involved in the central control of the interdigestive gastric motility and that these effects are not related to the stimulation of the hypothalamo-pituitary adrenocortical (HPA) axis.

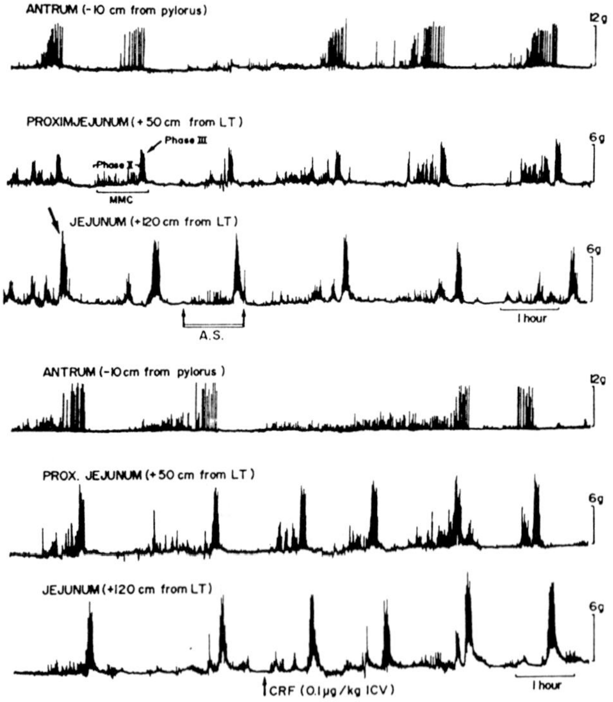

Fig. 1. Comparative influence of intracerebroventricular (ICV) administration of CRF and acoustic stress (AS) produced by one hour hearing of intense music in a fasted dog. *Note that both central CRF and AS inhibited selectively the gastric migrating myoelectric complex.*

These effects depend on the digestive state and similar ICV picomolar doses of CRF injected post prandially in dogs do not affect phase III activity of the antral while they increase both the amplitude and frequency of jejunal contractions. This lack of effects of CNS administration of CRF on antral motility in fed dogs contrasts with the dose-related inhibition of antral motor activity observed in fed sheep (RUCKEBUSCH et al., 1986) ; however in this last species, the antral motility is always organized in MMC independently of the digestive state (BUENO et al., 1975).

Similarly in rats GARRICK et al. (1988) have shown that intracisternal (IC) administration of CRF inhibits the antral motor response to IC administration of the TRH analog RX77368 but in contrast, at similar doses ICV it enhances the late phase II like activity associated with the postprandial state when injected 1 to 2 hours after the meal (unpublished observations).

At higher doses, CRF injected centrally is also able to delay the occurrence of MMCs on the duodenum and the proximal jejunum in fasted dogs (BUENO et al., 1986_a, BUENO et al., 1986_b) as well as in fed sheep (RUCKEBUSCH et al., 1986). The neurohumonal mechanisms through which central CRF alters gastrointestinal contractility are unknown although it may involve the parasympathetic outflow in rats and dogs (1986) since they are respectively blocked by atropine and are supprened after vagotomy (BUENO et al., 1986a ; GARRICK et al., 1988).

Table 1. Effects of CNS administration of CRF on gastrointestinal motility

SPECIES	ROUTE	STATE	STOMACH	SMALL INTESTINE	COLON	REFERENCES
Dog	ICV	fasted fed	inhibition (MMC) no effect	no effect stimulation	____ ____	BUENO et al (1985) BUENO et al (1986)
Sheep	ICV	fed	inhibition (MMC)	no effect	____	RUCKEBUSCH et al (1986)
Rat	IC	stimulation (TRH/2 DG)	inhibition	____	____	GARRICK et al (1988)
Rat	ICV	fed	increase	no effect	increase	(unpublished)

- *Transit measurements*

Both gastric emptying and intestinal transit are altered by central administration of CRF in rats, mice and dogs. In rats intracisternal or intracerebroventricular injection of CRF and related peptides such as sauvagine reduce gastric emptying of a non-nutritive liquid meal associated with a decrease in small bowel transit and an enhanced colonic transit and fecal output (LENZ et al., 1988 ; TACHE et al., 1987 ; BROCCARDO et al., 1982 ; WILLIAMS et al., 1987). Similarly in dogs, CRF injected in the 3rd ventricle also delays gastric emptying of a liquid protein meal (LENZ et al., 1987) while, in contrast in mice ICV injection of CRF increases gastric emptying of a milk meal (GUE et al., 1987, BUENO and GUE, 1988).

Pretreatment with a ganglionic or noradrenergic blocker (TACHE et al., 1987, LENZ et al., 1988a) as well as vagotomy suppress the CRF-induced delay in gastric emptying and intestinal transit while only vagotomy is able to prevent the effects of CRF on colonic transit (LENZ et al., 1988a).

Table 2. Influence of CRF on gastrointestinal and colonic transit

SPECIES	ROUTE	STATE	GASTRIC EMPTYING	INTESTINAL TRANSIT	COLONIC TRANSIT	REFERENCES
Rat	IC	fasted (saline)	inhibition	_____	_____	TACHE et al 1987
Dog	ICV	fasted (saline)	no effect	_____	_____	PAPPAS et al 1987
Mice	ICV	fed (milk)	stimulation	no effect	_____	GUE et al 1987
Rat	ICV (IV)	fasted (water)	inhibition	inhibition	stimulation	WILLIAMS et al 1987
Rat	ICV	fasted (NNM)	inhibition	inhibition	stimulation	LENZ et al 1988

All these results suggest that the centrally mediated effects of CRF on gastrointestinal motility are not univocal, they depend at least of the species and the digestive segment considered but also of the basal motor state. They also differ from proposed pathways for mediating CRF-induced inhibition of gastric acid secretion which involve efferent fibers of sympathetic nervous system and in part a vasopressin dependent pathway but not the parasympathetic nervous system, adrenal epinephrine release or opiate-sensitive pathways (DRUGE et al., 1989).

2. ROLE OF CRF IN STRESS-IDUCED MOTOR ALTERATIONS

Stress-induced alterations of intestinal motility was known from the beginning of the century since CANNON (1902) noted changes in the contour and flow of intestinal contents in cats confronted by a growling dog. Attemps to elucidate the mechanisms by which stress affects intestinal motor activity have led to conflicting results, possibly because different stress models were used in different studies.

- Motility studies

In humans, centrally acting stressful stimuli induce changes in gastroduodenal motility in fed (THOMPSON et al., 1982, 1983, STANGHELLINI et al., 1983, 1984) and fasted (Mc. RAE et al., 1980, KUMAR et al., 1985) states. While both naloxone or a combination of α- and ß adrenergic blockers suppress the inhibition of antral feeding activity induced by stressful stimuli, they do not prevent some effects produced by labyrinthine stimulation (STANGHELLINI et al., 1984).

In 1980, FIORAMONTI et al. showed that in fasted rats submitted to cold restraint stress gastric motility was transiently increased (1-2 hours) and then was dramatically inhibited, such an hypomotility preceding the macroscopic evidence of gastric ulceration.

In conscious dogs, acoustic stress produced by a 1-hr hearing of intense music through earpieces (< 100 dB) inhibits the occurrence of next gastric MMC similarly to the effects of oCRF injected ICV (GUE et al., 1987b) without affecting intestinal motility (fig. 1). These motor effects which are associated with a significant rise in plasma cortisol level, are not blocked by previous treatment with opiate antagonists and adrenergic blockers. The fact that such effects of AS on one hand are prevented by treatment with diazepam, a benzodiazepine or muscinol, a GABAergic agonist, both affecting the CNS release of CRF (MAKARA et al., 1974 ; NINAN et al., 1982) and on other hand that they are suppressed after vagotomy strongly suggests that they are reated to the central release of CRF. Such hypothesis was recently reinforced by numerous results obtained in other species through the evaluation of gastric emptying, intestinal and colonic transit.

- *Transit studies*

In mice both acoustic (AS) and cold exposure (CS) stress increase gastric emptying of a nutritive (milk) meal in mice, an effect mimicked by ICV administration of oCRF (GUE et al., 1987a). Similarly most of the stressors associated with the release of CRF such as noise, wrap restraint, ether exposure water swim or psychic stress (NAKANE et al., 1985; HASHIMOTO et al., 1988), decrease gastric emptying of a non nutritive meal and intestinal transit corresponding to fasted state in rats and dogs (WILLIAMS et al., 1988 ; TACHE et al., 1988 ; ENCK et al., 1988). In contrast cold restraint stress has been shown in rats to have a biphasic effect on gastric emptying increasing the rate of flow during about 60 min, followed by a strong slowing associated with hypothermia (KOO et al., 1985)/ Some of these stressors have also being reported to increase colonic transit in experimental animals (WILLIAMS et al., 1987 ; LENZ et al., 1988) as previously described in humans (WELGAN et al., 1985). These alterations of gastrointestinal transit observed in rats are also similar to those elicited by intracerebroventricular administration of CRF i.e. a decrease in gastric emptying of a non-nutritive meal (TACHE et al., 1987 ; LENZ et al., 1988b), a slowing of intestinal transit (WILLIAMS et al., 1987 ; LENZ et al., 1988) and an increase in colonic transit (WILLIAMS et al., 1987 ; LENZ et al., 1988).

Table 3. Evidence for CRF involvement in stress-induced alterations of transit

SPECIES	STRESSFUL STIMULUS	METHOD	ROUTE	GASTRIC EMPTYING	INTESTINAL TRANSIT	COLONIC TRANSIT	REFERENCES
Rat	W.R.S.	α-helical	IV/ICV	____	unblocked	blocked	WILLIAMS et al., 1987
Mice	A.S. + A.S.	Antiserum	ICV/IV	blocked	blocked	____	BUENO et al., 1988
	A.S. + C.S.	α-helical	ICV	blocked	blocked	____	GUE et al., 1988
Rat	P.R.S.	α-helical	ICV	blocked	blocked	blocked	LENZ et al., 1988
Rat	S.S.	α-helical	ICV	blocked	____	____	TACHE et al., 1988

A.S. : Acoustic Stress ; **C.S.** : Cold Stress ; **W.R.S.** : Wrapping Restraint Stress ;
P.R.S. : Partial Restraint Stress ; **S.S.** : Surgical Stress.

Finally, the evidence that CNS release of CRF is directly involved in the initiation of digestive motor disturbances induced by different stressors was obtained mice (BUENO et al., 1988). In this species, preatment with ICV administration of antiserum against rat CRF (BUENO et al., 1988) as well as α-helical. CRF_{9-41} (GUE et al., 1988a) considered as a CRF antagonist (RIVIER et al., 1984) are able to prevent the increase of gastric emptying of a milk meal induced by acoustic and cold stress in mice at doses that block the effects produced by ICV administration of CRF.

This result was confirmed in rats (LENZ et al., 1988b) on which cerebroventricular administration of α helical CRF_{9-41} but not of the CRF fragment CRF_{1-20}, prevents the gastrointestinal secretory and motor (transit) responses elicited by partial body restraint. Moreover α-helical CRF_{9-41} also prevents the abdominal surgery-induced inhibition of gastric emptying (TACHE et al., 1988).

- *Mechanisms involved*

CRF released by stressful stimuli seems to act directly on the supraspinal structures controlling gastric and intestinal motility and not through a stimulation of the HPA system as systemic administration of ACTH or corticosteroids at doses which mimick plasma increases in stress-conditions, does not affect gastric emptying in mice (GUE et al., 1988c) as well as gastrointestinal motility in dogs (BUENO et al., 1986a) and ACTH and ß endorphin do not affect intestinal transit in rats (WILLIAMS et al., 1988). Furthermore neither adrenalectomy nor hypophysectomy prevent slowing of intestinal transit induced by wrapping-restraint stress (WILLIAMS et al., 1988). In acoustic stress in dogs, opiate antagonists as well as α and ß adrenergic blockers are unable to prevent the alterations of gastric motility (GUE et al., 1986) ; similarly in rats both naloxone and phentolamine do not prevent alterations of gastric emptying induced by acoustic and cold stress but propranolol is efficient suggesting the involvement of central and(or) peripheral ß-adrenergic receptors and(or) pathways in their induction. Such hypothesis is supported by observations showing that a ß-adrenergic antagonist atenolol, but not α-blockers reduces the CS-induced acceleration of the orocaecal transit in humans (O'BRIEN et al., 1985).

Blockade of the effects of stress on gastric motility after vagotomy in dogs (GUE et al., 1987) as well as the inefficiency of central CRF to alter gastric emptying in vagotomized rats strongly suggest that the vagus are involved. Central administration of CRF modulates the parasympathetic outflow from the brain regulating gastric functions (BROWN et al., 1982) and similarly stressful stimuli are known to produce vagal excitation but the lack of preventing effects of CNS administration of atropine or pirenzepine on AS-induced gastric motor inhibition (unpublished observations) is not in agreement with this hypothesis.

Finally, if it is well-established that CRF released at CNS level plays a major role in the genesis of stress-induced gastrointestinal and colonic motor alterations induced by stressful stimuli, the effects observed are not univocal and mostly depend on the digestive status suggesting that they are mediated through different neural or hormonal pathways which remain to be elucidated.

REFERENCES

Broccardo, M., Improta, G., and Melchiorri, P. (1982) : Effect of sauvagine on gastric emptying in conscious rats. *Eur. J. Pharmacol.* 85: 111-114.

Brown, M., Fisher, L., Rivier, J., Spiess, J., Rivier, C. and Vale, W. (1982) : Corticotropin-releasing factor : effects on the sympathetic nervous system and oxygen consumption. *Life Sci.* 30: 207-210.

Brown, M.R., Fisher, L.A., Webb, V., Vale, W.W., and Rivier, J.E. (1985) : Corticotropin-releasing factor : a physiologic regulator of adrenal epinephrine secretion. *Brain Res.* 328: 355-357.

Buéno, L., and Ferré, J.P. (1982) : Central regulation of intestinal motility by somatostatin and cholecystokinin octapeptide. *Science* 216: 1427-1429.

Buéno, L., and Fioramonti, J. (1986a) : Effects of corticotropin-releasing factor, corticotropin and cortisol on gastrointestinal motility in dogs. *Peptides* 7: 73-77.

Buéno, L., and Gué, M. (1988) : Evidence for the involvement of corticotropin-releasing factor in the gastrointestinal disturbances induced by acoustic and cold stress in mice. *Brain Res.* 441: 1-4.

Buéno, L., Fargeas, M.J., Gué, M., Peeters, T.L. Bormans, V., and Fioramonti, J. (1986) : Effects of corticotropin-releasing factor on plasma motilin and somatostatin levels and gastrointestinal motility in dogs. *Gastroenterology* 91: 884-889.

Buéno, L., Ferré, J.P., Fioramonti, J., and Hondé, C. (1983) : Effects of intracerebroventricular administration of neurotensin, substance P and calcitonin on gastrointestinal motility in normal and vagotomized rats. *Regul. Pept.* 6: 197-205.

Buéno, L., Fioramonti, J., and Ruckebusch, Y. (1975) : Rate of flow of digesta and electrical activity of the small intestine in dogs and sheep. *J. Physiol.* 249: 69-85.

Cannon, W.B. (1902) : The movements of the intestines studied by means of the Roentgen rays. *Am. J. Physiol.* 6: 251-77.

De Souza, E.B. (1987) : Corticotropin-releasing factor receptors in the rat central nervous system : characterization and regional distribution. *J. Neurosci.* 7: 88-100.

Drüge, G., Raedler, A., Greten, H., and Lenz, J. (1989) : Pathways mediating CRF-induced inhibition of gastric acid secretion in rats. *Am. J. Physiol.* 256: G214-219.

Esch, F., Ling, N., Bohlen, P., Baird, A., Benoit, R., and Guillemin, R. (1984) : Isolation and characterization of the bovine hypothalamic corticotropin-releasing factor. *Biochem. Biophys. Res. Commun* 122: 899-905.

Fioramonti, J., and Buéno, L. (1980) : Gastrointestinal myolectric activity disturbances in gastric ulcer disease in rats and dogs. *Dig. Dis. Sci.* 25: 575-580.

Garrick, T., Veiseh, A., Sierra, A., Weinel, M., and Tache, Y. (1988) : Corticotropin-releasing factor acts centrally to suppress stimulated gastric contractility in the rat. *Regul. Pept.* 21: 173-181.

Gué, M., and Buéno, L. (1986) : Diazepam and muscimol blockade of the gastrointestinal motor disturbances induced by acoustic stress in dogs. *Eur. J. Pharmacol.* 131: 123-127.

Gué, M., and Buéno, L. (1988) : Involvement of CNS corticotropin-releasing factor in the genesis of stress-induced gastric motor alterations in Nerves and the gastrointestinal tract. SINGER and GOEBELL eds, p. 217-225.

Gué, M., Fioramonti, J., and Buéno, L. (1987) : Comparative influences of acoustic and cold stress on gastrointestinal transit in mice. *Am. J. Physiol.* 253: G124-G128. (a)

Gué, M., Fioramonti, J., Frexinos, J., Alvinerie, M., and Buéno, L. (1987) : Influence of acoustic stress by noise on gastrointestinal motility in dogs. *Dig. Dis. Sci.* 32: 1411-1417. (b)

Guillemin, R., and Rosenberg, B. (1955) : Humoral hypothalamic control of anterior pituitary : A study with combined tissue cultures. *Endocrinology* 57: 599-607.

Harris, G.W. (1937) : The induction of ovulation in the rabbit, by electrical stimulation of the hypothalamo-hypophysial mechanism. *Proc. Roy. Soc. Biol. Sci.* 122: 374-394.

Hashimoto, K., Suemaru, S., Takao, T., Sugawala, M., Makino, S., and Ota, Z. (1988) : Corticotropin-releasing hormone and pituitary-adrenocortical responses in chronically stressed rats. *Regul. Pept.* 23: 117-126.

Koo, M.W.L., Ogle, C.W., and Cho, C.H. (1985) : The effect of cold-restraint stress on gastric emptying in rats. *Pharmacol. Biochem. Behav.* 23: 969-972.

Kumar, D., and Wingate, D. (1985) : The irritable bowel syndrome : a paroxysmal motor disorder. *Lancet* 2: 973-977.

Lenz, H.J., Burlace, M., Raedler, A., and Greten, H. (1988a) : Central nervous system effects of corticotropin-releasing factor on gastrointestinal transit in the rat. *Gastroenterology* 94: 598-602.

Lenz, H.J., Raedler, A., Greten, H., Vale, W.W., and Rivier, J.E. (1988) : Stress-induced gastrointestinal secretory and motor responses in rats are mediated by endogenous corticotropin-releasing factor. 95: 1510-1517.

Lenz, HJ., Raedler, A., Greten, H., and Brown, M.R. (1987) : CRF initiates biological actions within the brain that are observed in response to stress. *Am. J. Physiol.* 252 (Regul. Int. Comp. Physiol. 21): R34-9.

Makara, G.B., and Stark, E. (1974) : Effect of gamma-aminobutyric acid (GABA) and GABA antagonist drugs on ACTH release. *Neuroendocrinology* 16: 178-190.

McRae, S., Thompson, D.G., Wingate, D.L., and Younger, K. (1980) : Changes in the pattern of fasting jejunal motor activity during mental stress. *J. Physiol.* (London) 308: 25P.

Nakane, T., Audhya, T., Kanie, N., and Hollander, C.S. (1985) : Evidence for a role of endogenous corticotropin-releasing factor in cold, ether, immobilization and traumatic stress. *Proc. Natl. Acad. Sci.* (USA) 82: 1247-1251.

Ninan, D.J., Insel, T.M., Cohen, R.M., Cook, J.M., Skolnick, P., and Paul, S.M. (1982) : Benzodiazepine receptor-mediated experimental "anxiety" in primates. *Science* 218: 1332-1334.

O'Brien, J.D., Thompson, D.G., Day, S., Burnham, W.R., and Walker, E. (1985) : Stress induced disturbances of human postprandial antroduodenal motility and orocaecal transit. The contribution of adrenergic pathways. *Dig. Dis. Sci.* 30: 785A (Abstract).

Patthy, M., Horvath, J., Mason-Garcia, M., Szoke, B. Schlesinger, D.H. and Schally, A.V. (1985) : Isolation and amino acid sequence of corticotropin-releasing factor from pig hypothalami. *Proc. Natl. Acad. Sci.* (USA) 82: 8762-8766.

Porter, J.C., Vanatta, J.C. and Dillon, H.T. (1955) : Effect of plasma obtained from hypothalamo-hypophysial portal vessel blood on urinary electrolyte excretion by the rat. *Fed. Proc.* 14: 116-118.

Rivier, C., Rivier J., and Vale, W. (1982) : Inhibition of adrenocorticotropic hormone secretion in the rat by immunoneutralization of corticotropin-releasing factor. *Science* 218: 377-379.

Rivier, J. Spiess, J. and Vale, W. (1983) : Characterization of rat hypothalamic corticotropin-releasing factor. *Proc. Natl. Acad. Sci.* (USA) 80: 4851-4855.

Rivier, J., Rivier C., and Vale, W. (1984) : Synthetic competitive antagonists of corticotropin-releasing factor : effect on ACTH secretion in the rat. *Science* 224: 889-891.

Ruckebusch, Y., and Malbert, C.H. (1986) : Stimulation and inhibition of food intake in sheep by centrally-administered hypothalamic releasing factors. *Life Sci.* 38: 929-934.

Saffran, M., Schally, A.V., and Benfey B.G. (1955) : Stimulation of the release of corticotropin from the adenohypophysis by a neurohypophysial factor. *Endocrinology* 57: 439-444.

Smith, J.R., Lahann, T.R., Chestnut, R.M., Carion, M.A., and Horita, A. (1977) : Thyrotropin releasing hormone : stimulation of colonic activity following intracerebroventricular administration. Science *216*: 1424-1427.

Stanghellini, V., Malagelada, J.R., Zinsmeister, A.R., Go, V.L.W., and Kao, P.C. (1984) : Effect of opiate and adrenergic blockers on the gut motor response to centrally acting stimuli. *Gastroenterology* 87: 1104-1113.

Stanghellini, V., Malagelada, J.R., Zinsmeister, A.R., Go, V.L.W., and Lao, P.C. (1983) : Stress-induced gastroduodenal motor disturbances in humans : possible humoral mechanisms. *Gastroenterology* 85: 83-91.

Swanson, L.W., Sawchenko, P.E., Rivier, J., and Vale, W.W. (1983) : Organization of ovine CRF immunoreactive cells and fibers in the rat brain : an immunohistochemical study. *Neuroendocrinology* 36: 165-186.

Taché, Y., Goto, Y., Gunion, M., Rivier, J., and Debas, H. (1984) : Inhibition of gastric acid secretion in rats in dogs by corticotropin-releasing factor. *Gastroenterology* 86: 281-286.

Taché, Y., Kolve, E., Stephens, R., and Rivier, J. (1988b) : Role of brain CRF in mediating surgical stress induced inhibition of gastric function in the rat. *7th Int. Symp. GI Hormones.*

Taché, Y., Maeda-Hagiwara, M., and Turkelson, C.M. (1987) : Central nervous system action of corticotropin-releasing factor to inhibit gastric emptying in rats. *Am. J. Physiol.* 253: G241-G245.

Taché, Y., Stephens, R.L., and Ishikawa, T. (1988a) : Stress-induced alterations of gastrointestinal function : involvement of brain CRF and TRH. In *New Frontiers of Stress Research*, Weiner, H., Florin, I., Hellhammer, D., and Murison, M. eds.IV. . : Hans Huber, 1-11.

Thompson, D.G., Richelson, E., and Malagelada, J.R. (1982) : Perturbation of gastric emptying and duodenal motility through the central nervous system. *Gastroenterology* 83: 1200-1206.

Thompson, D.G., Richelson, E., and Malagelada, J.R. (1983) : Perturbation of upper gastrointestinal function by cold stress. *Gut* 24: 277-283.

Vale, W., Spies, J. Rivier, C., and Rivier, J. (1981) : Characterization of a 41-residue ovine hypothalamic peptide that stimulates the secretion of corticotropin and ß-endorphin. *Science* 213: 1394-1397.

Welgan, P., Meshkinpour, H., and Hoehler, F. (1985) : The effect of stress on colon motor and electrical activity in irritable bowel syndrome. *Psychosom. Med.* 47: 139-149.

Williams, C.L., Peterson, J.M., Villar, R.G., and Burks, T.F. (1987) : Corticotropin-releasing factor directly mediates colonic responses to stress. *Am. J. Physiol.* 253: G582-G586.

Williams, C.L., Villar, R.G., Peterson, J.M., and Burks, T.F. (1988) : Stress-induced changes in intestinal transit in the rat : a model for irritable bowel syndrome. *Gastroenterology* 94: 611-621.

The effects of repeated acoustic or hypothermic stress on smooth muscle and enteric nerve function *in vitro* in the rat; a model for studying hyperresponsiveness in irritable bowel syndrome

Stephen Collins, Dianne Vermillion, Patricia Blennerhassett and Barry Randall

Intestinal Diseases Research Unit, McMaster University Medical Center, Hamilton, Ontario L8N 3Z5, Canada

INTRODUCTION.

There are numerous studies illustrating the effects of various stressful stimuli on motor responses throughout the gut in several animal species and in man. The majority of these studies assess the motor response to a single or acute stressful stimulus, and do not measure the impact of chronic or repeat stress on motor function.

Stress has been implicated in a variety of gastrointestinal diseases in which motility disturbances occur, and these include Inflammatory Bowel Disease (Collins, 1988), and Irritable Bowel Syndrome (Collins et al., 1988). These conditions are usually chronic, and it is not presently known how stress contributes to the pathogenesis of such disorders.

Stress may alter motility on an immediate basis by influencing neural or hormonal modulation of motor function at a central or peripheral level. In situations of acute stress, it is generally believed that these influences cease when the stressful stimulus is removed, permitting the motor system of the gut to return rapidly to a state of normal function and appropriate responsiveness.

In this study, we examined the effect of repeated acoustic or hypothermic stress on smooth muscle and enteric nerve function in vitro in the rat.

METHODS.

Male Sprague Dawley rats (280-300g) were housed in separate cages; they were allowed food and water ad libitum until just prior to each stress session when they were removed from their home cages.

<u>Acoustic Stress:</u> rats were placed in a sound-proof wooden box measuring 54x38x40cm and lined with 2cm of styrofoam. Two speakers

were placed adjacent to the box and delivered a selection of modern music ("punk or heavy metal") at 90dB for 2h using a Yorx Model BP-04R AM/FM stereo cassette player. Rats received two 2h concerts per day at random, for a total number of 1-4 days. Forty five minutes after the final period of acoustic stress, rats were stunned and euthanized by cervical dislocation. Age matched rats not subjects to AS were used as controls.

Hypothermic Stress: rats were removed from home cages and forced to walk across a slurry of ice water 2" deep in a plastic tray 18 x 24" on two occasions at random each day for a total of 1 to 4 days. Between exposures to the ice-slurry, animals were maintained in a cold room at 8C. This procedure was based on that described by Kita et al. (1975).

In Vitro Experiments: Approximately 45min after the final period of AS or HS, animals were sacrificed and the jejunum removed. The mucosa, submucosa and the circular muscle were removed, leaving the myenteric plexus and the longitudinal muscle layer. Strips were cut along the longitudinal axis and suspended in an organ bath and isometric tension recorded as described previously by us (Vermillion & Collins, 1988). Tension was expressed in grams per mm^2 cross sectional area of muscle. Unless stated otherwise, responses were obtained at L_o (the muscle stretch at which maximum active tension is generated, and in the presence of the neuronal blocker tetrodotoxin. Enteric nerve function was assessed by measuring the release of ^{3}H-acetylcholine from longitudinal muscle/myenteric plexus preparations preincubated with ^{3}H-choline as described by Szerb (1975) and modified by Collins et al. (1989). ACh release was evoked by adding KCl (50mM), or veratidine (50uM) to the superfusate or by electrical field stimulation (30v, 10Hz, 0.5ms), and measured as a fraction F of the total radioactivity present in the tissue at the time of stimulation.

Statistical analysis: Each point represents the mean of at least 3 separate experiments on different rats. Student's t test for unpaired data was used to compare two mean values, and a one-way analysis of variance used to compare three or more means. P values of less than 5% were considered significant.

RESULTS

Muscle strips were stretched to various increments of resting length and isometric tension was measured on adding carbachol 50uM. The length at which muscle produced maximal tension to carbachol is referred to as optimal stretch (L_o) and is expressed as the percentage increase in length over the original resting length. Values for Lo for rats stressed on one occasion only (Day 1), and twice daily for 2 and 4 days are shown in Table 1.

Table 1

Control	58.7%
Day 1	58.6%
Day 2	55.0%
Day 4	40.0% *

There was no significant change in L_o within the first 48hrs of AS. However, L_o was significantly reduced by 32% in rats receiving AS twice daily for 4 days. All subsequent studies were performed at the L_o appropriate for the experimental condition. We next examined the maximum tension generated by carbachol after different periods of AS. After one period of stress (Day 1), there was a 24% increase in carbachol-induced contraction, but this change was not significantly different from control. However, after two days of AS, maximum tension induced by carbachol was significantly increased by 45.5% above control, and remained increased at 39% above control after 4 days' stress. Analysis of full dose-response data showed that although the maximum tension induced by carbachol was increased, there was no change in the ED_{50} for carbachol-induced contraction.

Changes observed after 1 or 2 days' stress were readily immediately reversible (data not shown). The maximum reduction in L_o induced by AS occurred after 4 days (L_o=40%). However, after a one day recovery period, in which rats remained in their home environment and did not receive AS, L_o became even further reduced at 30%, and remained less than control at 43% when allowed to recover for 48h after four days of stress. In contrast, the maximum response to carbachol returned to control values when rats were allowed to recover 24h after 4 days of AS.

Acoustic stress had no significant effect on ^{3}H-ACh release from the myenteric plexus of rats stressed for as long as 6 days. Responses to 50mM KCl were unchanged whereas the evoked release of ACH by field stimulation or veratidine was slightly increased.

The contractile responses were generally similar to those observed with AS. After 2 days of stress, carbachol-induced contraction was almost 3-fold greater than in controls, and increased further after 4 days' stress. When rats were allowed to recover for two days, carbachol-induced contraction of muscle remained significantly greater than control.

DISCUSSION.

There are several lines of evidence suggesting that the observed responses are not the consequence of the most recent stress period before the animals were sacrificed. Had this been the case, one would have expected to see the largest response after the first application of the stressor (day 1), with subsequent reductions in response thereafter. In contrast, responses appeared to increase in a step-wise time-dependent manner, suggesting that they reflect the duration of stress. Furthermore, muscle properties remained abnormal after animals had been allowed a 48h stress-free interval following 4 days' of stress; carbachol-induced contraction remained 2-fold increased above control, and the muscle length at which carbachol induced maximal tension (L_o) remained lower than control 48h after 4 days' HS and AS respectively.

We found no significant change in ACh release from repeated acoustically stimulated rats. There was a small trend towards an increased release of the neurotransmitter in response to veratidine or EFS. However, the sample size (3 rats) may not have been sufficient to identify a statistically significant increase. It is possible that the response to KCl was already large and further increases might be difficult to see. The absence of a reduction in the release of this important excitatory neurotransmitter indicates, however, that changes in smooth muscle function do not occur as a consequence of functional denervation. We cannot rule out, however, that other changes occur in the myenteric plexus but are either too small or inappropriate to our technique.

In a study using repeated cold stress for up to 6 days, Uchida et al. (1978) demonstrated a reduction in the contractile response of duodenal muscle to acetylcholine in the mouse. These findings were accompanied by a decrease in the total specific binding of ^3H-QNB to muscarinic receptors, but no change in K_D, and could be prevented by treatment of the mice with norepinephrine or a tricyclic antidepressant. The same workers found a decrease in acetylcholinesterase activity and an increase in the total acetylcholine content of the duodenum, raising the possibility that the smooth muscle findings may have reflected down regulation of muscarinic receptors (Kita et al., 1986). Differences between these results and those reported in the present study may also reflect differences in the hypothermia protocols.

Our results show stress-induced changes in the fundamental properties of muscle cells. Following repeated, but not single AS or HS, a change in the intrinsic property of smooth muscle was observed (decreased L_o indicating altered stretch-tension relationship), and was accompanied by an increase in the maximum tension induced on pharmacologic stimulation by the muscarinic agonist carbachol. In addition, the changes persisted after cessation of the stress.

This model may be relevant to certain conditions in which stress has been implicated and where motility disturbances are known to occur, and these include IBD and IBS.

Acknowledgements. Mr.B.Randle was a recipient of a summer studentship from the American Gastroenterological Association.

REFERENCES.

Collins, S.M. (1988): The Irritable Bowel Syndrome. *Can. Med. Assn. J.* 138, 309-314.

Collins, S.M., Huizinga, J.D. and Vermillion,D.L. Smooth muscle function in the inflamed bowel. In *Recent developments in Inflammatory Bowel Disease*, ed. H. Freeman. Boca Raton, Florida USA: CRC Press Inc. USA. in press.

Collins, S.M., Blennerhassett, P.A., Blennerhassett, M.G., and Vermillion, D.L. Impaired acetylcholine release from the myenteric plexus of Trichinella-infected rats. *Am. J. Physiol.* In press.

Kita, T., Hata, T., Yoneda, R. and Okage, T. (1975): Stress state caused by alteration of rhythm in environmental temperature, and functional disorders in mice and rats. *Folia. Pharmacol.*

Japan. 71, 195-120.

Kita, T., Hata, T., Higashiguchi, T., Itoh, E., and Kawabata, A. (1986): Changes of total acetylcholine content and the activity of related enzymes in SART (Repeated Cold Stressed rat brain and duodenum. Japan. *J. Pharmacol.* 40, 174-177.

Szerb, J.C. (1975). Storage and release of labelled acetylcholine in the myenteric plexus of the guinea pig ileum. *Can. J. Physiol. Pharmacol.* 53, 566-574.

Uchida, S., Takeyasu, K, Noguchi, Y., Yoshida, H., Hata, T. and Kita, T. (1978): Decrease in muscarinic acetylcholine receptors in the small intestine of mice subjected to repeated cold stress. *Life Sci.* 22, 2197-2204.

Vermillion, D.L. and Collins, S.M. (1988): Increased Responsiveness of jejunal longitudinal muscle in Trichinella spiralis-infected rats. *Am. J. Physiol.* 254, G124-129.

Postprandial hormonal status and gastric emptying in stressed dogs

Theo Peeters, Michele Gué*, Inge Depoortere, Lionel Bueno*, and Gaston Vantrappen

*Gut Hormone Lab, Department of Medical Research, University of Leuven, B-3000, Leuven, Belgium and *Department of Pharmacology, INRA 31300 Toulouse, France*

INTRODUCTION

Conflicting results have been reported on the effect of stress on gastric emptying. In mice acoustic and cold exposure stress increase the gastric emptying rate of a fat meal (Gué et al.1987a) but in rats restraint stress has an opposite effect on the gastric emptying of a non-nutritive meal (Lenz et al., 1988). In man cold water stress delays gastric emptying (Thompson et al.,1983) but dichotomous listening has no effect (Cann et al.,1983).

One may assume that the effects of stress are mostly mediated by the nervous system, but a hormonal component may also be involved. We have shown that in fasting dogs acoustic stress inhibits the occurence of gastric migrating motor complexes (MMC) (Gué et al., 1987b) and that this effect is mimicked by the intracerebroventricular (icv) administration of corticotropin-releasing factor (CRF). Interestingly, icv administration of CRF also lowered peripheral plasma levels of motilin (Bueno et al.,1986), the peptide which has been implicated in the generation of gastric MMCs (Poitras, 1984; Peeters et al.,1988) suggesting a link between stress, gut hormone secretion and motility.

The present study was designed to extend our observations on the effect of acoustic stress upon gastrointestinal motility and hormone secretion in dogs, to the postprandial state. Thus gastric emptying of the liquid and solid phases of a standard meal and plasma levels of motilin and of three digestive hormones (gastrin, pancreatic polypeptide (PP) and somatostatin) were monitored under control conditions and acoustic stress.

MATERIAL AND METHODS

Animal preparation

In four female adult mongrel dogs weighing 12-16 kg, a Thomas cannula was placed on the great curvature of the gastric body, about 10 cm from the pylorus, under halothane anesthesia. The cannula was brought out through, and fixed to, the left abdominal wall at 5 cm from the midline. A silicone catheter was also inserted into the jugular vein and was brought subcutaneously to the back of the neck. The animals were allowed 3 weeks to recover before starting the experiments.

Experimental protocol

Dogs were fasted from 5.00 pm until the following morning 10.00 am when they received a test meal consisting of 400 g canned food (Fidele, Quaker, France) mixed with dog ovine liver labeled with ^{57}Co-cyanocobalamine and 100 ml of tap water containing 50 mg polyethyleneglycol 4000 and 0.5μCi ^{14}C-PEG (NEN Research Products, Specific activity 1 $\mu Ci.mg^{-1}$). The labeled liver was obtained from sheep given an iv injection of 10 μCi ^{57}Co-cyanocobalamine (Amersham, Paris, France) and killed 24 hours later. The meal was eaten in less than 5 minutes, and immediately after the meal the animals were submitted to acoustic stress which was applied during two hours. The acoustic stress consisted of prerecorded modern music (80-90 dB broad frequency noise) delivered through miniature earpieces inserted into the ears one hour before the meal. Controls were obtained with a blanck tape. Heart rate was monitored using skin electrodes and acoustic stress was considered as effective when an increase of heart rate was obtained within 10 minutes after the start of the music. All four animals were responsive.

Gastric contents were collected at 30, 60 or 120 min. Blood samples were taken 40 and 20 minutes before feeding, at the time of feeding (0 minutes) and 15,30,45,60,90,120,180 and 240 minutes after feeding during the experiments when the gastric contents were collected at 120 min.

The four animals were studied three times under stress and three times under control conditions, for each emptying period (30, 60, 120 min). Stress and control experiments were applied in random order.

Measurement of gastric emptying

The total contents of the stomach was blenderized after determination of the total weight and volume, and two series of 5 samples (4-5 ml) were rapidly taken. Each sample of the first series was weighed and ^{57}Co was counted using a gammacounter (MR 252, Kontron, Switzerland). The second series was prepared for ^{14}C-PEG determination using a liquid scintillation system (Beta V, Kontron). The percentages of gastric emptying of liquid and solid phases were calculated, as previously described (Gué et al., 1988).

Hormonal dosages

Plasma motilin, pancreatic polypeptide and somatostatin were determined by radioimmunoassay as previously described (Peeters et al., 1980 ; 1981; Janssens et al., 1982), using antimotilin antiserum from Dr.P.Poitras (Montreal, Canada), PP-antibody obtained from Dr.R.E. Chance (Eli-Lilly, Indianapolis, USA) and antisomatostatin antiserum raised in rabbits. These antisera exhibited no cross-reaction with other known regulatory peptides. The smallest amount of peptide detectable with 95 % confidence was for canine motilin 9 pg/ml, for PP 16 pg/ml and for somatostatin 8 pg/ml. Gastrin was measured using reagents commercially available (Becton Dickinson, Orangeburg, NY, USA). In our hands the sensitivity of this assay was 10 pg/ml.

Statistical analysis

The gastric emptying rates of both the liquid and solid phases were expressed as a percentage of the meal emptied. The effect of acoustic stress on gastric emptying were evaluated using Student's paired t test. Changes in plasma levels of the peptides studied, were evaluated by two-way analysis of variance. Significance was accepted at the 5% level. Values are always given as means ± S.E.M.

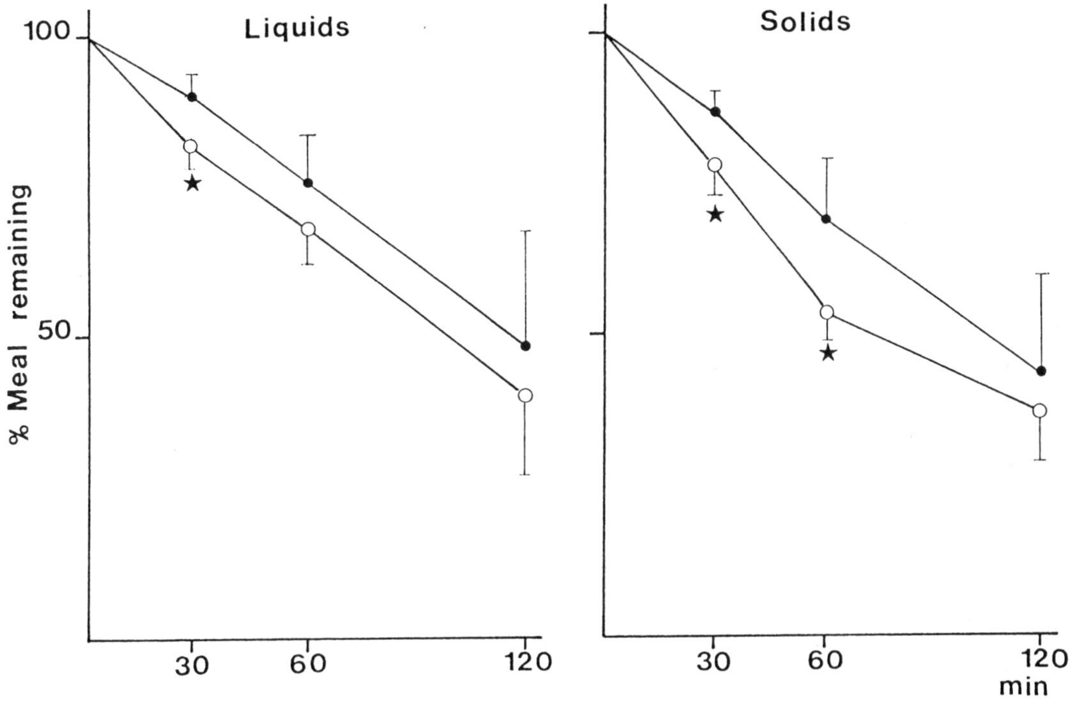

Figure 1. Gastric emptying of the liquid and solid phase of a standard canned food meal in dogs under control conditions (●) or under acoustic stress (○). Values are mean ± S.E.M. Asterisks indicate significant differences ($P<0.05$).

RESULTS

The percent of the volume of the liquid phase or of the weight of the solid phase of the meal, remaining in the stomach at the different time intervals, is shown in figure 1 for both stress and control conditions. As can be seen the emptying rate was slower under stress and the differences were significant at 30 minutes for the emptying of liquids (82 ± 3 % versus 90 ± 3 % for respectively control and stress conditions; $P<0.05$), and at 30 and 60 minutes for the emptying of solids (78 ± 5 versus 87 ± 3; 53 ± 4 versus 69 ± 10).

The changes in plasma levels of the four peptides are shown in figures 2, 3, 4, and 5. To facilitate the comparisons of the extent of these changes and to eliminate variations of basal levels, the average of the three basal, fasting sampling periods was substracted from all other values for each experiment. Under control conditions plasma PP, gastrin and somatostatin rose, motilin fell. The rise was most pronounced for PP, least pronounced for gastrin, and the maximum level for PP, somatostatin and gastrin (respectively +787 ± 85, +32 ± 8 and +19 ± 2 pg/ml) was reached almost simultaneously after 45 minutes. In contrast motilin reached a minimum (-104 ± 12 pg/ml) after 120 min only.

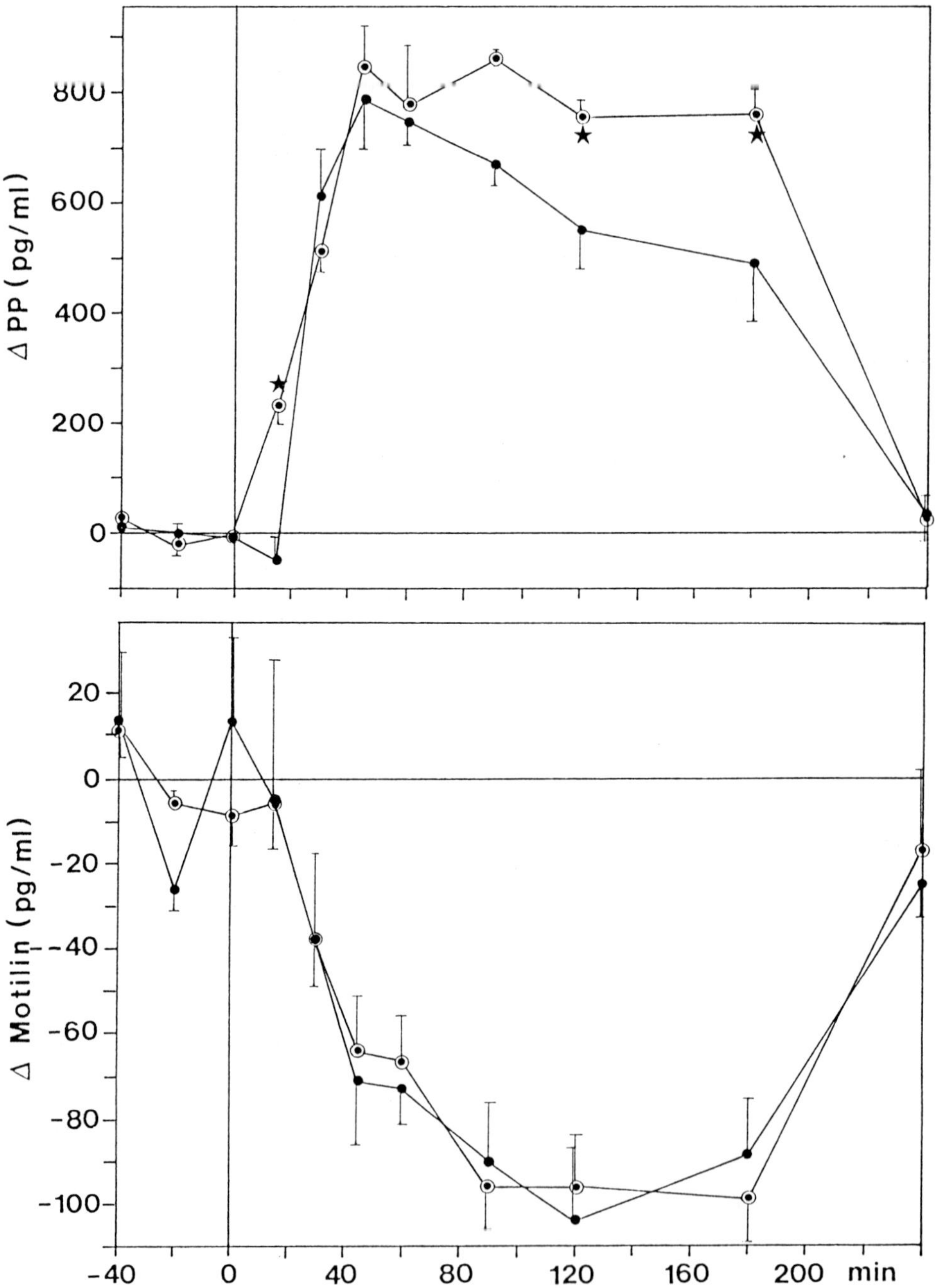

Figure 2 (Top). Changes in plasma PP levels induced by a meal under control (●) or under stress (◉).
Figure 3 (Bottom). Changes in plasma motilin levels induced by a meal under control (●) or under stress (◉).
The results are expressed as the difference with the mean level during the fasting period (mean ± S.E.M.; 4 dogs each studied three times). Asterisks indicate significant differences ($P<0.05$).

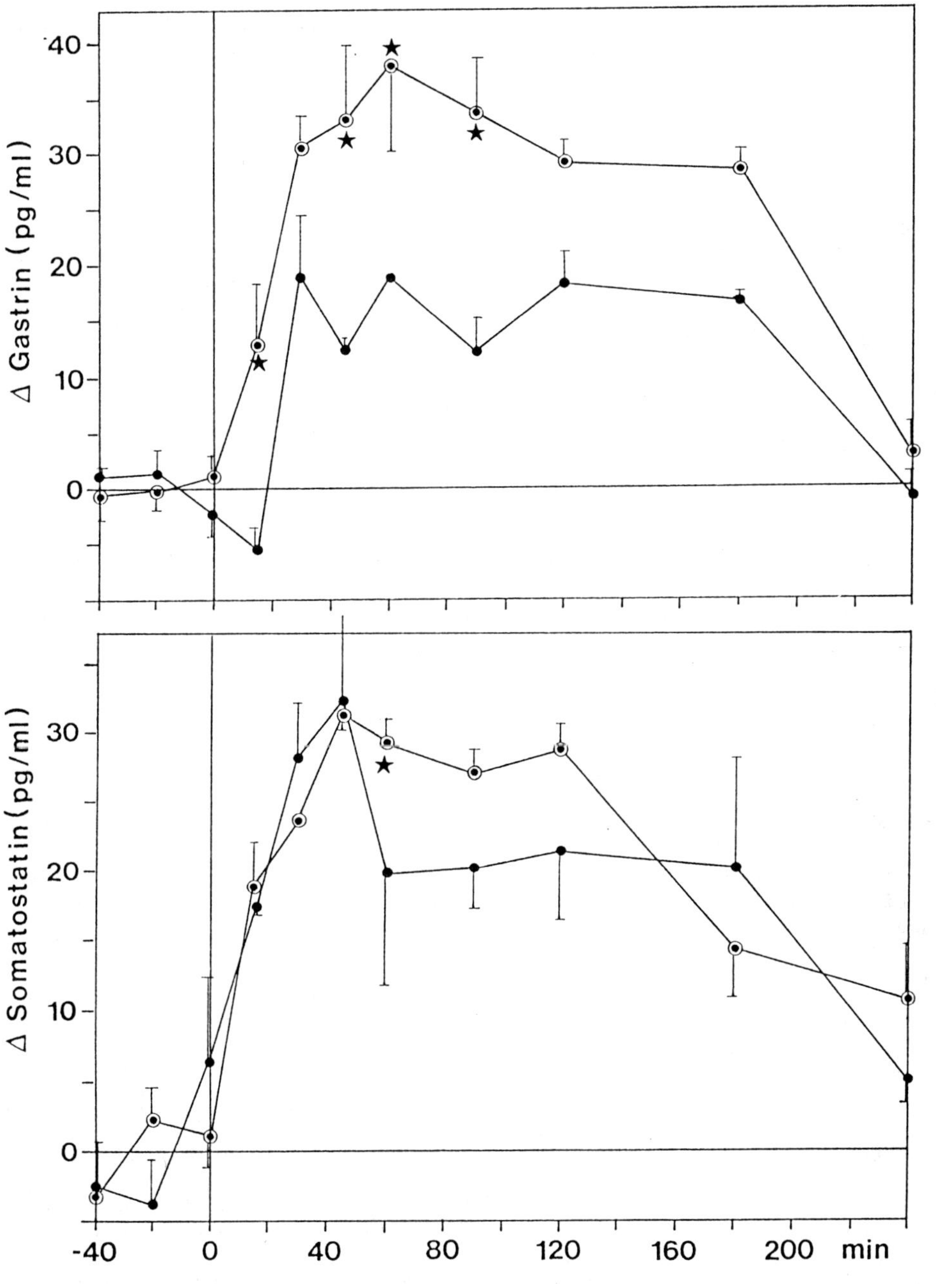

Figure 4 (Top). Changes in plasma gastrin levels induced by a meal under control (●) or under stress (⊙).

Figure 5 (Bottom). Changes in plasma somatostatin levels induced by a meal under control (●) or under stress (⊙).

The results are expressed as the difference with the mean level during the fasting period (mean ± S.E.M.; 4 dogs each studied three times). Asterisks indicate significant differences ($P<0.05$).

During acoustic stress the same release patterns were preserved. For motilin (figure 5) the extent of the decrease was almost identical (stress: -95 ± 11; control -104 ± 12 pg/ml), and over the different time periods no significant differences were observed. However, for PP, gastrin and somatostatin the rises were enhanced during stress. Quite pronounced differences were obtained for gastrin (figure 3), where a significant difference was obtained at 15, 45, 60 and 90 min after stress, with a peak of +38 ± 12 pg/ml after 60 minutes (+19 ± 4 under control conditions). PP showed an earlier rise after stress (figure 2). At 15 min after the meal the elevation in PP levels under stress was already +232 ± 30 pg/ml while under control conditions only a small change was observed at that moment (-49 ± 40 pg/ml). Peak PP values did not differ significantly, but plasma values remained for a longer time at an elevated level, with the difference between control and stress reaching significance again at 120 and 180 min. Somatostatin (figure 4) rose in a similar way in control and in stressed animals, but as for PP its elevation was more pronounced during stress. The late increase of plasma somatostatin level was significantly enhanced to +29 ± 2 pg/ml at 60 min in stressed animals, compared to +20 ± 1 pg/ml in controls.

DISCUSSION

This work establishes that acoustic stress, a centrally acting stressful stimulus, affects the rate of gastric emptying of a solid meal in dogs and the postprandial release of PP, gastrin and somatostatin but not of motilin. Under stress gastric emptying is slower and the release of PP, gastrin and somatostatin is enhanced.

One way by which stress may enhance the release of these two peptides is by vagal stimulation. It has been shown that stress, produced by electrical stimulation of the sciatic nerves at low intensity in cats, leads to an activation of the vagal nerves and to a subsequent release of gastrin and cholecystokinin (Uvnas-Möberg et al., 1986). Although not determined, one may presume that PP was elevated as well in this study because it is well known that PP release is under vagal control to the point that it is considered an indicator of vagal tonus (Schwartz, 1978). Uvnas-Möberg et al.,(1986) did not find a release of somatostatin but Woussen-Colle et al., (1988) noted that the initial postprandial response (0-30 min) of somatostatin was reduced after vagotomy, indicating that vagal stimulation elicits somatostatin secretion. In our experiments no significance was obtained during that period. Vagal stimulation could therefore only explain the rise of gastrin and PP, although it must be said that it is generally accepted that stress affects the sympathetic rather than the parasympathetic system.

Another mechanism by which stress could affect peptide release is via CRF. There is considerable evidence that this peptide is involved in the response to stress. For example, it has been demonstrated that CRF mediates the gastrointestinal disturbances induced by acoustic stress in mice (Bueno & Gué, 1988) and the suppression of feeding behavior and of gastrointestinal emptying by restraint stress in rats (Shibasaki et al., 1988; Lenz et al., 1988). In dogs icv administration of CRF reduces plasma motilin levels (Bueno et al., 1986) and in vitro, ovine CRF is able to stimulate the release of somatastatin from dispersed cells of rat brain (Peterfreud & Vale, 1983). It should be noted that CRF may also be released from peripheral sources, as the peptide is also present in rat antrum, (Uohaka et al., 1986) and that systemic administration of CRF affects the release of PP. Indeed Lytras et al., (1984) found a rise of plasma PP, but not of gastrin, somatostatin and motilin, after iv CRF in human volunteers. Konturek et al., (1985) obtained similar results in dogs. However as judged from plasma cortisol increases, CRF is released only during the first 30-45 min of the acoustic stress application (Gué et al., 1987a) while plasma PP and plasma gastrin were enhanced for at least 2 hours.

Because PP, gastrin (Cooke et al., 1972) and somatostatin (Seal et al., 1982) have been shown to delay gastric emptying it is tempting to suggest a causal relationship between the inhibition of gastric emptying and the enhanced release of these peptides during stress. However the inhibition of gastric emptying is limited to the 30-60 min postprandial period, when PP and somatostatin levels did not differ significantly. Moreover PP and gastrin remained considerably elevated till 120 minutes when there was no significant difference in emptying rate. Therefore it seems unlikely that the reduction in gastric emptying was causally related to the observed changes in plasma peptide levels.

The hypothesis that CRF released in the CNS, or in peripheral tissues, may be directly responsible for the slowing of gastric emptying in stressed animals, independently of the induced hormonal changes, is also arguable. Its release is certainly better correlated in time with the reduction in gastric emptying. How CRF may alter gastric emptying is unclear since controversy exists about the effects of central CRF on gastric emptying depending on the composition of the test meal and on the species considered (Gué et al., 1987a; Taché et al., 1987). As was already noted for CRF's effect upon peptide release, a peripheral action (and release) of CRF should also be envisaged. In dogs it has been found that CRF given icv at doses active peripherally, did not alter gastric emptying (Pappas et al., 1985). Consequently a release of CRF at the periphery induced by a stressor may be directly involved in the slowing of gastric emptying by acoustic stress.

In conclusion, the present work demonstrates that acoustic stress affects transiently the gastric emptying of a standard nutritive meal in dogs and enhances the postprandial release of PP, gastrin and somatostatin. The mechanisms involved and the causal relationships between these postprandial alterations remain to be clarified.

REFERENCES

Bormans, V., Peeters, T.L., Janssens, J., Pearce, D., Vandeweerd, M., and Vantrappen, G. (1987): In man, only activity fronts that originate in the stomach correlate with motilin peaks. Scand. J. Gastroenterol. 22, 781-784.

Bueno, L., Gué, M. (1988): Evidence for the involvement of corticotropin-releasing factor in the gastrointestinal disturbances induced by acoustic and cold stress in mice. Brain Res. 44, 1-4.

Bueno, L., Fargeas, M.J., Gué, M., Peeters, T.L., Bormans, V., Fioramonti, J. (1986): Effects of corticotropin releasing factor on plasma motilin and somatostatin levels and gastrointestinal motility in dogs. Gastroenterology 91, 884-889.

Cann, P.A., Read, N.W., Cammack, J., Childs, H., Holden, S., Kashman, R., Longmore, J., Nix, S., Simms, N., Swallow, K., Weller, J. (1983): Psychological stress and passage of a standard meal through the stomach and small intestine in man. Gut 24, 236-240.

Cooke, A.R., Chvast, T.E., and Weisbrodt, N.W. (1972): Effect of pentagastrin on emptying and electrical motor activity of the dog stomach. Am. J. Physiol. 223, 934-839.

Gué, M., Fioramonti, J., Bueno, L. (1987a): Comparative influences of acoustic and cold stress on gastrointestinal transit in mice. Am. J. Physiol. 253, G1248.

Gué, M., Fioramonti, J., Frexinos, J., Alvinerie, M., Bueno, L. (1987 b): Influence of acoustic stress by noise on gastrointestinal motility in dogs. Dig. Dis. Sci. 32: 1411-1417.

Gué, M., Fioramonti, J., Bueno, L., (1988): A simple double radiolabeled tecnique to evaluate gastric emptying of canned food meal in dogs: application to pharmacological tests. Gastroenterol. Clin. Biol. 12: 425-430.

Janssens, J., Hellemans, I., Adrian, T.E., Bloom, S.R., Peeters, T.L., Christofides, N., Vantrappen, G. (1982): Pancreatic polypeptides is not involved in the regulation of the migrating motor complex in man. Regul. Pept. 3: 41-49.

Konturek, S.J., Bilski, J., Pawlik, W., Thor, P., Czarnobilski, K., Szoke, B., Schally, A.V. (1985): Gastrointestinal secretory, motor and circulatory effects of corticotropin releasing factor (CRF). Life Sci. 37, 1231-1240.

Lenz, H.J., Raedler, A., Greten, H., Vale, W.W., River, J.E. (1988): Stress Induced Gastrointestinal Secretory and motor Responses in Rats are mediated by endogeneous Corticotropin-releasing factor. Gastroenterology 95, 1510-1517.

Lenz, H., J., Burlaged, M., Raedler, A., Greten, H. (1988); Central nervous system effects of corticotropin-releasing factor in gastrointestinal transit in the rat. Gastroenterology 94, 598-602.

Lytras, N., Grossman, A., Rees, L., Schally, A., Bloom, S., Besser, G. (1984): Corticotropin-releasing factor: effects on circulating gut and pancreatic peptides in man. Clin. Endocrinol. 20, 725-729.

Peeters, T.L., Vantrappen, G.R., Janssens, J. (1980): Fasting plasma motilin levels are related to the interdigestive motor complex. Gastroenterology 79, 716-719.

Peeters, T.L., Depoortere, I., Vantrappen, G. (1981): Radioimmunoassay for somatastatin using a simple extraction method. Clin. Chem. 29, 888-891.

Poitras, P. (1984): Motilin is a digestive hormone in the dog. Gastroenterology 87, 909-913.

Peterfreud, R.A. & Vale, W.W. (1983): Onine corticotropin-releasing factor stimulates somatostatin secretion from cultured brain cells. Endocrinology 112, 1275-1278.

Schwartz, T. (1983): Pancreatic polypeptide: a unique model for vagal control of endocrine systems. J. Autonomic Nerv. Systems 9, 99-111.

Seal, A., Yamada, T., Debas, H., Hollinshead, J., Oasdchey, B., Aponte, G., Walsh, J. (1982): Somatostatin-14 and -28: clearance and potency on gastric function in dogs. Am. J. Physiol. 234, G97-G102.

Taché, Y., Maeda-Hagiwara, Turkelson, M. (1987): Central nervous system action of corticotropin releasing factor in inhibit gastric emptying in rats. Am. J. Physiol. 253, G241-G245.

Thompson, D.G., Richelson, E., Malagelada, J.R. (1983): Perturbation of upper gastrointestinal function by cold stress. Gut 24, 277-283.

Shibasaki, T., Yamauchi, N., Kato, Y., Masuda, A., Imaki, T., Hotta, M., Demura, H., Oono, H., Ling, N., Shizume, K. (1988): Involvement of corticotropin-releasing factor in restraint stress-induced anorexia and reversion of the anorexia by somatostatin in the rat. Life Sci. 43: 1103-1110.

Uehaka, A., Minamino, N., Towsend, M.H., Arimura, A. (1986): Corticotropin-releasing activity in the rat gastric antrum. Proc. Soc. Emp. Biol. Med. 183, 106-113

Uvnas-Möberg, K., Posloncec, B., Ahlberg, L.(1986): Influence on plasma levels of somatostatin, gastrin, glucagon, insulin and VIP-like immunoreactivity in peripheral venous blood of anaesthetised cats induced by low intensity afferent stimulation of the sciatic nerves. Acta Physiol. Scan. 126, 225-230.

Woussen-Colle, M.C., Lalieu, C., Simoens, C, De Graef, J. (1987): Effect of vagotomy and atropine on plasma somatostatin response to a meal in conscious dogs. Regul. Pept. 21, 29-36.

A novel stress model to investigate stress effects on gastro-intestinal transit in the rat

Paul Enck

University Hospitals, Department of Internal Medicine, Division of Gastroenterology, Moorenstr. 5, D-4000 Düsseldorf, Federal Republic of Germany

Investigations of stress effects on gastrointestinal transit in animals have produced conflicting results: an acceleration as well as a delay of transit after stress have been reported with respect to stomach emptying, oro-caecal transit, and to colonic transit (Gue et al., 1987; Lenz et al., 1987; Williams et al., 1988). Several reasons may account for this: 1) The stress models used confound psychological components such as fear, unpredictability, or uncontrollability due to restraint, open field, noise, or light, with physical stress components such as a change in body temperature by cold or heat, restricted respiration by wrapping, physical pain, or systemic arousal by motor activity. 2) Most of the measurement techniques require multiple handling of the animals prior to exposure to the experimental stressor, e.g. for oral gavage of the marker. Handling, however, is known to act as a stressor itself, causing sustained raises of plasma catecholamines and cortisol. 3) Transit studies in the upper gut are usually performed with colour or radio-isotope labelled markers in liquid carrier solutions for oral infusion or application through a chronic fistula. Gastric emptying of liquids, however, is known to be quite different from that of solid food. 4) Transit studies usually do not allow multiple measurements in individual animals since propulsion of the marker within the gut can only be controlled after the animal has been sacrificed.

To avoid some of these disadvantages a novel stress model was developed closely resembling a standard "passive avoidance" situation (Fig.1) and applied to the study of gastric emptying of solid food, oro-caecal transit, and to the study of colonic transit in female Wistar rats (Enck et al., 1989).

Animals were trained to eat a standard amount (up to 15 g) of solid food (dry food mixed with water, 1:1) within a given time period (5 to 30 minutes) for 8 days prior to the experiments.

During this restricted feeding schedule animals had free access to the food for two hours at day -7, for 1 hour at days -6 to -4, and for 30 minutes at days -3 to -1. Feeding time was always 9.00 a.m. The animals were fed individually in their home cages at days

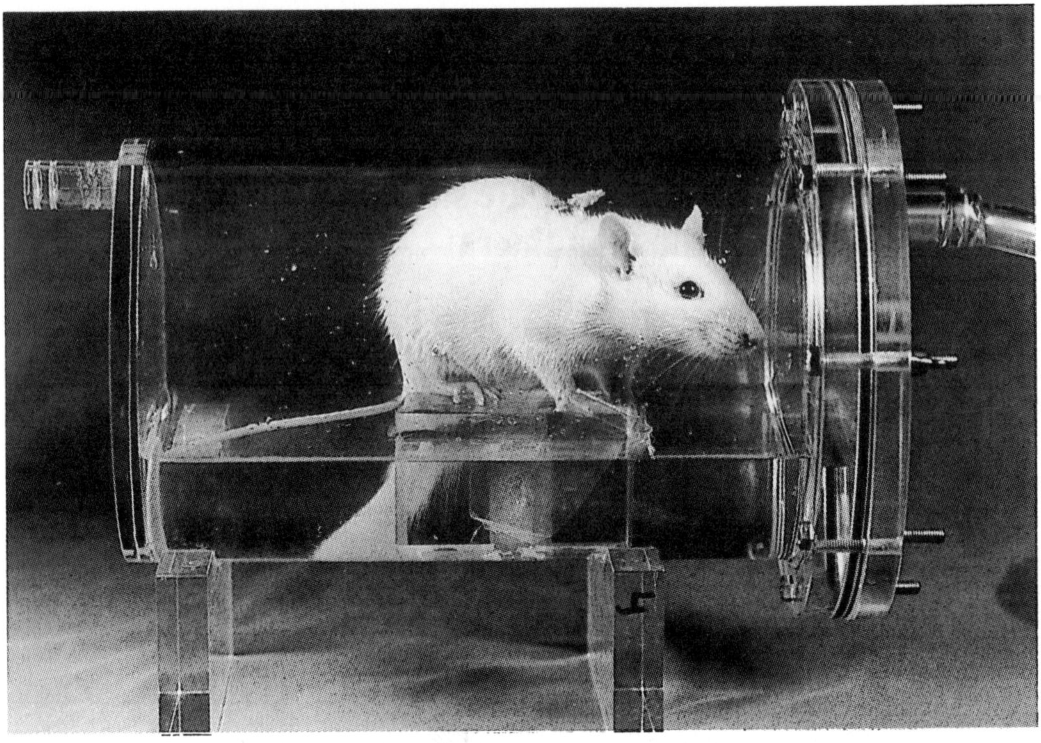

Fig.1: Stressor used in all experiments: The plexi glass box measuring 2500 cc is filled with 500 ml of water at body temperature. The "passive avoidance" situation allows the rat to avoid contact with the water by climbing onto a glass block measuring 3x4x5 cm. In control experiments the box remaines without water. The box can be safely closed to accumulate and determine the hydrogen concentration in the exhaled air for measurement of oro-caecal transit.

-8 to -5 and in the test box at days -4 to -1. During the pretraining and training period the rats received water ad lib. The animals were controlled daily for body weight. At the day of the experiment, gastric emptying was determined as gastric content (per cent of food consumed) after various periods of stress or rest. Oro-caecal transit was measured by breath hydrogen exhalation after the food had been labelled with 1 g of lactose (Brown et al, 1987). Colonic transit was determined by the arrival time of coloured faeces after infusion of a carmine red solution into the caecum via a chronically implanted catheter.
All animals easily learned to eat their daily food within a predefined time period and maintained their body weight after an initial drop. Gastric emptying showed a significant delay after stress exposure as compared to the rest condition (t/2: 2.66 and and 1.97 hours, respectively). Oro-caecal transit was signifi-

cantly accelerated from 131 min after rest to 86 min after stress. Colonic transit significantly decreased from 13.9 hours to 1.25 hours (s. Fig.2). We conclude that the same stressor may differentially affect transit in different compartments of the gastrointestinal tract. Furthermore, non-invasive and behavioural techniques which minimize additional stress exposure and allow for multiple measurement in individual animals are applicable in experimental stress re-search.

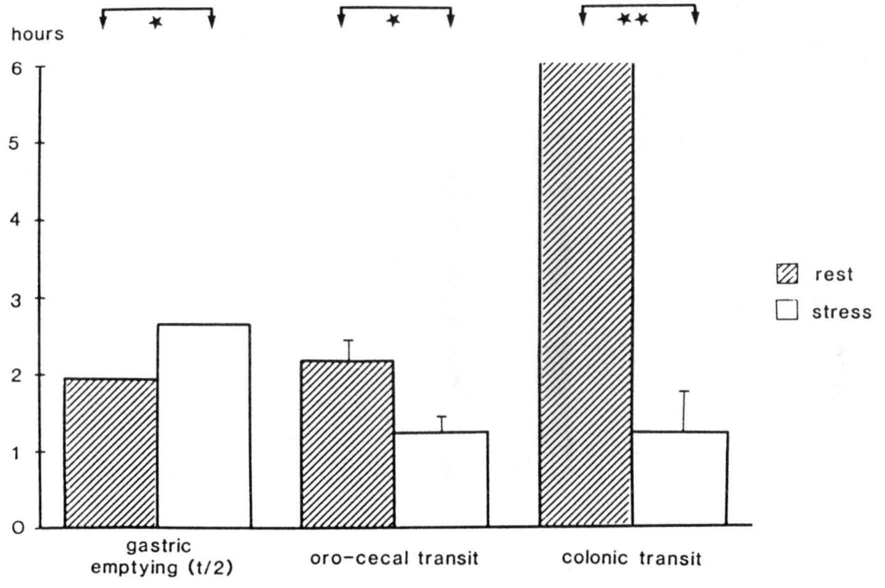

Fig.2: Stress effects on gastric emptying (t/2), orocaecal transit, and colonic transit (hours ± SEM, * $p < 0.05$; ** $p < 0.01$).

References:

Brown, N.J., Rumsey, R.D.E., and Read, N.W. (1987): Adaptation of hydrogen analysis to measure stomach to caecum transit time in the rat. Gut 28: 849 - 854.

Enck, P., Merlin, V., Erckenbrecht, J.F., and Wienbeck, M. (1989): Stress effects on gastrointestinal transit in the rat. Gut 30: (in press)

Gue, M., Fioramonti, J., and Bueno, L. (1987): Disturbance of gastric emptying and intestinal transit induced by acoustic and cold stress in mice. Am J Physiol 253: G124 - G128.

Lenz, H.J., Raedler, A., Greten, H., and Brown, M.R. (1987): CRF initiates biological actions within the brain that are observed in response to stress. Am J Physiol 252 : R34 - R39.

Williams, C.L., Villar, R.G., Peterson, J.M., and Burks, T.F. (1988): Stress-induced changes in intestinal transit in the rat: A model for irritable bowel syndrome. Gastroenterology 94:611 - 621.

(Supported by grants En 50/2 and Wi 285/5 from the Deutsche Forschungsgemeinschaft)

TRH and CRF injected into the brain have opposite effects on gastric contractility in the rat

T. Garrick, R. Stephens, H. Yang, H. Weiner and Y. Tache

Wadsworth VAMC, Center for Ulcer Research and Education, Brain Research Institute, University of California, Los Angeles, Ca 90073 U.S.A.

Thyrotropin resleasing hormone(TRH) and corticotropin releasing factor (CRF) in the brain may mediate the effects of experimental stress. The effects of these peptides on gastric contractility were evaluated in conscious or anesthetized rats.

Gastric contractility was measured with strain gauge force transducers sutured to the external surface of the corpus of the stomach in rats. Signals were collected and analyzed by computer. Peptides were injected into the cisterna magna (ic) or into specific brain nuclei using glass pipettes (50 um, 50-100 nl).

TRH, or its stable analogue RX77368 (260 pmol, ic), (unlike 0.9% NaCl) dose dependently stimulated gastric contractions in conscious rats 2-3x over basal levels (n=6) for greater than 1 h. Peptide action was inhibited by atropine (1 mg/kg) or vagotomy(1). RX77368 microinjected into the dorsal vagal complex(77 pmol, n=10), nucleus ambiguus(7.7 pmol, n=7), raphe pallidus(7.7 pmol, n=6), or raphe obscurus (7.7 pmol, n=5) nucleii closely associated with gastric function, also potently stimulated gastric contractility significantly over basal levels. Control (n=13) microinjections were non-stimulatory(2).

In contrast, ic CRF (6.3-210 pmol) dose-dependently inhibited gastric contractions stimulated by ic RX77368(260 pmol) or 2-deoxy-d-glucose(2-DG, 6 mg) but not iv. carbachol(200 mg/kg/hr). This effect is centrally mediated since iv CRF was much less potent or ineffective(3).

In sum, TRH (or its stable analogue, RX77368) and CRF have opposite CNS-mediated effects on gastric contractility. The inhibitory activity of CRF on centrally mediated stimulants of gastric contractility (TRH, RX77368, 2-DG) but not a peripheral stimulant (carbachol) suggests the action of CRF is centrally mediated involving vagal pathways. The inactivity of iv CRF in effecting similar actions supports this conclusion. Pharmacological and surgical evidence suggests that the mechanism through which CRF exerts its inhibitory effect may be related to the alterations of the autonomic nervous system. The sites at which each of these peptides are acting to inhibit each other is not clear from these studies.

These studies demonstrate that TRH is active at several medullary sites to stimulate gastric contractility. Although neural connections between these sites and the dorsal vagal complex has been documented previously, TRH appears active at each site but not in the brain parenchyma 100 nm from each nucleus or in some TRH containing nuclei such as the hypoglossal nucleus. Further experiments are necessary to detail specific sites of action for CRF to inhibit TRH stimulation of gastric contractility.
The presence of these peptides in medulla suggest a possible interaction in the medullary regulation of gastric contractility during stress.

References:

1. Garrick, T., Buack, S., Veiseh, A. and Tache, Y.(1987) Thyrotropin-releasing hormone (TRH) acts centrally to stimulate gastric contractility in the rat. Life Sciences 40:649-657.

2.Garrick, T., Stephens, T., Ishikawa, T., Sierra, A., Avidan, A., Weiner, H. and Tache, Y.(1989). Medulary sites for TRH analog stimulation of gastric contractility in the rat. American Journal of Physiology (In Press).

3. Garrick, T., Veiseh, A., Sierra, A., Weiner, H. and Tache, Y.(1988). Corticotropin-releasing factor acts centrally to suppress stimulated gastric contractility in the rat. Regulatory Peptides 221:173-181.

Inhibition of gastric motor function by circulating corticotropin-releasing factor in rats

Helen E. Raybould and Yvette F. Taché

Center for Ulcer Research and Education, VA West Los Angeles Medical Center, Department of Medicine and Brain Research Institute, University of California, Los Angeles, California 90073, U.S.A.

Corticotropin-releasing factor (CRF) is a 41 amino acid peptide originally isolated from ovine hypothalamus that plays a physiological role in regulating the secretion of proopiomelanocortin-derived peptides from the anterior pituitary (Vale et al, 1981; Rivier et al, 1983). It has been demonstrated that administration of CRF into the cerebrospinal fluid (CSF) elicits many of the endocrine, behavioral and cardiovascular responses associated with stress (Brown et al, 1986; Lenz et al, 1987). More recently, CRF has been implicated in mediating the stress-induced alterations of gastrointestinal secretory and motor function in the rat. CRF injected into the cerebrospinal fluid acts within the brain to decrease gastric motility and emptying of a non nutrient liquid meal, to delay small intestinal transit and to increase large bowel transit (Taché et al, 1989). These actions of CRF mimic the effects of stress on gastrointestinal transit and moreover, the CRF antagonist, α-helical CRF, injected into the cerebrospinal fluid prevented stress-induced changes in gastrointestinal transit (Taché et al, 1989a). In addition to its actions on gastrointestinal transit mediated at a central site, CRF has been shown to inhibit gastric emptying of a non nutrient liquid solution following peripheral injection in dogs (Pappas et al, 1985) and rats (Taché et al, 1987). We have investigated the changes in gastric motility that may underly the CRF-induced inhibition of gastric emptying and assessed the neurohumoral pathway by which peripheral administration of CRF alters gastric transit and motility.

Gastric motility was manometrically recorded in urethane-anesthetized rats using a catheter placed in the gastric corpus through the duodenum and secured at the pylorus (Raybould et al, 1987). The stomach was placed under 3-4 cmH_2O at the beginning of the experimental period to give a standardized baseline intraluminal pressure. Increasing doses of CRF (0.21-210 pmol) were given by bolus intravenous injections. CRF decreased baseline intraluminal pressure and inhibited phasic contractions of the gastric corpus; this decrease was dose-related and rapid in onset. The response was long lasting; the duration of the response following the 210 pmol dose was 10-60 min (29 ± 3; mean ± sem, n=5). Intravenous injection of CRF (210 pmol) in intact rats decreased intraluminal pressure by 1.3 ± 0.1 cm H_2O (n=5). The CRF response was significantly reduced to 0.5 ± 0.1 cmH_2O (t test $p<0.05$; n=4) and to 0.04 ± 0.04 cmH_2O ($p<0.01$; n=5) in subdiaphragmatically vagotomized and hexamethonium-treated (15 mg/kg intraperitoneally, 15 min pretreatment) rats respectively. Celiac/superior mesenteric ganglionectomy and bilateral adrenalectomy had no effect on the inhibition of gastric motility induced by peripheral administration of CRF (210 pmol, decrease in intraluminal pressure 1.5 ± 0.2 cmH_2O and 1.3 ± 0.2 cmH_2O respectively, n=6 in both groups). Thus the decrease in gastric corpus motility induced by peripheral administration of CRF seems partly dependent on the integrity of the vagus nerve and is completely abolished by hexamethonium, suggesting it is wholly mediated through a nicotinic synapse within the enteric nervous system. There is good evidence that vasoactive intestinal peptide (VIP) may be the putative transmitter of vagal non-adrenergic inhibitor of gastric smooth muscle in the enteric nervous system (Gillespie, 1982). We examined the effect of immunoneutralization of VIP using a polyclonal antibody (ab 7913, kindly donated by Dr J Walsh) on the CRF response. A 30 min pretreatment with the antibody (0.1 ml of 1:2 dilution) abolished the decrease in gastric motility induced by intravenous injection of VIP (33 pmol) but had no effect on CRF-induced (210 pmol i.v.) inhibition of gastric motility.

The neurohormonal pathway by which peripheral CRF inhibits gastric emptying was investigated by surgical and pharmacological lesion of the autonomic nervous system. Gastric emptying was measured using the method of Scarpignato et al. Briefly, the emptying of 1.5% methylcellulose solution was measured using a non-absorbable dye, phenol red. CRF or vehicle were injected intravenously through the jugular vein in 0.1 ml in rats lightly anesthetized with ether. The methylcellulose solution was delivered per orally by gavage 5 min later in conscious rats and gastric emptying measured after 20 min. Bilateral adrenalectomy or celiac/superior mesenteric ganglionectomy was performed under sodium methohexital anesthesia 24 h and 3-4 weeks respectively prior to experiments. Other groups of rats were pretreated with naloxone (1 mg/kg i.p.), hexamethonium bromide (10 mg/kg, i.p.), bretylium (25 mg/kg, i.p.) administered 15 min prior to intravenous administration of CRF. In animals injected with vehicle i.v. under light ether anesthesia 5 min before intragastric administration of the methylcellulose solution, 52 ± 3% (n=8) of the solution had emptied after twenty minutes. Intravenous injection of CRF (126 pmol) 5 min before intragastric administration of the methylcellulose solution reduced gastric emptying to 16 ± 4% (n=9), which represents an inhibition of 69% as previously reported (Taché et al, 1987). The percent inhibition produced by CRF i.v. was 74, 65, 78, 53 and 91% following adrenalectomy, sympathectomy and with bretylium, hexamethonium and naloxone treated respectively. Only the hexamethonium treatment produced a significant attenuation of the CRF response ($p<0.05$ ANOVA). None of the surgeries or different drug treatments had any significant effect on the rate of gastric emptying in vehicle-treated rats.

The present results demonstrate that picomolar amounts of CRF injected intravenously decreases gastric corpus motility and slows the gastric emptying of liquids in rats. The mechanism of action of CRF on gastric motility involves the vagus nerve and transmission at nicotinic synapses, presumably in the enteric nervous system. However, it is not clear which transmitter mediating non-adrenergic inhibition of gastric smooth muscle is involved, but from these preliminary results, it does not appear to be VIP. We have confirmed the inhibitory action of peripherally administered CRF on gastric emptying in rats. As gastric emptying of liquids seems to depend primarily on the pressure in the body of the stomach (Kelly, 1980), the ability of CRF to delay the gastric emptying of liquids may be ascribed to its action on proximal gastric motility described here. We have attempted to characterize the neurohormonal mechanisms by which CRF inhibits gastric emptying. Intravenous injection of CRF to rats induced release of proopiomelanocortin-derived peptides into the plasma, including β-endorphin (Vale et al, 1981). Peripheral administration of opiates has been shown to exert antipropulsive effects on the GI tract which are blocked by naloxone (Kostrisky-Pereira et al, 1984). However, the action of CRF reported here in rats was not blocked by naloxone as previously demonstrated in the dog (Pappas et al, 1988), suggesting the peptide is not acting via release of opioid-like peptides from the pituitary, adrenal gland or from the enteric nervous system. In addition, intravenous injection of CRF can increase plasma levels of epinephrine (Lenz et al, 1985). However, the delay in gastric emptying elicited by intravenous CRF was unaffected by adrenalectomy or noradrenergic blockade suggesting its action is not mediated by release of catecholamines from the adrenal gland or from postganglionic sympathetic neurons. In the dog, the delay in emptying in response to peripherally administered CRF was also found unmodified by ß-adrenergic blockade with propranolol (Pappas et al, 1988). A recent study also reported that i.p. CRF-induced delay in gastric emptying was not altered by bretylium or chlorisondamine in the rat (Lenz et al, 1988).

Taken together these results provide evidence that peripheral CRF-induced inhibition of motility and transit is not secondary to systemic endocrine alteration but requires vagal integrity and autonomic ganglionic transmission. Although specific binding sites for CRF have been demonstrated in peripheral tissues including primate sympathetic ganglia (Udelsman et al, 1986) and rat adrenal medulla (Dave et al, 1985) no study has investigated the presence of CRF receptors in the gastrointestinal tract. Immunoreactive CRF has been detected in rat plasma (Sumitomo et al, 1987) and antrum (Uehara et al, 1986). It has recently been demonstrated that intravenous injection of the CRF antagonist blocked stress induced increase colonic transit in the rat (Williams et al, 1987) and surgically-induced ileus (Taché et al, 1989a). These data may suggest a physiological role of CRF in the regulation of gastric motor function which remains to be further assessed.

REFERENCES

Brown, M.R., Gray, T.S. and Fisher, L.A. (1986): Corticotropin-releasing factor receptor antagonist: effects on the autonomic nervous system and cardiovascular function, Regul. Pept. 16, 321-329.

Dave, J.R., Eiden, L.E. and Eskay, R.L. (1985): Corticotropin-releasing factor binding to peripheral tissue and activation of the adenylate cyclase-adenosine 3',5'-monophosphate system. Endocrinology 116, 2152-2159.

Gillespie, J.S. (1982): Non-adrenergic non-cholinergic inhibitory control of gastrointestinal motility. In Motility of the gastrointestinal tract, ed. M. Weinbeck, pp 51-66. New York: Raven Press.

Kelly, K.A. (1980): Gastric emptying of liquids and solids: roles of proximal and distal stomach. Am. J. Physiol. 239, G71-G76.

Kostritsky-Pereira, A., Wouseen-Colle, M.C. and DeGraef, J. (1984): Effects of morphine, enkephalins and naloxone on postprandial gastric acid secretion, gastric emptying and gastrin release in dogs. Arch. Int. Physiol. Biochim. 92, 19-26.

Lenz, H.J., Fisher, L.A., Vale, W.W. and Brown, M.R. (1985): Corticotropin-releasing factor, sauvagine, and urotensin I: effects on blood flow. Am. J. Physiol. 249, R85-R90.

Lenz, H.J., Raedler, A., Greten, H. and Brown, M.R. (1987): CRF initiates biological actions within the brain that are observed in response to stress. Am.J. Physiol. 252, R34-R39.

Lenz, H.J., Burlace, M., Raedler, A. and Greten, H. (1988): Central nervous system effects of corticotropin-releasing factor on gastrointestinal transit in the rat. Gastroenterology 94, 598-602.

Pappas, T., Debas, H. and Tache, Y. (1985): Corticotropin-releasing factor inhibits gastric emptying in dogs. Regul. Pept. 11, 193-199.

Pappas, T.N., Welton, M., Tache, Y. and Rivier, J. (1988): Corticotropin-releasing factor inhibits gastric emptying in dogs: Studies on its mechanism of action. Peptides 8, 1011-1014.

Raybould, H.E., Roberts, M.E. and Dockray, G.J. (1987): Reflex decreases in intragastric pressure in response to cholecystokinin in rats. Am. J. Physiol. 253, G165-170.

Rivier, J., Spiess, J. and Vale, W. (1983): Characterization of rat hypothalamic corticotropin-releasing factor. Proc. Natl. Acad. Sci. USA 80, 4851-4855.

Scarpignato, C., Capovilla, T. and Bertaccini, G. (1980): Action of caerulein on gastric emptying of the conscious rat. Arch. Int. Pharmacodyn. 246, 286-294.

Sumitomo, T., Suda, T., Tomori, N., Yajima, F., Nakagami, Y., Ushiyama, T., Demura, H. and Shizume, K. (1987): Immunoreactive corticotropin-releasing factor in rat plasma. Endocrinology 120, 1391-1396.

Taché, Y., Maeda-Hagiwara, M. and Turkelson, C.M. (1987): Central nervous system action of corticotropin-releasing factor to inhibit gastric emptying in rats. Am. J. Physiol. 253, G241-G245.

Taché, Y.F., Garrick, T. and Raybould, H.E. (1989): Central nervous system action of peptides to influence gastrointestinal transit and motility. Gastroenterology, in press.

Taché, Y.F., Kolve, E., Stephens, R.L. and Rivier, J.E. (1989a): Role of corticotropin-releasing factor in mediating gastric ileus. Gastroenterology, in press.

Udelsman, R., Harwood, J.P., Millan, M.A., Chrousos, G.P., Goldstein, D.S., Zimlichman, R., Catt, K.J. and Aguilera, G. (1986): Functional corticotropin-releasing factor receptors in the primate peripheral sympathetic nervous system. Nature 319, 147-150.

Uehara, A., Minamino, N., Townsend, M.H. and Arimura, A. (1986): Corticotropin-releasing activity in the rat gastric antrum. Proc. Soc. Exp. Biol. Med. 183, 106-113.

Vale, W., Spiess, J., Rivier, C. and Rivier, J. (1981): Characterization of a 41-residue ovine hypothalamic peptide that stimulates secretion of corticotropin and β-endorphin. Science 213, 1394-1397.

Williams, C.L., Peterson, J.M., Villar, R.G. and Burks, T.F. (1987): Corticotropin-releasing factor directly mediates colonic responses to stress. Am. J. Physiol. 253, G582-G586.

Cold restraint and tail shock stimulate gastric contractility in the rat

T. Garrick , H. Weiner and P. Bass

Center for Ulcer Research and Education, West Los Angeles VA, University of California and Univeristy of Wisconsin, Madison, U.S.A.

Cold water immersion restraint(CR) or mild intermittent tail shock(TS) of awake rats reliably produces gastric injury. The present studies were performed to evaluate the effects of CR or mild intermittent TS on gastric contractility. Chronically implanted strain gauge force transducers were used to monitor gastric contractility. CR was performed at 20°C for three hours. Mild intermittent TS was performed for 1.5 hrs, followed by a three hour home cage rest using 100 - 1 ma 5s tail shocks presented in a variable interval (avg. 1 min) pattern.

CR was associated with the stimulation of persistent high amplitude gastric contractions having a prolonged duration (Fig.1). Average amplitude was not statistically different from the contractions stimulated by food ingestion (first 10 min postprandial) in 24 h fasted rats. High amplitude contractions continued for the duration of cold restraint. Duration of contractions increased 2.4 fold after two hr of cold restraint(1).

Mild intermittent TS also stimulated high amplitude contractions (after 30 min shock) but having a normal duration. On average, high amplitude contractions stimulated by shock was of the same magnitude as postprandial contractions(2). High amplitude contractions persisted for two hours after the animals were returned to their home cage(Fig.2).

Gastric erosion formation was observed with both procedures, but to a much lesser extent with TS. In cold restraint, high amplitude contractions occurring for one hour or less was not associated with mucosal erosion formation. Greater than one hour of high amplitude contractions were needed for the induction of mucosal injury(3). In the shock experiment, lesion areas were significantly correlated with cumulative contractility scores(2, $r=.36$, $p<0.05$). We conclude that the stimulation of high amplitude gastric contractions is associated with the induction of experimental stress and may be related to gastric injury in observed with these procedures.

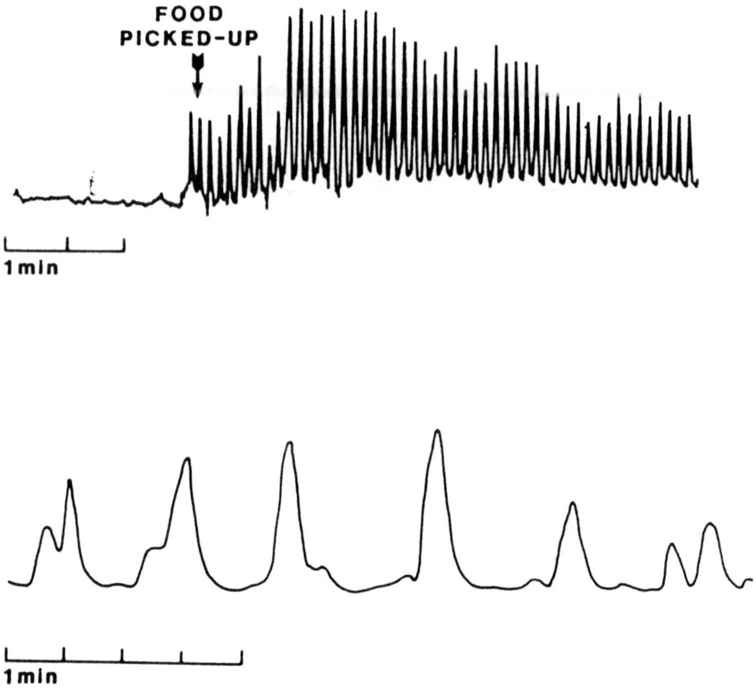

Fig. 1. Examples of recordings of gastric motility from the same animal.
Upper Panel: Gastric contractile activity when a 24 h fasted rat starts to eat.
Lower Panel: Gastric contractile activity following two hr cold water immersion restraint (21°C) in the same animal. 24 h fasted baseline prior to cold restraint is essentially the same as in the upper panel.

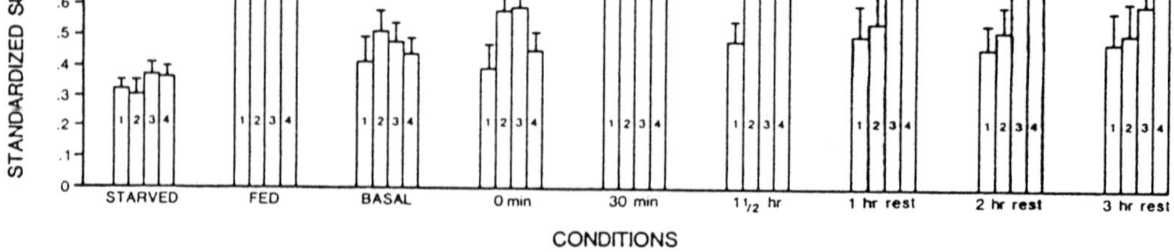

Fig. 2. Mean standardized contractile activity (± S.E.) before feeding, after feeding, at various times during tailshock and at three points during unrestrained postshock rest. All measures standardized to the fed state.

References:

1. Garrick, T., Buack S., and Bass, P.(1986):Gastric motility is a major factor in cold restraint-induced lesion formation in rats. American Journal of Physiology, 250, G191-G199.

2. Garrick, T., Minor, T.R., Buack, S., Weiner H., and Guth, P. (1989): Predictable and unpredicatble shock stimulates gastric contractility and causes mucosal injury in rats. Behavioral Neuroscience 103, 1-7.

3. Garrick, T., Leung, F.W., Buack, S., Hirabayashi, K., and Guth, P.H.(1986): Gastric motility is stimulated but overall blood flow is unaffected during cold restraint in the rat. Gastroenterology, 91:141-8.

4th SESSION :

Pharmacological and clinical observations

Moderators : *D. Thomson, J. Akkermans*

Involvement of opiate and adrenergic pathways on stress-induced gastrointestinal motor disturbances

Vincenzo Stanghellini, Roberto Corinaldesi and Luigi Barbara

1st Medical Clinic, University of Bologna, Ospedale S. Orsola, via Massarenti 9, 40138 Bologna, Italy

INTRODUCTION

The concept that stressful stimuli acting on the central nervous system markedly influence digestive motor activities dates back to the early 19th century, when Beaumont (1833) reported that emotions could delay gastric emptying. These anedoctical observations have been confirmed in recent years by quantitative techniques (Thompson et al., 1983). The motor abnormalities responsible for the delay of gastric emptying have also been elucidated by manometric tests (Thompson et al., 1982). No studies, however, had explored the possible pathways through which stressful stimuli may affect the digestive system. Endogenous opioids and catecholamines represent possible mediators, since they are released by physical (Bortz et al., 1981) and psychological stress (Danner et al., 1981; Dimsdale & Moss, 1980), and markedly affect gut motility (Silbiger & Donner, 1968; Elliot, 1905). Also, both opioid (Hollt and Wuster, 1978) and adrenergic receptors (Starke and Docherty, 1980; Gottrup et al., 1979) have been identified in the human gut.
Thus, we carried out a series of studies designed to verify whether catecholamines and opioids mediate the effects of centrally acting stimuli on gut functions.

GASTROINTESTINAL MOTOR ABNORMALITIES AND HUMORAL CHANGES INDUCED BY ACUTE SOMATIC STRESSES

Twelve healthy adult subjects took part in this study (Stanghellini et al., 1983). Fasting and postpandial gastrointestinal motor patterns were measured by a low compliance perfusion system connected to a multi-lumen open-tipped tube. The side openings were located so that a continuous recording of the distal antrum, antroduodenal junction, duodenum and proximal jejunum was obtained. Each subject was studied on one occasion and, ten minutes after the end of meal ingestion, was simultaneously exposed to two different stressful stimuli: labyrinthine stimulation, to produce vertigo, and cold pressure test, to produce pain. Both stimuli were either active (with cold water) or in their control forms (with water at body temperature) and were applied on the basis of a 2x2 factorial

design. During the studies, blood samples were drawn to assay β-endorphin and norepinephrine plasma levels. Both vertigo and cold-pain induced marked increases in circulating levels of both hormones.
Concomitantly, the two stressful stimuli profoundly disrupted the digestive gastrointestinal motor patterns. Antral contractility was significantly and similarly inhibited by the two stressful stimuli. Furthermore, in one third of the cases, vertigo interrupted the intestinal motor pattern and induced the appearance of a migrating phase III-like activity in the proximal small bowel.
Although suggestive, these observations did not necessarily indicate that humoral and motor events were linked to one another.

EFFECT OF ADRENERGIC AND OPIATE BLOCKERS ON STRESS-INDUCED GUT DISORDERS

In order to elucidate whether the increase in blood levels of opioids and catecholamines and the disruption of digestive motor activities were not merely two simultaneous effects of stressful stimuli, but that the hormones did in fact act as mediators through which vertigo and cold pain induced the motor disturbances, we carried out a further study in which we tried to prevent the stress-induced motor abnormalities by infusing opioid and adrenergic blockers (Stanghellini et al., 1984). Twenty-four healthy volunteers entered a 2x4 factorial experimental design. The procedure was similar to that of the study previously described, the only difference being that the stressful stimuli were preceded by intravenous administrations of either saline as a placebo, naloxone as an opioid blocker, phentolamine plus propanolol as adrenergic blockers, or a combination of naloxone, phentolamine and propanolol, in order to achieve a simultaneous inhibition of both the opioid and adrenergic systems.
Stressful stimuli still produced a significant overall increase of both β-endorphin and norepinephrine and neither naloxone nor adrenergic blockers modified their normal response to stress. However, the gastrointestinal motor patterns appeared to be markedly influenced by the drug infusions. Both naxolone and adrenergic blockers, when infused separately, prevented the inhibitory effect of stress on feeding antral contractility. Individual observations suggested that naloxone was particularly effective in blocking the inhibitory effect of either cold pain or labyrinthine stimulation, although the blocking effect seemed to weaken when stress was increased by administering both stimuli together. These observations suggest that stress-induced inhibition of feeding antral motility is at least partially mediated by endogenous opioids, although other inhibitory mechanisms seem to be involved. Adrenergic blockers antagonized the inhibitory action of cold pain on fed antral motor activity, but appeared to be much less effective in preventing the effects of labyrinthine stimulation. These differences could be explained by cold pain eliciting a greater sympathetic arousal than vertigo. Interestingly, the combination of the two blocking agents appeared to be unable to prevent the inhibitory effects of stress. This interaction between naloxone and andrenergic blockers could have been due to factors not measured in the study, such as corticosteroids that are known to enhance the potency of β-endorphin (Holaday et al., 1977).

The small bowel responded to pharmacological blockers in an altogether different manner than the stomach. Naloxone did not prevent the appearance of a migrating burst of phase III-like activity after feeding induced by vertigo. On the other hand, adrenergic blockers promoted the appearance of this abnormal intestinal motor activity. Indeed, such bursts of activity were recorded in all subjects exposed to labyrinthine stimulation receiving adrenergic blockers and even in one subject exposed to cold pain during a particularly marked adrenergic inhibition. Conversely, in the absence of adrenergic blockade, labyrinthine stimulation interrupts intestinal fed pattern in approximately 1/3 of subjects while no such event has ever been observed to be determined by painful stimuli in the absence of pharmachological interactions (Thompson et al., 1982; Stanghellini et al., 1983).

EFFECTS OF INFUSIONS OF ADRENERGIC AND OPIOID SUBSTANCES ON DIGESTIVE MOTILITY

Antagonism by adrenergic and opioid blockers is a necessary, though not sufficient criterion for demonstrating mediation of an event. Such events should also be mimicked by exogenous infusions of mediators stimulating adrenergic and opioid receptors.

Catecholamine infusions have been consistently demonstrated to produce a diffuse inhibition of gut motility (Elliot, 1905). Furthermore, exogenous administration of β-adrenergic agonists has been reported to induce motor effects resembling those caused by stress such as inhibition of gastric emptying (Rees et al., 1980) and bursts of intestinal motor activity (Summers et al., 1982).

We carried out a study to evaluate the effects of intravenous infusions of human synthetic β-endorphin on fed pressure activity in the human upper gut (Camilleri et al., 1986). Gastrointestinal manometry was studied in 45 healthy subjects by a 12-lumen probe with 10 recording sites (1 cm apart) positioned across the pyloric junction and 2 recording sites (20 cm apart) in the proximal small bowel. Six doses of human synthetic β-endorphin 0-2500 ng/kg/min) and four doses of naloxone (0-1140 ng/kg/min) were randomly infused, after ingestion of the test meal, on the basis of a 5x4 factorial design in which each subject was studied on only one occasion.

Intravenous β-endorphin induced a dose-related stimulatory effect on pyloric contractility, the response being essentially linear up to one infusion dose of 250 ng/kg/min. As to antral motility, lower and intermediate doses of β-endorphin produced an effect that paralleled that on the pylorus, while the highest dose markedly inhibited antral contractions. Intravenous β-endorphin doses of 250 and 2500 ng/kg/min interrupted normal intestinal fed motility and elicited an intense burst of rhythmic contractile activity that resembled phase III of the interdigestive motor complex, but appeared to occur simultaneously in the duodenum and proximal jejunum. These bursts of rhythmic activity were followed by a period of relative motor quiescence in the antrum and proximal small bowel before the normal fed pattern was restored.

Naxolone alone had no significant effect on antral and pyloric motility and only at the highest dose did it induce the appearance of a burst of rhythmic activity in one subject. Naxolone induced a dose-related inhibition of the effects on pyloric and antral motility induced by the dosages of β-endorphin that resulted in plasma levels within one order of magnitude of the physiological

range. Furthermore, the competitive opioid blocker significantly reduced the probability that intermediate and higher doses of β-endorphin infusion would result in intestinal phase III-like bursts of activity.
These data demonstrate that the effects of β-endorphin on motility are similar to those of other μ-opiate agonists. Indeed, morphine had been shown to induce gastric relaxation, the effect being blocked by naloxone (Lefebvre et al., 1981) and to trigger the onset of intestinal bursts resembling phase III of the interdigestive migrating motor complex (Sarna & Condon, 1984).

CONCLUSIONS

Substantial evidence has been produced to demonstrate that both opiate and adrenergic pathways participate in mediating the effects of centrally acting stressful stimuli on digestive motility. Different types of stressful stimuli elicit different digestive disturbances by acting, at least partially, through different pathways. Wolf and Wolff (1947) observed opposite effects of fear and anger on the vascularity of the gastric mucosa and the gastric contractility of their fistolous patient, Tom. Similarly, Canon (1911) reported that gastric motility was stimulated by fear, but inhibited by rage and anxiety, in the dog. In our studies, we observed that both vertigo and cold pain inhibited feeding antral contractions, but exerted different effects on the intestinal response to food ingestion.
Vertigo elicited the appearance of a burst of rhythmic contractions resembling phase III of interdigestive migrating motor complex in 30% of subjects, in the absence of pharmacological interactions, and in all subjects in whom adrenergic influences were inhibited by α+β blockade. On the contrary, the painful stimulus never induced such an intense disruption of postpandrial intestinal motility, except in one case in whom a particularly marked adrenergic block had been induced. These different peripheric effects are most likely attributable to different pathways followed by the different external stimuli. Painful stimuli induce a greater adrenergic arousal than vertigo, as demonstrated by extraintestinal autonomic functions. Vertigo, in turn, seems to more directly activate the opioid system via both endocrine and neural pathways. In fact, infusions of synthetic human β-endorphin produce disturbances of intestinal motility similar to those determined by labyrinthine stimulation, but not cold pain.
Circumstantial evidence suggests that neural pathways must concur to modulate the gut response to stress. Circulating β-endorphin levels required to disrupt antral and intestinal motility (Camilleri et al., 1986) are several orders of magnitude higher than those measured after stressful stimuli (Stanghellini et al, 1983; Stanghellini et al., 1984). Furthermore, temporary cooling of the cervical vagus nerves in dogs is known to interrupt the fed pattern and to result in phase III-like bursts of contractions similar to those induced by labyrinthine stimulation (Diamant et al., 1980). Vestibular fibers of the eighth cranial nerve link the labyrinth to the vestibular nuclei which are intimately connected to the vomiting center and chemoreceptor trigger zone which, in turn, are adjacent to the motor nucleus of the vagus trigger zone. It seems plausible to hypothesize that stressful stimuli may induce a temporary inhibition of the activity of vagal pathways.

Some aspects of these studies may be relevant to human disease. Antral hypomotility is responsible for delayed gastric emptying of solids (Malagelada, 1981) and opiate-induced intestinal bursts of rhythmic activity are associated with slowing of intestinal transit (Borody et al.). The association between emotions and digestive abnormalities have been anecdoctically recognised by physicians for centuries. Indeed, gastrointestinal motor abnormality (Malagelada & Stanghellini, 1985) and high levels of anxiety and neuroticism (Mendeloff et al., 1970; Malagelada & Stanghellini, 1985) are common findings in patients with idiopathic digestive functions. Thus, studies on the effects of acute and chronic stressful stimuli on gut functions can certainly shed some light on the important, although still nebulous field of digestive functional diseases.

REFERENCES

Beaumont, W. (1833): Experiments and observations on the gastric juice and the physiology of digestion, ed. F.P. Allen. Plattsburg.

Borody, T.J., Quigley, E.M.M., Phillips, S.F., Wienbeck, M., Tucker, R.L., Haddad, A.C. & Zinsmeister, A.R. (1985): Effects of morphine and atropine on motility and transit in the human ileum. *Gastroenterology*. 89, 562-570.

Bortz, W.M., Angwin, P., Mefford, I.N., Boarder, M.R., Noyce, N. & Barchas, J.D. (1981): Catecholamines, dopamine and endorphin levels during extreme exercise. *N. Engl. J. Med.* 305, 466-7.

Camilleri, M., Malagelada, J.R., Stanghellini, V., Zinsmeister, A.R., Kao, P.C. & Li, C.H. (1986): Dose-related effects of synthetic human β-endorphin and naloxone on fed gastrointestinal motility. *Am. J. Physiol.* 251, 6147-54.

Cannon, W.B. (1911): The mechanical factors of digestion, pp.217-220. New York: Longman's, Green & Company.

Danner, S.A., Endert, E., Koster, R.W. & Dunning, A.J. (1981): Biochemical and circulatory parameters during purely mental stress. *Acta Med. Scand.* 209, 305-8.

Diamant, N.E., Hall, K., Mui, H. & El-Sharkawy, T.Y. (1980): Vagal control of the feeding motor pattern in the lower esophageal sphincter, stomach, and small intestine of dog. In *Gastrointestinal motility*, ed. J. Christensen, pp. 365-70. New York: Raven Press.

Dimsdale, J.E.& Moss, J. (1980): Short-term catecholamine response to psychological stress. *Psychosom. Med.* 42, 493-7.

Elliott, T.R. (1905): The action of adrenalin. *J. Physiol.* 32, 401-67.

Gottrup, F., Ornsholt, J. & Andersen, D. (1979): Effect of two types of β-adrenergic blockade on gastric acid secretion during penta-gastrin stimulation in non-vagotomized gastric fistula dogs. *Scand. J. Gastroenterol.* 14, 857-64.

Holaday, J.W., Law, P.Y., Tseng, L.F., Loh, H.H. & Li, C.H. (1977): β-endorphin: pituitary and adrenal glands modulate its action. *Proc. Natl. Acad. Sci. USA.* 74, 4628-32.

Hollt, V. & Wuster, M. (1978): The opiate receptors. In *Developments in opiate research*, ed. A. Herz, Chap 1,pp. 2-65. New York: Marcel Dekker.

Lefebvre, R.A., Willems, J.L. & Bogaert, M.G. (1981): Gastric relaxation and vomiting by apomorphine, morphine and fentanyl in the conscious dog. *Eur. J. Pharmacol.* 69, 139-145.

Malagelada, J.R. (1981): Gastric, pancreatic, and biliary responses to a meal. In *Physiology of the gastrointestinal tract*. Vol. 2, ed. L.R. Johnson, pp. 893-924. New York: Raven Press.

Malagelada, J.R. & Stanghellini, V. (1985): Manometric evaluation of functional upper gut symptoms. *Gastroenterology*. 88, 1223-31

Mendeloff, A.I., Monk, M., Shegel, C.I. & Lillenfeld, A. (1970): Illness experience and life stresses in patients with irritable colon and with ulcerative colitis. *N. Engl. J. Med.* 232, 14-17.

Rees, M.R., Clark, R.A. & Holdsworth, C.D. (1980): The effect of beta-adrenoceptor agonists and antagonists on gastric emptying in man. *Br. J. Pharmacol.* 10, 551-4.

Sarna, S.K. & Condon, R.E. (1984): Morphine-initiated migrating myoelectric complexes in the fed state in dogs. *Gastroenterology*. 86, 662-669.

Silbiger, M. L. & Donner, M.W. (1968): Morphine in the evaluation of gastrointestinal disease. *Radiology*. 90, 1086-90.

Stanghellini, V., Malagelada,J. R., Zinsmeister, A.R., Go, V.L.W. & Kao, P.C. (1983): Stress-induced gastroduodenal motor disturbances in humans: possible humoral mechanism. *Gastroenterology*. 85, 83-91.

Stanghellini, V., Malagelada, J.R., Zinsmeister, A.R., Go, V.L.W. & Kao, P.C. (1984): Effect of opiate and adrenergic blockers on the gut motor response to centrally-acting stimuli. *Gastroenterology*. 87, 1104-1113.

Starke, K. & Docherty, J.R. (1980): Recent developments in α-adrenoreceptor-research. *J. Cardiovasc. Pharmacol.* 2 (Suppl. 3) S269-86.

Summers, R.W., Flatt, A., Yanda, R., Yamada, T. & Poitras, P. (1982): Evidence that somatostatin mediates isoproterenol-induced activity fronts in fed dogs (abstr). *Gastroenterology*. 82, 1190.

Thompson, D.G., Richelson, E. & Malagelada, J.R. (1982): Perturbation at gastric emptying and duodenal motility via the central nervous system. *Gastroenterology*. 83, 1200-6.

Thompson, D.G., Richelson, E. & Malagelada, J.R. (1983): Perturbation of upper gastrointestinal function by cold stress. *Gut*. 24, 277-83.

Wolf, S. & Wolff, H.G. (1947): Human gastric function. New York: Oxford University Press.

Central and peripheral opioid inhibitory pathways on stress-induced gastric motor alteration in fasted dogs : a pharmacological approach

J.L. Junien, M. Gue, X. Pascaud and L. Bueno

Jouveinal Laboratoires, B.P. 100, 94265 Fresnes, France
INRA, Department of Pharmacology, 31300 Toulouse, France

INTRODUCTION

Various stressful stimuli are known to activate endogenous opioid system (Amir et al, 1980, Cesselin et al, 1982, Le Bars et al, 1987). Opioids are involved in stressful conditions at cerebral and peripheral levels since they are known to modify behavior, to modulate hypothalamus pituitary adrenal axis at the brain level and to be released with cathecholamines from the adrenal glands. In regard to digestive tract motility, Stanghellini et al (1984) have reported that the inhibition of antral postprandial activity following labyrinthine stimulation in unfasted man is prevented by concomitant infusion of naloxone whereas induction of migrating duodenal bursts in the same stressful conditions is not. We have recently developed a model of acoustic stress in the fasted dog, based on the effects of loud noise on gastrointestinal motility (Gue et al, 1987). In such conditions, the gastric migrating motor complex (MMC) is delayed while jejunal MMCs occur at a normal frequency. As expected in a normal stress situation, heart rate and plasma cortisol are significantly increased. Following intravenous administration, diazepam and muscimol abolished the effect of stress while naloxone, phentolamine and propranolol were inactive. Corticotropin Releasing Factor (CRF) (100 mg/kg) given intracerebroventricularly (i.c.v.) also delayed the gastric MMC without affecting jejunal MMC and this effect was not antagonized by diazepam and muscimol. The effects of acoustic stress and CRF are suppressed by bilateral thoracic vagotomy indicating that the gastric motor inhibition by acoustic stress in the dog is due to the CNS release of CRF which affects, in turn, the vagal output to the stomach. This paper summarizes results with opioid agonists and antagonists using the acoustic stress model in dogs. The results show that during stress opioid systems alter gastrointestinal motility and hormonal responses at different levels including a direct action at the gut wall level itself.

METHOD

The method was similar to that used previously (Gue et al, 1987). Adult mongrel dogs weighing 15-18 kg were used for the experiments. Under halothane anesthesia, three strain gauge transducers were sewn on the stomach at 7 and 15 cm from the pylorus and on the proximal jejunum, 60 cm aborally to the ligament of Treitz. In addition, a stainless steel cannula was implanted into the right ventricle. The animals were allowed to recover 10-15 days before starting experiments. The dogs received a standard meal of 600g of canned food (Fido-Quaker, France) each day at 17h. Water was available ad libitum. Gastrointestinal mechanical activity was recorded for 23 h each day on a four channel Wheastone bridge amplifier (Vishay, Paris, France) connected to a potentiometer recorder. Amplitude calibration of each strain gauge was performed before implantation. The experiments were performed at 2 day intervals, 15 h after the last meal. The animals were exposed for 1h to music (80-90dB) via miniature earpieces previously inserted into the ears. The stress session of 1 hr began 40-50 min after the occurence of the last MMC. Blood samples for plasma cortisol measurements were taken from 20 min before to 60 min after acoustic stress. During this period heart rate was monitored using skin electrodes and the noise was considered to be an acoustic stress when a significant increase in heart rate compared to controls was obtained within 10 min after the beginning of the noise. I.c.v. and i.v. infusions of either kappa agonists (dynorpin, ethylketocyclazosine (EKC), U-50488) or mu agonists (DAGO) were given 10 min before the stress session, and oral administrations of EKC, U-50488, PD-117302 or morphine were given 30 min before. Opioid antagonists were injected i.v. simultaneously or before with agonists (naloxone, MR.2266). Motor effects were evaluated by measurement of the duration of gastric or jejunal cycles of contractions evaluated from the beginning of two consecutive phase III activities on the direct strain gauge recording.

RESULTS

In control animals, 1 hr of noise delayed the occurence of the next gastric MMC by about 110 per cent while the jejunum MMC was not changed. Plasma cortisol, which oscillated from 5 to 10 ng/ml in basal conditions was increased by more than 200 per cent after stress stimuli at 15 min. All animals responded with an increase in heart rate of more than 10 beats/min. The maximal rate was observed 8-10 min after the beginning of acoustic stress. This corresponded to a 33 per cent mean increase in heart rate.

I.c.v. administration (table 1)

When given i.c.v. at doses from 10 to 100 ng/kg, dynorphin abolished the lenghtening of gastric MMC cycle due to acoustic stress. At a higher dose (200 ng/kg), dynorphin decreased MMC frequency. The other kappa agonists, EKC and U-50488 both at 20 ng/kg also blocked the effect of stress on MMC. In contrast, DAGO either had no effect over the same dose range (20-100 ng/kg) or delayed MMCs at a higher dose (200 ng/kg). At doses effective against stress-induced hypomotility, both dynorphin (50 and 100 ng/kg) and EKC (10 and 20 ng/kg) reduced significantly the associated plasma cortisol increase (Fig. 1). As reported before, oCRF (100 ng/kg icv) delayed gastric MMC occurence (76 ± 36 min vs 213 ± 46 min). This effect of oCRF was neither inhibited by EKC nor by U50488. On the other hand, the plasma cortisol increase following intravenous injection of ACTH (5 IU/kg) was not modified by previous icv administration of dynorphin (100 ng/kg) or EKC (20 ng/kg). None of the drugs tested altered the stress-induced increase in heart rate.

Table 1. Comparative influence of i.c.v. dynorphin, EKC, U-50488 and DAGO on acoustic stress-induced lengthening of duration of gastric MMC cycle in fasted dogs

	Dose, ng/kg	Duration of gastric MMC Cycle, min	
		Control	Acoustic stress
Vehicle		76 ± 36	189 ± 46a
Dynorphin (1-13)	10	89 ± 10	146 ± 31a
	20	111 ± 24b	88 ± 27b
	50	84 ± 21	92 ± 29b
	100	106 ± 13	101 ± 16b
	200	207 ± 37a	
EKC	10	86 ± 17	91 ± 13b
	20	110 ± 31	108 ± 12b
	50	244 ± 49b	
U-50488	20	104 ± 16	105 ± 16b
DAGO	20	108 ± 17	199 ± 44a
	100	111 ± 18	176 ± 29a
	200	269 ± 34b	

Values are means ± SE for 6 dogs.
a = significantly different from corresponding control values
b = significantly different from values observed before acoustic stress.

Oral administration

Both EKC and U-50488, administered orally at a dose of 0.1 mg/kg, significantly lengthened the duration of gastric MMC; Each drug, however, exerted an opposite effect when given at a lower dose (0.01 mg/kg) (table 2).
U-50488 (0.01/0.05 mg/kg) and PD-117302 (0.01/0.05 mg/kg) inhibited the effect of stress; EKC (0.01/0.1 mg/kg) was partially active in the test table 2). Morphine did not antagonize acoustic stress at 1 mg/kg, a dose which did not modify gastrointestinal motility in control experiments; at a higher dose (3 mg/kg), morphine inhibited spontaneous motility of the stomach and initiated apparition of ectopic MMCs at jejunum level.

Table 2. Influence of orally administered kappa agonists on acoustic stress-induced lengthening of gastric MMC cycle in fasted dogs.

	Duration of gastric MMC cycle (min)		
	Basal	Acoustic Stress	
mg/kg		Before	After
Control	77 ± 25	87 ± 13	194 ± 30b
EKC			
0.01	92 ± 7	96 ± 11	131 ± 21a,b
0.1	139 ± 27a	-	-
U-50488			
0.01	101 ± 20	91 ± 19	102 ± 27a
0.05	92 ± 18	108 ± 21	117 ± 29*
0.1	186 ± 39a	-	-
PD 117302			
0.01	105 ± 33	98 ± 16	91 ± 18a
0.05	86 ± 28	109 ± 12	131 ± 33a
0.1	192 ± 11a	-	-

a = significantly different from corresponding control values
b = significantly different from values observed before acoustic stress
* n = 2

The effect of the opioid agonists drugs on plasma cortisol hypersecretion during stress session was investigated. (Fig. 1). U-50488 (0.1 mg/kg p.o.) did not affect basal cortisolemia but reduced by 71 per cent the acoustic stress-induced increase in plasma cortisol (9.0 ± 3.5 vs 34.9 ± 7.4 ng/ml). This effect was dose-related from 0.01 mg/kg to 0.1 mg/kg. Similarly, PD 117302 (0.05 and 0.1 mg/kg p.o.), also significantly reduced the cortisol response. In contrast, bremazocine (0.1 mg/kg) and morphine (1.0 mg/kg), did not modify basal plasma cortisol and its maximal increase induced by stress. When animals were submitted to acoustic stress 10 to 30 days after bilateral thoracic vagotomy, no inhibition of gastric MMC by acoustic stress was recorded (Gue et al, 1987), but cortisolemia was still increased at a similar extent to non-vagotomized dogs. In these animals, previous oral administration of U-50488 (0.1 mg/kg) was unable to prevent the rise of plasma cortisol as observed in non vagotomized stressed dogs.

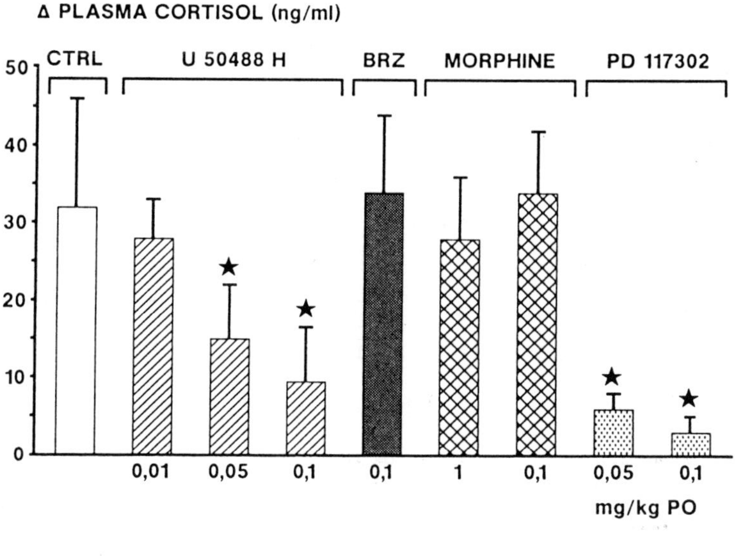

Fig. 1 - Effect of opioid agonists on stress-induced hypercortisolemia in dogs.

When injected 10 min prior to U-50488 (0.1 mg/kg p.o) both naloxone (0.1 mg/kg i.v.) and MR 2266 (0.1 mg/kg i.v.) abolished the effects of U-50488 on the plasma cortisol increase induced by stress (table 3). The effect of PD 117302 (0.1mg/kg) also was significantly decreased by naloxone or MR 2266 pretreatment. Naloxone alone increased basal cortisol to 28.2 ± 7.5 ng/ml although acoustic stress was still able to further increase values close to that normally recorded in non-treated dogs (64.9 ± 9.5 ng/kg). MR 2266 had no effect (table 3).

As after i.c.v. administration, U-50488 or PD 117302 (0.1 mg/kg) given orally were devoid of any effect on the rise of plasma cortisol due to oCRF(100 ng/kg) injected icv.

Table 3. Inhibitory effect of orally administered U-50488 on the cortisol increase induced by acoustic stress (AS) in dogs : Effects of the opioid antagonists naloxone and MR-2266.

	VEHICLE		
	Basal	AS max	max
Control (n = 12)	6.4±2.5	40.3±13.0	34.9±7.4
Naloxone (0.1 mg/kg, iv)	28.2±7.5b	64.9±9.5b	36.7±11.2
MR-2266 (0.1 mg/kg, iv)	9.7±4.3	54.3±7.6	44.6±10.2
	U-50488 (0.1 mg/kg, orally)		
	Basal	AS max	max
Control (n = 12)	8.2±3.8	17.2±7.8a	9.0±3.5a
Naloxone (0.1 mg/kg, iv)	21.9±7.5b	43.6±5.0b	21.7±2.9b
MR-2266 (0.1 mg/kg, iv)	7.6±4.1	44.8±7.5b	37.2±0.3b

Values are the mean ± SD.
Results are expressed in ng/ml.
a = Significantly different ($P \leq 0.05$) from corresponding vehicle value by t test.
b = Significantly different ($P \leq 0.05$) from corresponding control value by t test.

I.v. administration

Morphine and U-50488 did not alter the effect of stress at doses between 0.01 and 1mg/kg. At higher doses, morphine spontaneously inhibited gastric motility and induced jejunal phase 3. U-50488 delayed both gastric and jejunal MMC. In regard to plasma cortisol, U-50488 (0.01/0.05 mg/kg) neither affected basal nor stress-induced increases. At 0.1 mg/kg, U-50488 increased basal cortisol to 47.8±6.9 ng/ml, a value similar to that measured after acoustic stress in control animals.

DISCUSSION

Previous studies have demonstrated that diazepam and muscimol attenuated the acoustic stress-induced alteration of gastric motility in dogs (Gue et al, 1987). In contrast to the findings in man using a different stress stimulus (Stanghellini et al, 1988), the present experiments demonstrate that naloxone did not prevent the gastric effect of stress. Opioid agonists, however, administered either centrally or orally were able to protect gastric motility against acoustic stimuli. It is now well established that the view of a "general adaptation syndrome" to stress postulated by Selye (1936) is rather simple and that various specific neuro-hormonal mediators can be activated both in the brain and subsequently at the periphery depending on the type of stress stimulus (Gaillard and Al-Damluji, 1987).

After i.c.v. administration, only the kappa agonists dynorphin, EKC and U-50488 were able to inhibit motility and cortisol response to stress. oCRF mimicks the effects of acoustic stress on gastric motility and cortisol and kappa agonists did not suppress these effects. The results show that kappa opioids probably act at a locus prior to CRF release or on CRF release itself. Kappa agonists reduce central cholinergic activity (Cheney et al, 1974), a system known to be activated during stress events which stimulates adrenergic networks responsible for most of the behavioral and neuroendocrine responses to stress (Janowsky et al, 1984). On the other hand, it has been demonstrated that dynorphin, an endogenous ligand for kappa receptors reduces in vitro the release of CRF from rat hypothalamus (Yajima et al, 1986). Modulation of the hypothalamo pituitary adrenal axis (HPA) activity has been reported in many studies but results differ among many opioids and species. In man, acute injection of morphine stimulates the release of ACTH, while chronic administration inhibits the response (Buckingham 1982, Gibson et al, 1979). The opiate antagonist naloxone stimulates the HPA axis in man and dog (Volavka et al, 1979), the present study suggesting that endogenous opiates have an inhibitory effect on HPA activity. In rodents, endogenous opioids such as β-endorphin and enkephalin stimulate the HPA axis (Gibson et al, 1979, De Souza et al, 1982). However, dual effects of enkephalin on the CRF-ACTH system have been described recently (Hashimoto et al, 1987). Together, these results comfirm that mu, delta, kapppa and endogenous opoids modulate the HPA axis and play an important role at this level in the physiological control of stress.

Oral administration of kappa agonists also blocked the effect of stress on gastric motility and cortisol. The inhibition was clearly established at low doses which is poorly compatible with a systemic diffusion of the drugs although no pharmacokinetic data have been available. The absence of inhibitory activity of these drugs on motility and hormonal stress response after iv injection or higher oral doses and the lack of effect on stress-induced cortisol increase in vagotomized dogs suggest a direct effect of kappa opioids on receptors located in the intestinal wall. The hypothesis of an inhibitory reflex on the adrenal gland secretion through the medulla may be excluded since cortisol release induced by icv administration of oCRF was not blocked by U-50488 administered orally. These observations strongly suggest that activation of peripheral kappa receptors may activate inhibitory afferent pathways affecting the release of CRF. In agreement with the hypothesis of a local primary site of action there is now substantial evidence that opiate receptors of different classes are present in the gastric and intestinal wall, in the myenteric plexus and in gastric smooth muscle (Nishimura et al, 1986). Moreover, the dog is a species with opiate enkephalin and dynorphin peptide immunoreactive nerve cells in the submucosal plexus, muscularis mucosae, and villi of the stomach, pylorus and proximal intestine (Daniel et al 1987). Accordingly, it has been shown that oral administration of kappa agonists increases gastric emptying of a solid meal in dogs while similar doses given i.v. are ineffective (Gue et al, 1987). In addition, injection of delta or kappa agonists to the pylorus produces a dose-dependent motor inhibition (Allescher et al, 1988). More recently, kappa receptors located in the gastric wall have been shown to play an important role in gastric relaxation induced by feeding in dogs (Gue et al, 1989).

REFERENCES

Amir, S., Brown, Z.W. and Amit, Z. (1980). The role of endorpins in stress : evidence and speculation, Neurosci. Biobehav. Rev. 4, 77-80.

Allescher, H.D., Ahmad, E., Daniel, E.E., Dent, J., Kostolanska F. and Fox, J.E.T (1988): Inhibitory opioid receptors in canine pylorus. Amer. J. Physio, 255, G.352-360..

Buckingham, J.C. (1982): Secretion of corticotropin and its hypothalamic releasing factor in response to morphine and opoid peptides. Neuroendocrinology, 35, 111.

Cesselin, F., Oliveras J.L., Bourgoin, S., Sierralta, F., Michel, R., Besson, J.M. and Hamon M. (1982): Increased levels of Met-enkephalin-like materiel in the CSF of anesthethized cats after touth pulp stimulation. Brain Res. 237., 325-

Cheney, D.L., Trabucchi M., Racagni, G., Wang, C. and Costa, E. (1974): Effect of acute and chronic morphine on regional rat brain acetylcholine turnover rate. Life. Sci. 15., 1977-90.

Daniel, E.E., Fox J.E.T., Allescher, H.D., Ahmad, S. and Kostolanska, F. (1987): Peripheral actions of opiates in canine gastrointestinal tract : actions on nerves and muscles. Gastroenterol. Clin., Biol., 11, 35.

Gaillard, R.C. and Al-Damluji, S. (1987): Stress and the pituitary-adrenal axis. Balliere's Clinical Endocrinology and Metabolism., 1, 2319-354.

Gibson, A., Guinsburg, M., Hall, M. and Hart, S.L. (1979): The effects of opiate receptor agonists on the stress-induced secretion of corticosterone in mice. Br. J. Pharmacol., 65, 139.

Gue, M., Fioramonti, J., Frexinos, J., Alvinerie, M. and Bueno, L.(1987): Influence of acoustic stress by noise on gastrointestinal motility in dogs. Dig. Dis. Sci., 32, 12, 1411-1417.

Gue, M., Fioramonti, J., Junien, J.L. and Bueno, L. (1988): Orally administered kappa but not mu opiate agonists enhance gastric emptying of a solid canned food meal in dogs. J. Pharm. Pharmacol. 40, 873-875.

Gue, M., Junien, J.L. and Bueno, L. (1989). Central and peripheral opiod influences on gastric relaxation induced by feeding in dogs. Accepted for publication in J. Pharm. Exp. Ther.

Hashimoto, K., Suemaru, S., 1Ono, N., Hattori, T., Inoue. H, Takoa.T, Sugawara, M., Kagemaya, J. and Ota, Z (1987): Dual effects of (D-Ala3,Met5) enkephalinamide on CRF and ACTH secretion. Peptides, 8, 113.

Janowski, D.S., Rich, S.C. and Ziegler, M. (1984): Central Tacetylcholine in stress and affective disorders. Clin. Neuropharmacol. 7, suppl. 1, 958-59.

Le Bars, D.S., Bourgoin, S., Clot, A.M., Hamon, M. and Cesselin, F. (1987). Noxious mechanical stimuli increase the release of Met-enkephalin like material heterosegmentally in the rat spinal cord. Brain Res., 402, 188.

Nishimura, E., Buchan A.M.J. and McIntosh C.H.S. (1986): Autoradiographic localization of mu and delta type opioid receptors in the gastrointestinal tract of the rat and the guinea pig. Gastroenterology, 91, 1084.

Stanghellini, V., Malagelada, J.R., Zinsmeister, A.R., Go, V.L.M., Kao, P.C. (1984): Stress-induced effect of opiate and adrenergic blockers on the gut motor response to centrally acting stimuli. Gastroenterology, 87, 1104-1113.

Volavka, J., Chod, D., Mallya, A., Baumn, J., Pevnick, J., Reker, D., James, B. and Dornbusch, R. (1979): Naloxone increases ACTH and cortisol levels in man. N. Engl. J. Med., 300, 1056.

Yajima, F., Sud, T., Tomori, N., Takashi, S., Nakagami, Y., Ushiyama, T, Demura, H. and Shizume, K. (1986): Effects of opioid peptides on immunoreactive CRF release from the rat hypothalamus in vitro. Life Sci., 39, 181-186.

The effect of dopamine antagonists on stress-induced alterations of intestinal motor activity

D. Kumar, R.M. Valori, D.L. Wingate

Gastrointestinal Science Research Unit, London Hospital Medical College, London E1 2AJ, England

It is generally assumed assumed that the stomach (Wolf and Wolf, 1947) and the colon (Almy, 1951) are the regions of the digestive tract that are most susceptible to the effects of psychological stress; this assumption is supported by numerous anecdotal reports in the literature, but not, until recently, by controlled studies. It is at first sight surprising that the first demonstration (McRae et al, 1981) of the effect of controlled stress on gastrointestinal motility was on the small intestine; not an organ generally thought to be susceptible to stress.

The problems to be solved in the study of the effects of stress on digestive motor activity were, first, the detection of reproducible patterns of motor activity in the region under study, and second, the development of techniques for recording such activity that are not so inherently stressful that the application of an external stressor is a relatively inadequate stimulus. The discovery of stereotypic fasting motor activity in the small intestine in the form of the migrating motor complex (MMC), and the development of techniques of prolonged monitoring of human small bowel motor activity (Thompson et al, 1981) provided the required technology for the study of motor activity, while advances in experimental psychology, stimulated by a worldwide interest in the effects of stress, offered a number of protocols that included suitable psychological stressors.

The original study (McRae et al, 1982) indicated that a prolonged psychological stress inhibited MMC incidence, but the protocol was limited by the available technology, which did not allow the subjects to be freely mobile during the study. Further developments (Browning et al, 1981, 1982) in monitoring, utilising twin pressure sensitive radiotelemetric capsules (RTCs) conferred mobility on subjects under study, allowing a wider choice of stressors, and using 3 such stressors, Valori and Wingate (1983) confirmed and extended the results of the previous study.

At that point, it seemed reasonable to see whether 'prokinetic' drugs - agents that appear to stimulate gut motility and transit - might reverse the stress-induced inhibition of MMCs. As perhaps the most widely-used of such agents, metoclopramide was an obvious choice. Metoclopramide, however, acts on the CNS as well as at the level of the gut, and therefore it was decided to compare its action on stress-induced alterations of motility with domperidone, a newer gut-selective dopamine antagonist with diminished activity in the CNS.

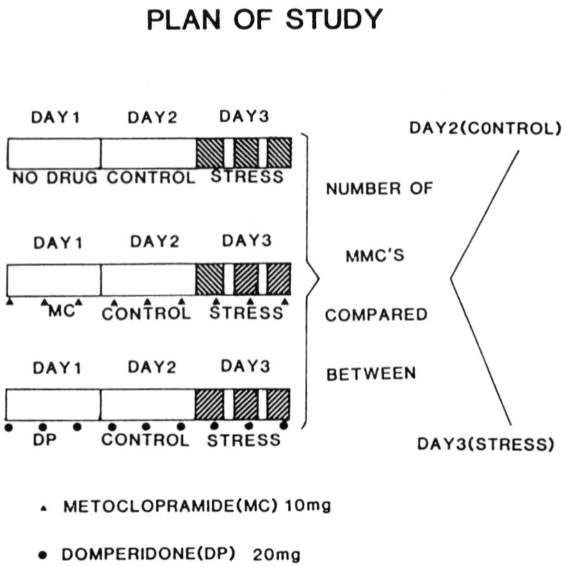

Figure 1: Plan of study.

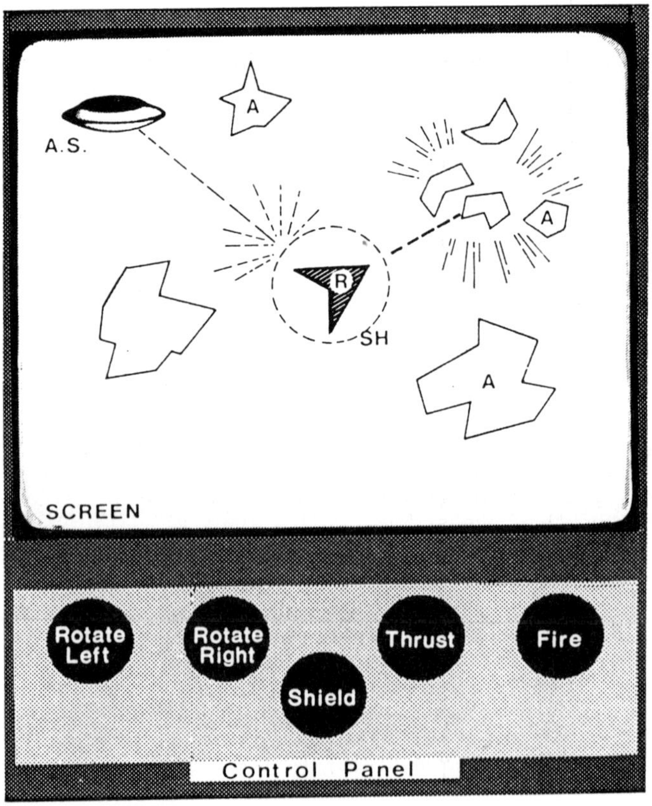

Figure 2: Video display and control panel of "Asteroids de Luxe", showing the rocket ship (R), controlled by the player, attacking an asteroid (A) while being attacked by an alien spaceship (AS), both controlled by the machine.

The design of the study is illustrated in Fig 1. On Day 1, subjects in each of two groups were started on medication with either metoclopramide 10 mgm tds or domperidone 20 mgm tds, and this medication was continued for three days. At the beginning of the second day, subjects swallowed the twin RTCs, and continuous recording of upper small bowel motility was started when the RTCs were in place at the level of the duodenojejunal flexure, and continued until the end of the study. On the first day, no stressors were applied, and subjects were free to engage in activities of their choice; on this day, however, and the subsequent day, the subjects until the evening. On the following morning (Day 3), the subjects were exposed to psychological stressors for three 2-hour periods, each stressor being followed by a 1-hour rest period. The study was then terminated. Fig 1 illustrates the plan of the study, and as shown in the figure, the incidence of MMCs on the rest day (Day 2) was compared with the incidence of MMCs on the stress day (Day 3).

The data from the drug studies were compared with data obtained from a control group who followed the same protocol but received no medication. The level of stress in each subject was assessed objectively from serial measurements of pulse and blood pressure, and subjectively by asking subjects to mark their level of discomfort on visual analogue scales; these scales utilised bipolar values such 'drowsy/active' and 'peaceful/tense'.

Three different stressors were used in this study. The first required the subject to play a video arcade game ("Asteroids de Luxe") for two hours. The game, normally coin-operated but free for this study, requires the player to sit at a console facing a video screen (Fig 2), and to use controls to manoeuvre a space craft out of the range of predatory asteroids and other enemies; the game adjusts to the expertise of the operator, becoming more difficult as the player becomes more skilled. The second stressor was delayed audio feedback (DAF), requiring the subject to read aloud from a text into a microphone while hearing his own voice coming through stereo headphones with a 0.25 second delay; this is more difficult that the description suggests. The third stressor was driving a car through heavily congested streets. These stressors resemble the stresses of working life in an urban society; sitting at VDUs, wrestling with often recalcitrant telephone systems and commuting in heavy traffic.

As shown in Fig 3, domperidone did not prevent the inhibition of MMC incidence induced by psychological stress; the results in the domperidone-treated group were identical with the changes seen in the control (no drug) group (not illustrated). Surprisingly, however, metoclopramide appeared to block completely the effect of stress (Fig 4); in the metoclopramide-treated group, there was no reduction in MMC incidence on the stress day. Neither drug affected MMC incidence on the rest day of the study; MMC incidence on the rest day was identical with that found in the drug-free control group. Again outside the period of stress, neither drug altered the postprandial interruption induced by the evening meal, suggesting that gastric emptying was unaltered (Fig 5).

The effect of stressors on bowel motility can only be detected by monitoring motility; there is no subjective correlate, and the stress-induced inhibition of MMCs is not associated with gastrointestinal symptoms. However, although metoclopramide blocked the effect of stress on bowel motility, it did not block the effect of stress on the cardiovascular system, or on the subject's perception of stress (Fig 6).

DOMPERIDONE AND STRESS

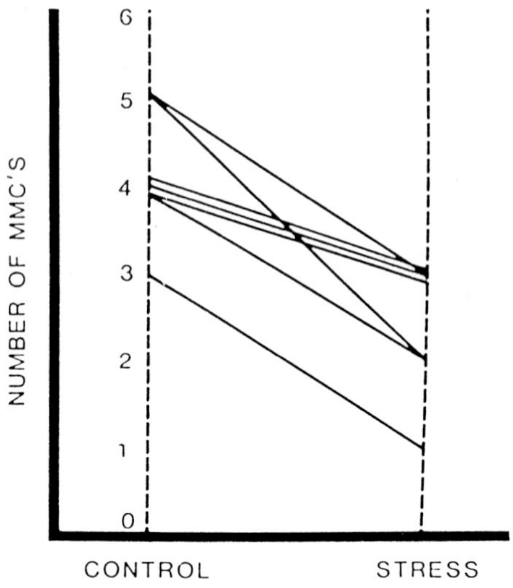

Figure 3: Incidence of MMCs in domperidone-treated subjects on the rest day (left), and the stress day (right). Lines connect data from each subject

METOCLOPRAMIDE AND STRESS

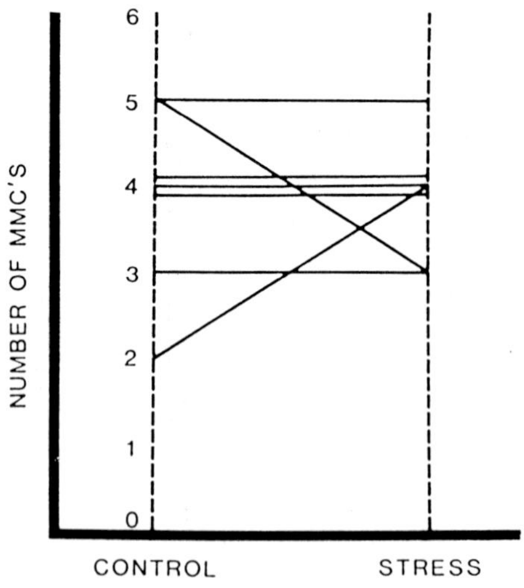

Figure 4: Incidence of MMCs in metoclopramide-treated subjects.

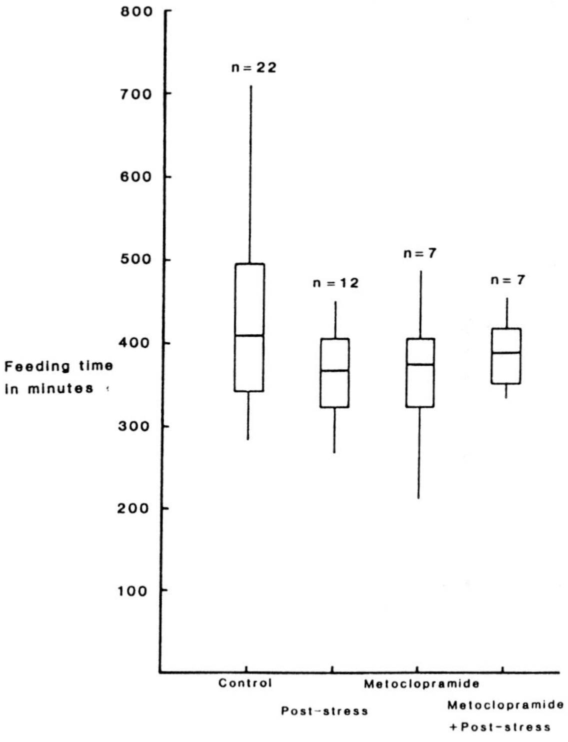

Figure 5: "Box and whisker" plot of the duration of postprandial (feeding) motor activity following evening meals during the study. Each box is divided by the median value, and the box and vertical line above and below the median indicate the interquartile ranges. The two columns on the left are for the evenings before and after exposure to stress in drug-free controls; the two columns on the right show similar data for the metoclopramide-treated group.

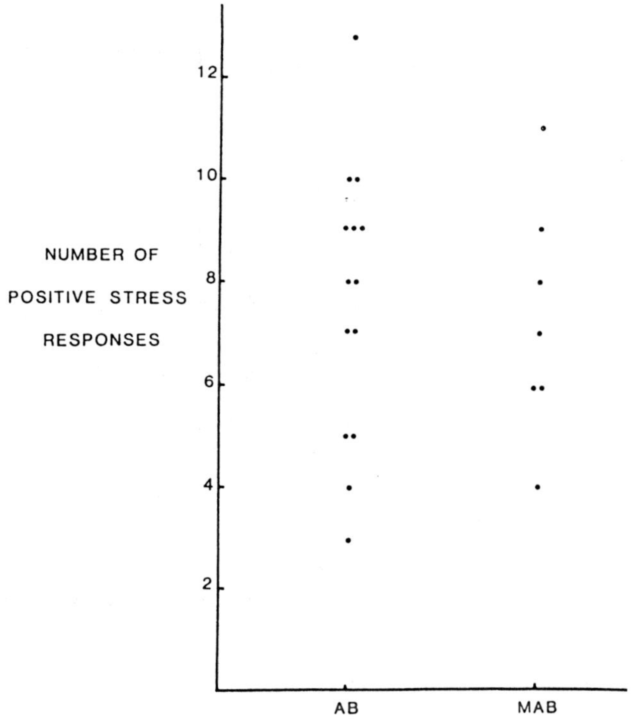

Figure 6: Comparison of positive cardiovascular and subjective stress responses in untreated subjects (AB - left) and metoclopramide-treated subjects (MAB right). Stress scores are aggregated for each subject, the maximum possible being 15. It will be seen that the response in the metoclopramide-treated subjects lies within the range of the untreated subjects.

These data shed some light upon the possible pathways involved in the modification of motility by stressors. Taking the effects of both drugs into account, there would appear to be two alternative explanations. Metoclopramide has both central and peripheral dopamine antagonist actions, whereas the action of domperidone as a dopamine antagonist is predominantly peripheral. Thus one possible explanation is that the effects of stress on the gut are mediated through central, but not peripheral, dopaminergic pathways.

Metoclopramide is, however, not only a dopamine antagonist; it is also a cholinergic agonist, whereas domperidone does not share this property. This provides an alternative explanation or our findings, which is that stress inhibits cholinergic activity in the gut which can be reversed by metoclopramide but not by domperidone. If such inhibition is produced by adrenergic stimulation, it is unlikely to be the mechanism for the drug action that we have demonstrated, since metoclopramide failed to modify the cardiovascular or perceptual response to stress.

Clearly, there is no way of distinguishing between the two possible explanations without more evidence on the effects of these and other related pharmacological agents, nor do these data carry any useful clinical implications. But there implications from this study which may be of importance in the design and the interpretation of studies that are yet to be done. The first and most important point is that there may be dissociation between different types of physiological response to stress -in our case, cardiovascular and enteric - and that different aspects of the stress response may be selectively blocked or enhanced by appropriate chemical modulation. The second, of wider significance in the therapy of stress-induced disorders, is that blockade of stress effects may be possible at the level of the CNS rather than at the level of the gut effectors (smooth muscle, secretory cells) or their control neurones in the enteric nervous system.

Research in the pharmacology of gut function has always been directed towards the identification of gut-selective compounds that act at the enteric level and do not affect the CNS. Apart from the benefit of avoiding unwanted CNS effects, such an approach makes sense in the treatment of enteric disorders - but only when the lesion or dysfunction is at the enteric level, Where dysfunction is CNS-induced, the possibility has to be considered that intervention at the level of the CNS may be a more promising therapeutic avenue. Indeed, one may extend this approach even further, to the actual perception of stress. Stressors are not absolute; while some stressors are so severe that they will be perceived as such by everyone who is exposed to them, most stressors are only perceived as stressful because of factors such as the expectation and experience of the subject; for example, apprehension of a visit to the dentist is greater in individuals who have had a previous adverse experience of dentistry. This phenomenon was well illustrated by a patient with irritable bowel syndrome who completed the protocol used in this study. Somewhat to our surprise - because she complained of being upset by stress - no alteration of function was induced by our three stressors. On being questioned, she said that she didn't feel stressed during the study, "but then," she remarked, "you have to remember that the stress of this study was trivial compared with my normal job as teacher in a primary school with thirty noisy and active six-year olds to look after all day." Just as beauty is in the eye of the beholder, so is psychological stress in the mind of the subject, and it is there that stress intervention may be most effective.

REFERENCES

Almy TP. (1951): Experimental studies on the irritable colon. Am J Med, 10:60-67

Browning C, Valori RM, Wingate DL & McLachlan D. (1981): A new pressure-sensitive ingestible radio-telemetric capsule. Lancet, ii:504-505

Browning C, Valori RM & Wingate DL. (1982): Receiving, decoding and noise-limiting systems for a new pressure-sensitive ingestible radio-telemetric capsule. J Biomed Eng, 5:262-266

McRae S, Younger K, Thompson DG & Wingate DL. (1982): Sustained experimental stress alters human jejunal motor activity. Gut, 23:404-409

Thompson DG, Wingate DL, Archer L, Benson MJ, Green WJ & Hardy RJ, (1981): Normal patterns of human upper small bowel motor activity recorded by prolonged radiotelemetry. Gut, 21:500-506

Valori RM & Wingate DL (1983). Stress, distress, and the migrating motor complex. Gastroenterology, 84:1340

Wolf S & Wolff HG (1947). Experimental study of changes in gastric function in response to varying life experiences. Rev Gastroenterol, 14:419-426

Environmental stress, psychiatric disorder and functional abdominal pain

Francis Creed*, Tom Craig**

**University Department of Psychiatry, Rawnsley Building, Manchester Royal Infirmary, Oxford Road, Manchester M13 9WL, UK*

***Department of Policy and Social Science, Bedford College, University of London, UK*

INTRODUCTION

In order to make an accurate assessment of the relationship between environmental stress, psychiatric disorder and functional abdominal pain the researcher has three requirements; a) a standardised clinical interview to assess psychiatric disorder, b) a standardised interview to assess environmental stress, and c) a group of patients with clear onset of pain so that the dates of onset of pain and exposure to stress can be compared. In the absence of these factors the conclusions reached may not be scientifically valid (Creed and Guthrie 1987).

Standardised Clinical Interviews for Psychiatric Illness.

There have now been several studies which have used standardised clinical interviews on patients with functional abdominal pain and these have established that psychiatric disorder is 2-3 times more common among such patients than among patients with organic gastro-intestinal disease (Table 1). These instruments classify individual patients as cases of psychiatric disorder if they have sufficient symptoms of adequate severity. For example, the Present State Examination, which we have used, classifies a patient as psychiatrically ill if a sympton score of 11 is reached during an interview covering 40 psychiatric symptoms (Wing et al 1974). A score of 1 would be recorded if the symptom is present in mild form, 2 if marked. So difficulty in getting off to sleep, for example, must have been present for at least ten nights over the last month and is scored mild (1) if it is one hour or more, or marked (2) if it is two hours or more. Different instruments have different criteria but have produced similar results.

Since these studies used standardised clinical interviews, and not self-administered questionnaires, the results are reliable but the interpretation is difficult. Among clinic patients psychiatric disorder might be a *consequence* of the abdominal pain, rather than its cause, unless it can be demonstrated that the psychiatric disorder preceded the onset of abdominal pain. Only two studies have distinguished patients with such disorder and the proportion remains significantly greater than those with organic disease (Table 1).

Table 1 *Prevalence of psychiatric disorder (as per cent), assessed using standardised interviews, among patients attending gastro - enterology clinics (a) with functional abdominal pain and (b) with organic gastro-intestinal disease.*

	No.		Functional abdominal pain	Organic disease
McDonald and Bouchier(1980)	32	CIS	53	20
Colgan et al (1988)	37	CIS	57	6
Craig and Brown (1984)	79	PSE	42(34)	18(16)
Ford et al (1987)	48	PSE	42(31)	6(0)

CIS = Clinical Interview Schedule.
PSE = Present State Examination.
Figures in parentheses refer to psychiatric disorder that was present ***before*** *the onset of the abdominal pain.*

Standardised interview to assess life events

There have been very few studies that have used a similarly systematic method to assess whether life events occur before the onset of abdominal pain. Some researchers have tried to use self-administered questionnaires, but one such questionaire includes the item: "Over the last six months, have you experienced concern over the health or behaviour of a family member (major illness, accidents, etc.)?"
This leaves the patient to decide who is a family member, which illnesses should be considered major and the result is only dated to the nearest six months. So if the patient's pain developed three months ago and a relative became ill two months ago this questionnaire would give an inaccurate impression that the life event contributed to the cause of the abdominal pain.

To ensure a truly objective and reliable measure of environmental stress we use the life events and difficulty schedule (LEDS; Brown & Harris 1978). This defines at the outset exactly which relatives and other individuals are to be considered and the exact nature of life events. For example "being of work" through illness is included only if the patient himself is off for at least four weeks, the breadwinner in the family is off for a minimum of eight weeks, or there is objective evidence of marked financial hardship. The accurate dating of an event means that any events occurring *after* the onset of abdominal pain are excluded from the analyses.

The objective threat of the event is rated by a group of experienced raters to whom the circumstances of the event are presented. This procedure is necessary because otherwise a distressed, tearful patient describing a brief tiff with her husband might be given a higher rating of threat than the stoical patient whose mother has recently died - we have been concerned only with objective, not subjective assessment of threat. Each event is rated on two four point scales; the immediate (short-term) threat, and on the long term threat - that which remains after one week. A severe event is one which is rated 1 or 2 on long term threat - examples are bereavement, marital separation and the break-up of a close heterosexual relationship (these are referred to as severe events).

SUBJECTS AND METHOD

In order to assess whether environmental stress or psychiatric disorder preceded or followed the onset of pain it was necessary to select patients with a recent onset of abdominal pain which could be accurately dated. The first study (Creed 1981) chose patients aged 17-30 years undergoing appendicectomy, over one third of whom had an appendix that was classified as not acutely inflamed. The second study (Craig & Brown 1984) included patients aged 18-60 years attending a gastroenterology clinic who had a clear onset or recurrence of abdominal pain within one year of the clinic attendance. In each case patients with organic gastro-intestinal illness were used as a control group.

The assesssment of psychiatric disorder and life events was made before it was known whether the patient had an organic diagnosis (such as appendicitis or peptic ulcer) or a "functional" one (appendix not acutely inflamed or irritable bowel syndrome), so that both patient and experimenter were "blind" to the eventual diagnosis at the time that environmental stress was measured.

In each study psychiatric disorder was assessed for the month prior to onset of abdominal pain using the PSE (Wing et al 1974), and environmental stress was measured using the Life Events and Difficulties Schedule (LEDS) (Brown and Harris 1978).

The results of a third study (Farmer & Creed 1988) are included for comparison because the same measures were used on patients aged 17-35 years who were admitted to hospital following an overdose, since it is well-known that these patients have undergone recent crises and become distressed. Each of the abdominal pain groups had a community comparison group.

<u>Life event results</u> are expressed as the proportion of subjects who had experienced a severely threatening event during the preceding thirty eight weeks. This time period is important in the aetiology of depression; it is long enough to include those severe events, such as bereavement, which may affect the individual for some months afterwards, but not so long that distorted data might result from poor recall.

Statistical significance of differences between groups has been assessed using the chi-square test.

RESULTS

The first two studies are not strictly comparable because the patients attending the gastroenterology clinic were older than those undergoing appendicectomy and a greater proportion were married. In both studies there was a predominance of females in the functional abdominal pain groups so adjustment for sex was necessary. There were no significant differences between the demographic characteristics of the subjects in the deliberate self harm group and those of the community comparison group for the appendicectomy study.

The commonest diagnoses in the gastroenterolgoy clinic sample were peptic ulcer (41%) for the organic group; irritable bowel syndrome (35%), dyspepsia (18%) abdominal pain (44%) for the functional group. For convenience hereafter "organic" refers to organic gastroenterology clinic patients and acute appendicitis patients, whereas "functional" refers to the remaining clinic patients and those with a not acutely inflamed appendix.

All the groups considered were similar in the proportion who had experienced any kind of life event over the previous 38 weeks. This result is important because it demonstrates that all groups were interviewed with similar intensity.

However, when we considered only those events rated as severely threatening in the long term (severe events) a distinct pattern emerged: the functional abdominal pain groups had experienced these severe events in a proportion similar to the self-poisoning group and significantly greater than either the organic ($p<0.01$) or healthy comparison ($p<0.0001$) groups (Fig. 1). Analysis by sex did not affect these findings. The high rate of severe events is very similar to that found in depressed patients Brown & Harris (1978).

As a further check in reliability I was able to interview a number of siblings of the patients undergoing appendiciectomy; for those with a not acutely inflamed appendix 11 of 15 patients had experienced a severe event compared to four out of 15 of the healthy siblings ($P<0.05$).

The most frequent type of severe event in the case of the functional abdominal pain group involved a major disruption of close relationships; a marital separation, a family member leaving home or break-up of a serious girl-boyfriend relationship (Fig 2). Since these events almost always included arguments we have called them "row" events, which occurred in the functional abdominal pain groups approximately 5 times as often as the organic illness and healthy comparison groups, and nearly as often as those in the overdose group.

I indicated earlier that approximately one third of the functional abdominal pain group had symptoms of depression sufficiently severe

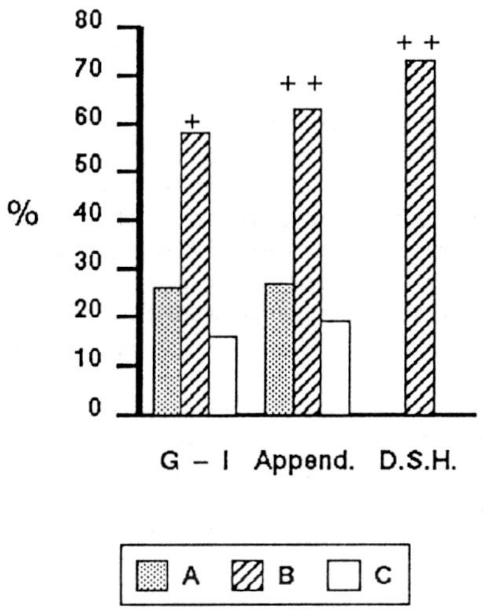

Fig 1 Proportion of subjects (as percentage) who had experienced a severe life event during 38 weeks before onset of abdominal pain or before interview for community comparison group.
G-I = patients attending a gastro-enterology clinic, Append= patients undergoing appendicectomy, DSH = patients admitted following deliberate self-harm.

A=organic g-i dis/append'tis
B=functional abdominal pain
C=community comparison gp.

+= p< 0.01, ++= p<0.0001 compred to community group.

to be classified as a "case" of psychiatric illness that had developed prior to the onset of the abdominal pain. It is therefore appropriate to consider whether the excess of severe life events found in the function pain group is attributable to those with depression - such events are known to be associated with the onset of depression.

To our surprise this was not the case. Table 2 indicates that even those patients with functional abdominal pain who did *not* have psychiatric disorder had a clear excess of severe life events compared to the organic and community comparison groups. They were similar to those patients who take an overdose but do not have severe depression.

Prognosis

In their classic description of the irritable bowel syndrome Chaudhury and Truelove (1962) reported prognosis over two years; the proportion who became symptom free was greatest in those without psychological problems and with a history of dysentery. The patients who had psychological problems and had no history of dysentery had the worst prognosis. The patients in the present appendicectomy study were classified according to the presence or absence of psychiatric disorder during the month leading up to the

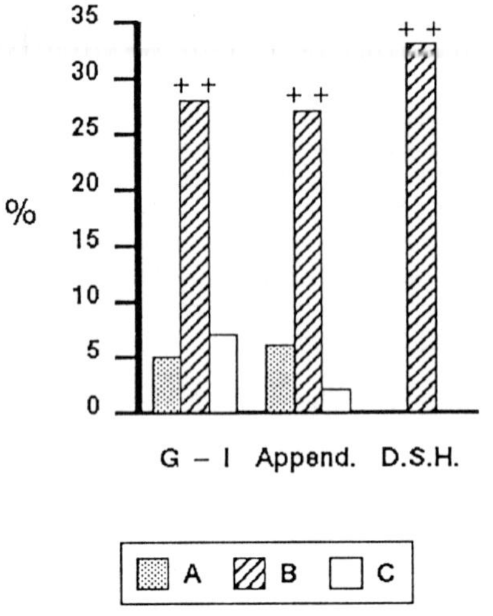

Fig 2 Proportion of subjects (as percentage) who had experienced a severe row event during 38 weeks before onset of abdominal pain or before interview for community comparison group.
G-I = patients attending a gastro-enterology clinic, Append= patients undergoing appendicectomy, DSH = patients admitted following deliberate self-harm.

A=organic g-i dis/append'tis
B=functional abdominal pain
C=community comparison gp.

++= p< 0.0001 compared to community comparison group.

Table 2 *Proportion of subjects (per cent) who had experienced a severe event by group and psychiatric illness*

G-I Clinic			Appendicectomy			Delib. Self Harm.	
Psych. Dis;	Yes	No		Yes	No	Yes	No
Organic (N=56)	67	17	Ac. Inflamed. (N=63)	40	25	68	73
Functional (N=79	70 *	65 *	No Ac. Infl. (N=56)	78 *	53 *	68	73
Community Comparison (N=135)	64	11	Community Comparison (N=63)	40	16		

key; * = p<0.01 or greater compared to organic and community comparison groups

operation to see whether this predicted continuing pain at follow-up one year after the appendicectomy.

The proportion at follow-up with abdominal symptoms severe enough to keep them off work and/or to seek treatment from the doctor was 10% of those with clear appendicitis and no psychiatric disorder at time of the operation, compared to 44% of those with an appendix not acutely inflamed who had psychiatric disorder at the time of appendicectomy ($p<0.01$). Many were describing typical IBS symptoms at follow-up.

The patients whose appendix was not acutely inflamed and who also had psychiatric disorder at the time of apendicectomy were also significantly different from the whole cohort in the following respects; their treatment for abdominal pain had been initiated by others rather than by the patient themselves ($p< 0.01$), they stayed in hospital longer ($p< 0.05$), and they reported more trivial bodily symptoms (both within and outside the gasto-intestinal tract) at the time of appendicectomy and one year later ($p<0.05$). Two days after their appendicectomy their estimate of how long they would be in hospital and how long they would be off work tended to belonger. These factors are likely to indicate illness behaviours as none could be related to objective post-operatve complications which were evenly distributed across the whole cohort.

DISCUSSION

Using accurate measures we have shown that severely threatening life events commonly precede functional abdominal pain whether or not psychiatric disorder is present. When psychiatric disorder is present the patient is more likely to show illness behaviour.

One limitation of these studies was the selection of patients with an acute onset of functional abdominal pain. This was necessary to ensure that we only included environmental stress and psychiatric disorder that *preceded* the onset of abdominal pain. However, many of the patients undergoing appendicectomy, whose appendix was not acutely inflamed, developed clear IBS one year later. Others have reported that 30-50% of patients attending the gastrointestinal clinic with IBS have had a normal appendix removed previously (Chaudhury and Truelove 1962, Lane 1973, Keeling and Fielding 1975) and many IBS patients report the original onset was in their late teens or early twenties (Waller and Misiewicz 1969, Harvey et al 1987)

Two other life events studies have reported similar findings. Ford et al (1987) also used the LEDS, although they limited their study to anxiety and ignored depression. They found that the weighted life event scores for the functional pain group were twice that of the events experienced by the organic group. Canton et al (1984) used another life events measure but found that patients having a normal appendix removed had experienced life events very similar to a group of depressed patients attending a psychiatrist.

Canton et al (1984) al documented the fact that patients having a

8

normal appendix removed were likely to show illness behaviour. Joyce et al (1986) similarly found increased anxiety and abnormal illness behaviour among those patients admitted with acute abdominal pain for which no organic cause could be found. There have been a nuber of reports of abnormal illness behaviour among IBS patients but this is likely to reflect accompanying psychiatric disorder rather than an aspect of the disorder itself (Colgan et al (1988).

However, environmental stress preceding the onset of functional abdominal pain is *not* confined to those with psychiatric disorder. It may be that the experience of such stress directly alters colonic motility (Almy et al 1951, Chaudhury and Truelove 1961, Wangel and Deller 1964), so the experience of a severe life event may lead to painful contractions of the colon in those who are constitionally predisposed to develop them. In addition, where psychiatric symptoms are present, depression or anxiety may lead to a lowered pain threshold and this may contribute to the experience of abdominal pain.

Since our studies have been confined to hospital samples an alternative explanation is the possibility that the experience of environmental stress leads to treatment seeking for symptoms which would otherwise not have been brought to the hospital. However, our current psychological treatment study suggests that reduction of psychological distress does more than reverse treatment-seeking; the symptoms improve also.

REFERENCES

Almy, T.P. (1951): Experimental studies on the irritable colon. *Am. J. Med.* 10, 60-67.

Bass, C. (1986): Life events and gastro-intestinal symptoms. *Gut* 27, 123-126.

Brown, G.W. & Harris, T. (1978): *Social origins of depression.* London: Tavistock.

Canton, G., Santonastaso, P. and Fraccon, I.G. (1984): Life events, abnormal illness behaviour and appendectomy. *Gen. Hosp. Psych.* 6, 191-195.

Chaudhury, N.A., and Truelove, S.C. (1961): Human colonic motility: a comparative study of normal subjects, patients with ulcerative colitis, and patients with irritable colon syndrome. *Gastroenterology* 40, 27-36.

Chaudhury, N. A. and Truelove, S.C. (1962): The irritable colon syndrome. *Quart. J. Med.* 31, 307-322.

Colgan, S., Creed, F.H., and Klass, S. H. (1988): Psychiatric disorder and abnormal illness behaviour in patients with upper abdominal pain. *Psychol Med.* 18, 887-892.

Creed, F.H. (1981): Life events and appendicectomy. *Lancet* 1, 1381-1385.

Creed, F.H. and Guthrie, E. (1987): Psychological factors and the irritable bowel syndrome. *Gut* 28, 1307-1318.

Craig, T.K. and Brown, G.W. (1984): Goal frustrating aspects of life event stress in the aetiology of gastrointestinal disorder. *J. Psychosom. Res.* 28, 411-421.

Farmer, R. and Creed, F.H. (1988): Life events, hostility and self-poisoning. *Brit. J. Psychiat.* (In press).

Ford, M.J., Miller, R. McC., Eastwood, J. and Eastwood, E.A. (1987): Life events, psychiatric illness and the irritable bowel syndrome. *Gut* 28, 160-165.
Harvey R.F., Mauad E.C., Brown A.M., (1987): Prognosis in the irritable bowel syndrome. A 5 year prospective study. *Lancet*, 1, 963-5.
Keeling, P.W.N. and Fielding, J.F. (1975): The irritable bowel syndrome: a review of 50 consecutive cases. *J.Ir. Coll.Phys. Surg.* 4, 91-94.
Lane, D. (1973): The irritable colon and right iliac fossa pain. *Med. J. Austr.*, 1. 66-67.
Macdonald, A.J. and Bouchier, P.A.D. (1980): Non-organic gastro-intestinal illness: a medical and psychiatric study. *Brit.J. Psych*. 136, 1276-283.
Waller S.L, and Misiewicz J.J. (1969); Prognosis in the irrritable bowel syndrome. *Lancet*. 2, 753-6.
Wangel, A.E. and Deller, D.J. (1964): Intestinal motility in man. III. Mechanism of constipation and diarrhoea with particular reference to irritable colon syndrome. *Gastroenterology* 48, 69-84.
Wing, J.J., Cooper, J.E. and Sartorius, N. (1974): *The measurement and classification of psychiatric symptoms: an instruction manual for the Present State Examination and CATEGO Programme.* (London Cambridge University Press).

Acknowledgements

This research was performed while Francis Creed held a Mental Health Leverhulme Research Fellowship and Tom Craig held a Medical Research Council Grant. We are grateful to Roger Farmer for the results concerning the deliberate self harm patients.

Simultaneous measurement of intraluminal pressure and transit; a newly developed technique for the study of colonic function under different conditions

William J. Snape, Jr., S. Narasimha Reddy, Gabrielle Bazzocchi*, Javier Villanueva-Meyer**, Ismael Mena** and Eduardo Moreno-Osset***

Departments of Medicine and Nuclear Medicine, Harbor-UCLA Medical Center, 1124 W. Carson St, Torrance CA 90502, U.S.A.

**Via Mongardino N°9, 40044 Sasso Marconi, Bologna, Italy*

*** Department of Nuclear Medicine, Harbor-UCLA Medical Center, 1000 W. Carson Street, Box 23, Torrance, Ca 90509, U.S.A.*

**** Isabel La Catolica 1, 22ª, 46004 Valencia, Spain*

INTRODUCTION

Emotionally stressful situations alter the bowel habit in people who have no gastrointestinal complaints and in patients who have functional complaints referable to the gastrointestinal tract. Stressful stimuli delivered in a controlled environment affect the motor function of the small intestine (2) and the colon (5). Colonic motility increases during the stressful stimuli, including those which are painful and those which require difficult cognitive skills (5). The preadministration of chlordiazepoxide decreases stress stimulation of the colonic motility.

Eating stimulates an increase in colonic motility in healthy subjects and in patients with the irritable bowel syndrome (7). Patients who have an abnormality in their bowel habit also may have an altered postprandial increase in colonic motility (6,7). The correlation between the observed motility disorder and the clinical abnormality in the bowel habit is unknown. The purpose of the present study is to correlate the changes in colonic motility with the transit of intraluminal contents in human subjects.

METHODS AND MATERIALS

Studies were performed on 11 healthy volunteers who had no gastrointestinal symptoms or previous gastrointestinal surgery, 16 patients with constipation and 8 patients with diarrhea. Each of the patients with constipation had less than 3 bowel movements per week. Each of the patients had greater than 3 bowel movements per day. The patients and healthy subjects were taking no medications at the time of the study.

All subjects fasted at least 12 hours before the study. Each subject drank 1 gallon of a balanced electrolyte solution containing polyethylene glycol (Colyte R) between 4PM and 7PM of the preceding day. No additional colonic preparation was used on the morning of the study.

A nine-lumen manometric catheter was used to record intraluminal pressure and to inject the radionuclide. It consisted of seven ports, each 15 cm apart. The most proximal port was located 5 cm from the catheter's distal tip. One port was used for instillation of radioisotope.

Colonoscopy was performed using minimal air insufflation. After reaching the proximal transverse colon, a soft-tipped Teflon biliary guidewire was inserted through the colonoscope. The guidewire was positioned and the colonoscope was withdrawn, leaving the guidewire in position. The manometric catheter was advanced over the guidewire. The guidewire was then removed and the tube was fixed to the patient's thigh using tape.

The subjects were placed supine under a gamma camera which was equipped with an all purpose parallel hole collimator and was interfaced with a dedicated acquisition computer. Scintigraphic data acquisition was made by taking a sequence of 24 frames, 1 minute images every 5.8 minutes, on a 64x64 matrix. The data were stored in floppy disks for future analysis.

The position of the manometric catheter was confirmed by the gamma camera after introducing a test dose of technetium into the dead space of the catheter. The position of the port for instillation of the radioisotope into the splenic flexure was checked and adjusted on the basis of its 30cm distance from the most proximal port. The position of the camera was adjusted to include in the field of view the transverse, descending, and proximal sigmoid colon.

With the instillation port placed in the splenic flexure, four of the seven pressure ports were positioned in the distal half of the transverse colon, the splenic flexure, and descending and proximal part of the sigmoid colon. The pressure catheters were continuously perfused at 0.5 ml/min with distilled water using a low-compliance capillary system. Pressure was recorded on a 8-channel rectilinear recorder.

A 5 mCi dose of Tc-99m-DTPA was instilled into the splenic flexure, and the catheter was flushed with 6 ml of saline. The total volume, 8 ml, was injected slowly. Scintigraphic data acquisition and pressure recording began immediately and images were gathered during a 60 min basal period and for 100 min postprandial period. The meal (100 Kcal) was completely consumed in less than 10 min.

Time activity curves were generated for two non-overlapped regions of interest (ROI's): 1)the entire transverse colon, and 2) the distal portion of the descending colon and the proximal sigmoid colon (Figure 1). The curves represented counts per pixil per minute in the ROI's. The size of both ROI's were similar. Care was taken not to include in the ROI's portions of the splenic flexure, which contained significant amounts of activity.

A colonic motility index was calculated by measuring the area under the pressure records for each 30-min period using a computerized planimeter. Patterns of colonic motor contractions were identified by analyzing the records visually. Non-propagating contractions were defined as contractions that did not propagate a least 15 cm between the recording ports. Propagating contractions travelled at least 30 cm and involved 3 recording ports.

Non-parametric methods were used to analyze the data. The Wilcoxon signed ranks test was used to compare the differences between variables during the baseline period and each postprandial period of interest. Results were expressed as mean + SEM.

RESULTS

Healthy Subjects

During fasting there was no movement of the tracer that was placed in the splenic flexure in healthy subjects. Eating a 1000 kCal meal stimulated transit of the marker from the splenic flexure to both the transverse colon and the descending colon in healthy subjects (Fig. 2). The increased level of the tracer remained stable in the transverse and descending colon for 120 min after eating the meal in each of the patients.

Figure 3 shows the change in motility before and after eating the meal in healthy subjects. During fasting there was minimal phasic intraluminal pressure. Within 15 minutes of eating, there was an increase in the pressure in each region of the colon. The increase was greatest in the upper descending colon ($p<0.05$). The intraluminal pressure decreased to fasting levels approximately 45 minutes after eating.

Figure 4 shows the effect of pretreatment with 8 mg diazepam on colonic motility in 3 subjects. The postprandial increase in intraluminal pressure was not changed by diazepam in any region of the colon. The scintigraphic studies were also similar.

Propagating contractions occurred 68.8+10.1 minutes after eating in healthy subjects. There were 1.8+0.3 propagating contractions per individual. These propagating contractions were associated with the rapid movement of intraluminal contents from the transverse colon to the sigmoid colon.

Constipated Patients

Similar to the healthy subjects, patients with constipation had no movement of the marker in the splenic flexure during fasting. After eating the standard meal, 9/16 patients had both retrograde and antegrade movement of the intraluminal marker. The other patients had no movement of the marker from the splenic flexure.

In the patients who had movement of the marker, there was an increase in the postprandial intraluminal pressure. However, the increase in pressure was lower in the patients with constipation than in the healthy subjects ($p<0.05$), except in the sigmoid colon where the pressure was greater in the constipated patients. The intraluminal pressure did not increase after eating in the patients who had no movement of the marker.

Neither group of patients with constipation had postprandial propagating contractions.

Diarrheal Patients

During fasting there was a high level of tracer in the transverse and descending colon in patients with diarrhea compared to the healthy controls ($p < 0.05$). The values for the tracer fluctuated in both areas of the colon before and after eating. Instead of the plateau for radioactive contents that was present in the healthy subjects, there was a rapid decline in the intraluminal contents in both areas of the colon. The marker collected in the rectum, which was outside the field of the collimator.

There was no increase in the postprandial contractions in the diarrhea patients in transverse, descending, and sigmoid colon. However there were more propagating contractions which occurred before and after eating. The propagating contractions occurred more rapidly after eating than in the normal subjects.

The propagating contractions were the primary mediator of intraluminal transit in the patients with diarrhea. The propagating contraction were more numerous and so more intraluminal contents was transported distally compared to the healthy controls.

DISCUSSION

In healthy subjects who have a normal bowel habit, there is no increase of motility nor a movement of intraluminal contents during fasting. However, after eating there is an increase in non-propagating contractions and in transit of intraluminal contents proximally and distally into the transverse and descending colon. There are also propagating contractions initiated approximately one hour after eating.

Diazepam did not affect the colonic motility before or after eating the meal. This is important because colonic motility can be more easily performed in patients with irritable bowel syndrome, who are sensitive to distention of the bowel.

The present study demonstrates the importance of the normal pattern of motility in the maintenance of normal bowel habit. In constipation the absence of propagating contractions is the major defect that is present. Although frequency and amplitude of non-propagating contractions can be altered in some patients with constipation, absence of propagating contractions appears to be a more important defect in these patients. The increase in the propagating contractions that occurs in the patients with diarrhea suggests that the propagating contraction may be important for the normal control of bowel habit.

The mechanism for the initiation of the propagating contraction is unclear. In the patients with constipation there may be two mechanisms which differ and may require distinct therapy. In the patients with a postprandial increase in the colonic motility, the decrease in the propagating contractions may be secondary to an afferent sensory defect. The reflux of contents into the transverse colon may not initiate the propagating contraction. In the patients without the reflux into the transverse colon, the lack of transverse colonic distention may be responsible for the lack of a propagating response.

The increase in the propagating contractions that occurs in patients with diarrhea provides additional data that the change in bowel habit is associated with the propagating contraction. In other studies laxatives stimulate propagating contractions (1,3). The mechanism by which the propagating contractions are stimulated in diarrhea or after a laxative is still unknown.

Characterization of the normal and pathological motility and transit will allow the study of patients with stress related changes in their bowel habit. These future studies are important, since many patients with the irritable bowel syndrome may have stress-related alterations in their bowel habit.

REFERENCES

1. Fioramonti, J., Staumont, G., Garcia-Villar, R., and Bueno, L. (1988): Effect of sennosides on colon motility in dogs. Pharmacology 36:23-30.
2. Kumar, D., and Wingate, D.L. (1985): The irritable bowel syndrome: a paroxysmal motor disorder. Lancet 1:973-977.
3 Hardcastle, J.D., and Mann, C.V. (1968): Study of large bowel peristalsis. Gut 9:512-520.
4. Hardcastle, J.D. and Wilkins, J.L. (1970): The action of sennosides and related compounds on human colon and rectum. Gut 11:1038-1042.
5. Narducci, F., Snape, W.J. Jr., Battle, W.M., London, R.L., and Cohen, S. (1985): Increased colonic motility during exposure to a stressful situation. Dig. Dis. Sci. 30:40-44.
6. Snape, W.J., Jr. (1983): Colonic motility in health and disease. In Proceedings of International Symposium on Functional Bowel Disease, edited by W. Chey, pp 287-291. Raven Press
7. Sullivan, M.A., Cohen, S., and Snape, W.J. Jr. (1978): Colonic myoelectrical activity in irritable bowel syndrome: effect of eating and anticholinergics. N. Engl. J. Med. 298:878-883.

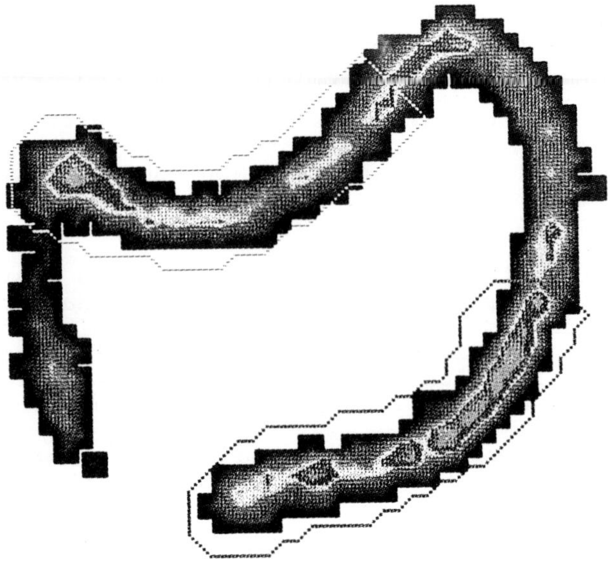

SNAPE ET AL

FIGURE 1

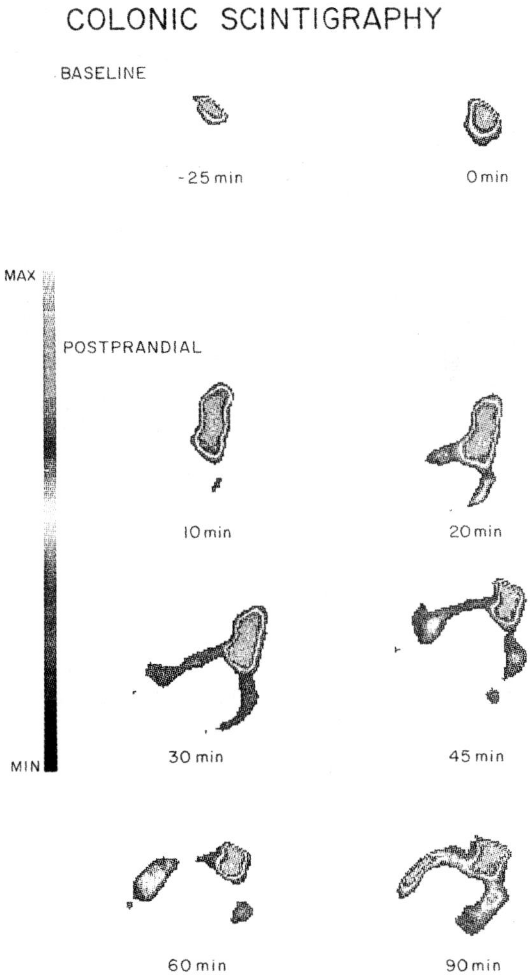

SNAPE ET AL

FIGURE 2

LEGENDS

Figure 1. A scintigram that outlines the areas of the transverse and descending colon that were used for counting intraluminal marker. This scintigram was obtained during the insertion of the test dose of the radionuclide.

Figure 2. Colonic scintigram from a healthy subject before and after eating a meal. The intraluminal marker does not move during fasting, but moves retrograde and antegrade soon after eating a meal.

Figure 3. The change in motility in the transverse colon, splenic flexure, descending and sigmoid colon before and after eating a meal in healthy subjects. The meal was eaten at time 0 min.

Figure 4. The effect of 8 mg of diazepam on colonic motility in healthy subjects.

ACKNOWLEDGEMENT

We thank Connie Madrigal for secretarial assistance. These studies were supported by the National Institutes of Health 3 RO1 DK31147 and the Inflammatory Bowel Disease Center 5P30-DK-36200.

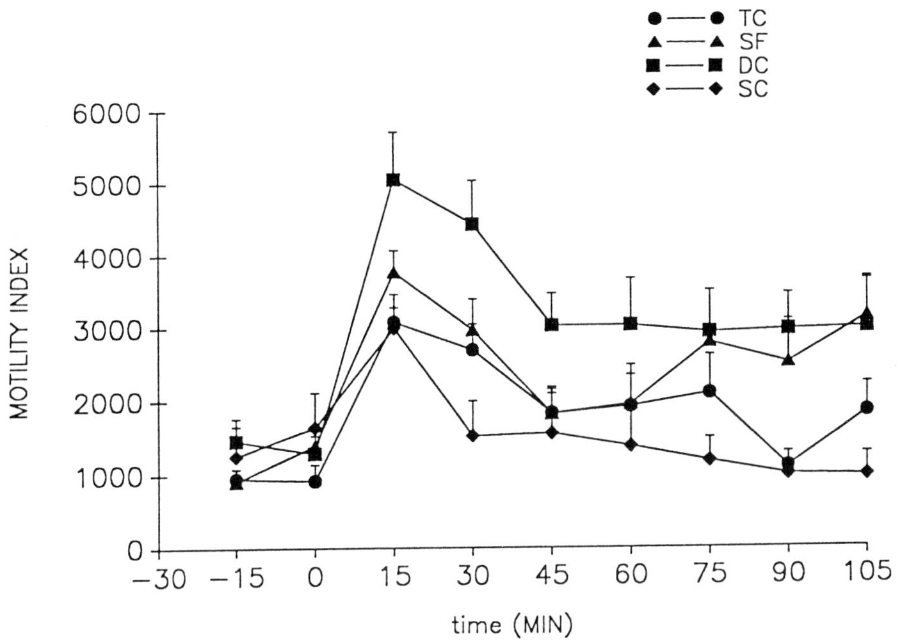

SNAPE ET AL

FIGURE 3

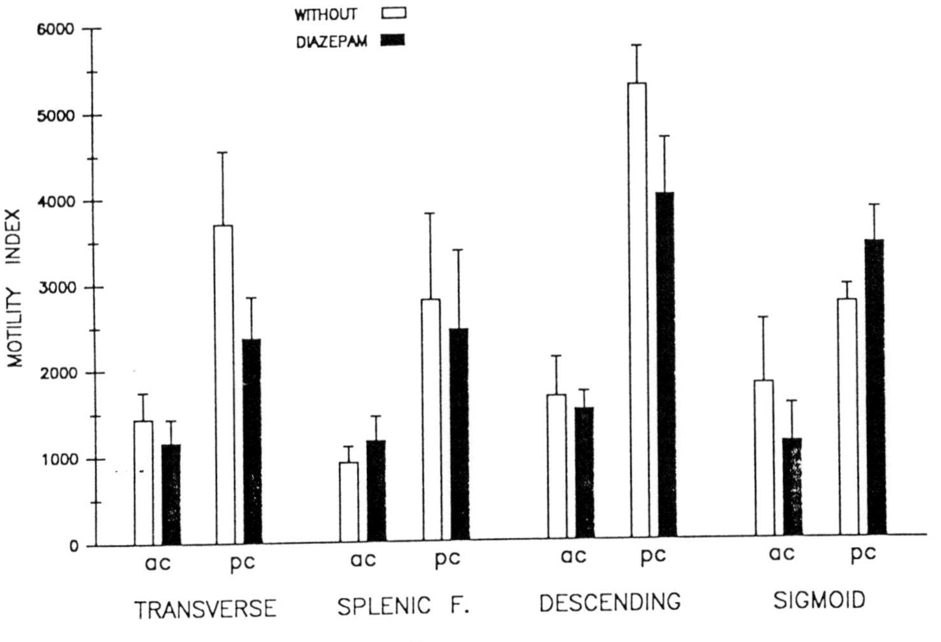

SNAPE ET AL

FIGURE 4

Evaluation of the effect of stress on the gut; clinical implications

Professor N.W. Read and Dr. Alison Prior

Department of Gastrointestinal Physiology and Nutrition, Royal Hallamshire Hospital, Floor K, Sheffield S10 2JF, U.K.

INTRODUCTION

It is common knowledge the psychological stress can influence gastrointestinal function. There can be few people who have not experienced nausea or frequency of defaecation in anticipation of a feared event, or abdominal pain during periods of intense emotions. The linkage between the mind and the gut is so strong in the popular mind that gastrointestinal terms are often used to describe emotions. For example, if we are apprehensive, we complain of butterflies in the stomach;a greater threat may 'give us the runs.' If we run away from the situation, we are said to have 'no guts' or to be 'lily-livered'. If we dislike something intensely, it may 'stick in our gorge' and we maybe unable to 'stomach' it.

The effects of continued stress on gastrointestinal function may be so intense as to result in 'disease'. Conditions such as irritable bowel syndrome and non-ulcer dyspepsia are thought by many to be stress disorders while stress may be a aetiological factor in some patients with ulcerative colitis and duodenal ulceration. Although many would intuitively accept that stress may cause gastrointestinal upset and acknowledge that stress is an important component in many if not all gastrointestinal diseases, the methods that have been used to study stress are not always the most appropriate. This chapter discusses the methods that have been used to gain insights into how stress affects the gut (table), and may cause or exacerbate gastrointestinal disease.

EXPERIMENTAL STRESSORS

These are ideally suited for laboratory based studies because the stress is stereotyped, can be repeated, and physiological measurements can be conducted at the same time. The disadvantages are the stress is often inappropriate in that it is unlikely to be encountered in the subject's daily life, and different stressors can have different effects on gastrointestinal motility.

One of the most commonly-employed stressors is the cold pressor test, in which pain is induced from plunging the hand and forearm into ice cold water for long periods of time. This painful stimulus inhibits gastric acid secretion (Thompson et al, 1983), inhibits antral and duodenal contractile activity (Stanghellini et al, 1983; O'Brien et al, 1985), induces tonic and phasic pyloric contractions (Fone et al, 1988) and delays gastric emptying (Thompson et al, 1983). In the small intestine, the cold pressor test delays small bowel transit (O'Brien 1987) and increases intestinal absorption. Barclay and Turnberg (1985) Wyatt and Read (Abstract in Gt 1984) reported a reduction in absorption. In the rectosigmoid colon, Narducci (1985) reported an increase in myoelectrical spike potentials and motor activity although subjects showed habituation to the cold stress.

Plunging the arm into ice-cold water is a potent stimulator of the sympathetic nervous system. It accelerates heart rate, increases blood pressure and releases catecholamines into the circulation [O,Brien 1987]. It is possible, therefore, that the effects that are observed on the gastrointestinal tract may be caused more by direct activation of sympathetic nerves rather than the psychic experience associated with the test. O'Brien et al (1985) have shown that the effects of cold stress on small intestinal transit and motility can be blocked by beta-adrenergic antagonists. The results of the cold pressor test bear little relationship to the effects of emotional stress, and may therefore provide a limited insight into the possible role of stress in gastrointestinal disease (unless the patient happens to be an inadequately equipped polar explorer).

Mental stressors are arguably more relevant to the patients experience. The dichotomous listening test attempts to mimic everyday effects of mental harrassment that are familiar to people working in business or trying to cope with running a home and several children. Subjects are equipped with stereo-headsets and have to listen to two pieces of information coming simultaneously through each ear and answer questions on either one or the other source of information when triggered by bells and buzzers. The effects of this stressor on gastrointestinal function differ from the cold pressor test. For example, it has no effect on gastric emptying (Cann et al, 1983 it accelerates small bowel transit time of a meal (Cann et al, 1983) and it reduces intestinal absorption and in some instances causes net secretion (Barclay et al, 1987, Wyatt and Read, (Abstract in Gut 1984) .

A variety of other tests have been used to investigate the effect of stress on gastrointestinal function. They include delayed auditory feedback, in which the patient attempts to read whilst listening through headphones to his own voice which as been delayed by upto 0.17 seconds, the Stroop word test in which subjects must read in fast sequence 50 cards on which the name of a colour (green etc.) is written in another colour (blue etc.) and white noise. Wingate's group has shown that most mental stressors alter the fasting motor activity of the small intestine in a characteristic fashion, decreasing the incidence of phase III and increasing phase II of the interdigestive migrating motor complex (Valori1986 McCrae 1982). An important consideration is whether such tests investigate the effects of stress or the effects of arousal?. Sleep is associated with a marked reduction in phase II activity and an increased frequency of phase III (Kumar et al 1988). Our experience with the dichotomous listening test is that subjects adapt to it remarkably quickly and do not necessarily appear 'stressed', while my nine-year-old son would hardly regard computer games as a stress.

Stress has come to be regarded in popular terminology as synonymous with the emotional effects of that stress. We talk about somebody 'showing signs of stress', when strictly speaking, we mean that he or she is showing signs of strain. There are no characteristic signs of stress; indeed some people are happier and arguably more healthy when exposed to the sort of situations that the 'so-called' stress tests attempt to simulate; they 'thrive on stress'. When we talk about the effects of stress on disease, are we really talking about the general arousal brought about by demanding situations? Or are we talking about effects of the failure to cope with stress? I suspect it is the latter. If that is the case, should we really be studying the relationship between the emotional responses to stress and the physiological changes? This was what Thomas Almy was trying to do when he conducted stress interviews on his patients (Almy 1949 a).

STRESS INTERVIEWS

The studies of Thomas Almy reported in the 1940's provide the most extensive documentation of the relationship between emotion and gastrointestinal function. With balloon sensors in the distal colon or tubes in the stomach, Almy encouraged his patients to discuss the most painful aspects of their private lives. He showed a clear and dramatic association between the emotional response of the patient and patterns of gastrointestinal motility. Moreover, he illustrated how in some patients, different emotional responses could be associated with different motor effects. Anger and intense anxiety, for example, was often accompanied by an increase in sigmoid motor activity while distress and weeping was associated with a reduction in motility. These results resemble direct observations on the stomach of patients with gastric fistulae. Colonel William Beaumont, working for the U.S. Cavalry Army described over 150 years ago, how when his volatile patient, the fur trapper Alexis St Martin, became angry, the stomach lining became red and engorged, secreted more fluid and increased its' motor activity, which fear and depression was associated with a blanching of the mucosa, and reductions in secretion and motor activity (Baumont 1833). Stewart Wolf made similar observations in his patient 'Tom', who was given a gastric fistula after he mistook a pan of boiling clam chowder for beer and stenosed his oesophagus (Wolf 1965) . As a corollary to this, Cannon 1929 observed that the stomach of became hite and hypomotile when dogs with gastric fistulae were confronted with a posturing and hissing cat. An important insight into the emotional state of the dog; I wonder what the cat's stomach looked like! Sadler and Orton (1969) observed how anger and rage could increased the motor activity of a Thiry Vella loop in humans, while sadness depressed it and his ' fear' on being told the diagnosis of carcinoma of the larynx abolished it completely. In a recent work, Welgan and his colleagues [1988] studied the effect of inducing anger either by making patient ith IBS or normal subjects wait for a long time in the clinic or appearing to disbelieve their statements. Anger was associated with an increase in colonic motor activity and patients with the Irritable Bowel Syndrome showed a greater emotional and manometric response than normal volunteers. This study provides useful data on the correlation between emotional state and physiological change. It does not necessarily tell us that IBS patients are particularly irritable people. They may well be, but their heightened response to the experimental provocation employed by Welgan may be related to the fact that the patients were giving their time free for research,and had a vested interest in the outcome, while the volunteers were being paid to do a test.

Almy has discussed how changes in the blood flow to the face, sweating and lacrimation are all autonomic responses that betray our emotional condition. We use them as protective device to signal our emotions (or to indicate the emotions that continued action by a parent, lover or aggressor might provoke). Autonomic nerves supply all of the viscera and it is logical therefore to propose that the stomach will 'blush', the intestine may be contorted by muscular contraction and the rectum may secrete 'tears' of mucus.

<u>The nature study or the provocative study.</u>

Techniques of ambulatory recording of gastrointestinal activity have now become so advanced that multiple channels of data can be recorded for up to 24 hours on tape while the patient pursues his or her normal life style. These studies offer the opportunity to investigate the effect of normal life events and correlate the responses to them with changes in gastrointestinal motility and symptoms. The patients can record their psychic or physical experiences on the same record. This technique has been used to great effect in studies on hypertension and is only just recently been applied to gastrointestinal motility disorders. Wingate's group have used ambulatory recordings to show how driving through heavy traffic can induce a change in small intestinal motor activity [Kumar 1985, Valori 1987]. Clearly, the demonstration of a relationship between a real life event and a change in gastrointestinal motility has more validity in evaluating the relationship between stress and patient's symptoms than any contrived situation in a laboratory, but there are some limitations. First motility can only be recorded for a few hours. Secondly, the patient is aware of being studied and may be unlikely to expose himself to a situation that threatens his emotional equilibrium. And finally, interpretation of the data depends on accurate recording by the patient of both the event and the emotion it provokes.

CLINICAL STUDIES

Stressful Life Events in Irritable Bowel Syndrome

Of all gastrointestinal conditions, the irritable bowel syndrome is most commonly thought to be related to life stress and emotional disturbance. Studies on life events and psychopathology in IBS patients only partly support this belief. Many studies have shown that stressful life events are common in the IBS population (Waller and Misiewicz 1969, Chaudhany and Truelove 1962, Svedlund 1983) However, stressful life events are also common in control groups of patients without IBS (Ford et al, 1987; Fava et al, 1976; Mendeloff et al, 1970). Unlike other gastrointestinal disease however, exacerbations of IBS do appear more likely to be preceded by stressful life events, especially if these provoked anxiety (Hislop 1971, Ford et al, 1987; Craig et al, 1984).

Psychopathology in Irritable Bowel Syndrome

Many studies have shown that patients with IBS attending hospital have a higher incidence of anxiety, depression than patients with organic disease.(Hislop 1971, Palmer et al 1974, Young and Alpers 1976, Ford et al 1987). However, it is now well recognised that most people with IBS in the general population do not seek medical advice (Thompson and Heaton 1980, Drossman et al

1982) and it may be therefore that in hospital we see a small subset whose very neurosis might have taken them to a physician. This was supported by Greenbaum (1983) who showed that subjects with IBS symptoms attending a doctor had more psychopathology than those not attending. However, Welch and colleagues (1985) found that reporters and non-reporters with IBS both exhibited psychopathological behaviour more frequently than normal controls. An alternative explanation has that those subjects attending a doctor just have more severe symptoms, Lowman et al (1987).

Stress reduction, behavioural psychotherapy and hypnotherapy of Irritable Bowel Syndrome.

Both Svedlund (1983) and Hislop (1980) found psychotherapy effective in reducing symptoms. Hislop reported that about half of his patients were asymptomatic 8 to 33 months after commencing psychotherapy. Whitehead (1985) used biofeedback training to decrease rectal contractions induced by distension, but this did not result in any change in symptoms.

The results of hypnotherapy in reducing symptoms of IBS are particularly encouraging. Whorwell (1984, 1987) reported that 85% of his patients were well three years after a course of hypnotherapy and a recent paper from Bristol reported good results in 65% of patients with IBS. The mechanism by which hypnotherapy exerts it effect is unclear, but the clinical results have sugessted that its effect is not just via stress reduction.

Psychotherapeutic Drugs

Psychotherapeutic drugs are often prescribed to patients with IBS although the results of controlled trials have largely been disappointing. Whereas Greenbaum et al (1987) showed an impovement with desipramine in pain and bowel habit in diarrhoea predominant patients, Heefner (1978) found only an improvement in well being. A similar improvement in overall well being was reported for Motival (fluphenazine and nortriptyline) (Ritchie and Truelove 1980) whereas amitriptyline was found to produce no significant changes in any parameters measured (Steinhard et al 1981), and trimipramine improve only vomiting and sleeplessness (Myren et al 1982). Tricyclic antidepressants have a direct action on smooth muscle and it is possible that not all of their effects in IBS are secondary to an action on the central nervous system.

Table 1.

Methods that have been used to study the effect of stress on the Gut.

Experimental Stress

Pain

Cold pressure test

Tightening Head Band

Arousal/Concentration

Dichotomous Listening Test

Stroop Word Test

Computer Games

Driving in heavy traffic

Delayed activity feedback

Noise

White Noise

Stress Inverviews

Inducement of Anger

Clinical Observations

Life Stress Inventory

Psychopathology Score

Responses to psychotherapy.

REFERENCES

Almy TP, Kern, F, Tulin N. Alterations in colinic function in man under stress. Gastroenterology, 1949, 12; 425 436.

Almy TP, Hinkel LE, Berle B, Kern F. Alterations in colonic function in man under stress. Gastroenterology 1949: 12: 437-449.

Barclay GR, Turnberg LA. Influence of physical and psychological stress on fluid and electrolyte absorption in the human jejunum in vivo. 1985, Gut 26; A554-555

Barclay GR, Turnberg LAM. The effect of psychological stress on salt and water transport in the human jejunum. Gastroenterology 1987; 93: 91-93.

Beaumont W. Experiments and observations on the Gastric Juice and Physiology of Digestin. Plattsburg, F>P> Allen 1833.

Cann PA, Read NW, Cammack J, Childs H. Holden S, Kashman R, Longmore J, Nix S, Simms N, Swallow K, Weller J. Psychological stress and the passage of standard meal through the stomach and small intestine in man. Gut 1983; 245: 236-240.

Cannon WB. Bodily changes in pain, hunger, fear and rage. New York, D. Appleton 1929.

Chaudhary NA, Truelove SC. The irritable colon syndrome. Quart J. Med. 1962, 31; 307-322.

Craig TKJ, Brown GW. Goal frustration and life events in the aetiology of painful gastrointestinal disorder. J. Psychosom. Res. 1984; 28: 411-421.

Drossman DA, Sandler RS, McKee DC, Lovitz AJ. Bowel patterns among subjects not seeking health care. Gastroenterology 1982; 83: 529-534.

Fava GA, Pavan L. Large bowel disorder. In. Illness configuration and life events. Psycholther. Pschosom 1976; 27: 93-99.

Fone D, Horowitz M, Maddox A, Akkerman L, Dent J, Read NW. Cold stress induces isolated pyloric pressure waves in healthy volunteers. Gastroenterology 1988, 94; A133.

Ford MJ, Miller P.McC, Eastwood J, Eastwood MA. Life events, psychiatric illness and the irritable bowel syndrome. Gut 1987; 28: 160-165.

Greenbaum DS, Abitz L, Van Egeren LE, Mayle JW, Greenbaum RB. Irritable bowel symptoms prevalence, rectosigmoid motility and psychometrics in symptomatic subjects not seeing physicians. Gastroenterology; 1983, 84: 1174A.

Greenbaum DS, Mayle JE, VanEgeren LE, Jerome JA, Mayle JW, Greenbaum RB, Matson RW, Stein GE, Dean HA, Halvorsen NA, Rosen LW. Effects of desipramine on irritable bowel syndrome compared with atropine and placebo. Dig. Dis. Sci, 1987, 32: 257-266.

Harvey RF, Hinton RA, Gunary RM, Barry RE. Individual and group hypnotherapy in treatment of refractory irritable bowel syndrome. Lancet. 1989; 1, 424-425.

Heefner JD, Wilder RM, Wilson ID. Irritable colon and depressino. Psychosmatics 1978; 19: 540-547.

Hislop IG. Psychological significance of the irritable colon syndrome. Gut 1971, 12; 452-457.

Hislop IG. Effect of very brief psychotherapy on the irritable bowel syndrome. Med. J. Aust. 1980; 2: 620-623.

Kumar D, Wingate DL. The irritable bowel syndrome: a paroxysmal motor disorder. Lancet, 1985: ii: 973-977.

Kumar D, Idzikowski C, Soffer EE, Siderfin C, Thompson P, Wingate DL. Do the brain and the gut sleep together? Gastroenterology 1988; 94: A241.

McCrae S, Younger K, Thompson DG, Wingate DL. Sustained mental stress alters human jejunal motor activity. Gut 1982; 23: 404-409.

Mendeloff AL, Monk M, Siegel CI, Lilienfeld A. Illness experience and life stresses in patients with irritable colon and with ulcerative colitis. N.Engl. J. Med. 1970; 282:14-17.

Myren J, Groth H, Larsen S. The effect of trimipramine in patients with the irritable bowel syndrome; a double blind study. Scand. J. Gastroneterol. 1982; 17, 871-875.

Narducci F, Snape WJ, Battle WM, London RL, Cohen S. Increased colonic motility during exposure to a stressful situation. Dig. Dis. Sci. 1985, 30: 40-44.

O'Brien JD, Thompson DG, Holly J, Burnham WR, Walker E. Stress disturbs human gastrointestinal transit via a beta-1-adrenoreceptor mediated pathway. Gastroenterology, 1985; 88: 1520.

O'Brien JD, Thompson DG, Brunham WR, Holly J, Walker E. The action of centrally mediated autonomic stimuli on human upper gastrointestinal transit: a comparative study of two stimuli. Gut, 1987,28;960-969.

Palmer RL, Crisp AH, Stonehill E, Waller SL, Misiewicz JJ. Psychological charactristics of patients with the irritable bowel syndrome. Postgrad. Med. J. 1974, 50: 416-419.

Ritchie JA, Truelove SC. Comparison of various treatments for irritable bowel syndrome. Br. Med. J. 1980, 281, 1317-1319.

Sadler HH, Orton AU. The complementory relationship between the emotional state aand the function of the ileum in the human subject. Am. J. Psychiatry 1968; 124: 1375-1384.

Stanghellini V, Malagelada J-R, Zinsmeister AR, Go VLW, Kao PC. Stress induced gastroduodenal motor disturbances in humans: possible humoral mechanisms. Gastroenterology 1983; 85: 83-91.

Steinhart MJ, Wong PY, Zarr ML. Therapeutic usefulness of amitriptyline in spastic colon syndrome. Int. J. Psychiatry Med. 1981-1982; 11: 45-57.

Svedlund J. Psychotherapy in irriable bowel syndrome. A controlled outcome study. Acta Psychiatr. Scand. 1983; 67: suppl 306: 1-86.

Thompson WG, Heaton KW. Functional bowel disorders in apparently healthy people. Gastroenterology, 1980; 79: 283-288.

Thompson DG, Richardson E, Malagelada J-R. Perturbation of upper gastrointestinal function by cold stress. Gut 1983; 24: 277-283.

Valori RM, Kumar D, Wingate DL. Effects of different types of stress and of 'prokinetic' drugs on the control of the fasting motor complex in humans. Gastroenterology 1986; 90: 1890-1900.

Waller SL, Misiewicz JJ. Prognosis in the irritable bowel syndrome. Lancet 1969; 2: 753-756.

Welch GW, Hillman LC, Pomare EW. Psychoneurotic sympatomatology in the irritable bowel syndrome; a study of reporters and non-reporters.Br. Med. J. 1985; 291: 1382-1384.

Welgan P, Meshkinpour H, Beeler M. Effect of anger on colon motor and myoelecric activity in irritable bowel syndrome. Gastroenterology 1988; 94: 1150-1156.

Whitehead WE.Psychotherapy and biofeedback in the treatment of irritable bowel syndrome. In: Irritable Bowel Syndrome. Read NW. Ed. Grune and Stratton, New York 1985 pp 245-266.

Whorwell PJ, Prior A, Faragher EB. Controlled trial of hypnotherapy in the treatment of severe refractory irritable bowel syndrome. Lancet 1984: ii: 1232-1234.

Whorwell PJ, Prior A, Colgan SM. Hypnotherapy in severe irritable bowel syndrome: further experience. Gut 1987, 28: 423-425.

Wolf S. The stomach. Oxford University Press. New York 1965.

Young ST, Alpers DH, Norland CC, Woodruff RA. Psychiatric illness and the irritable bowel syndrome; practical implications for the primary physician. Gastroenterology 1976, 70: 162-166.

Influence of sudden awakening on colonic contractile activity in man

Gabrio Bassotti, MD, Cesare Betti, MD, Antonio Morelli, MD

Laboratorio di Motilità Intestinale, Cattedra di Gastroenterologia, Istituto di Clinica Medica Generale e Terapia Medica I, Università di Perugia, Italy

There is at present convincing evidence that stress influences colonic motor activity in man (Almy 1951; Almy et al, 1949; Narducci et al, 1985; Welgan et al, 1988). However, the different type of stressors employed, chiefly represented by stress interview, are difficult to standardize (Schuster 1983) and other stimuli, such as mechanical distention of the rectum (Whitehead et al, 1980), are likely unphysiological. Moreover, all the above cited and other investigations on this argument have been conducted only either on the rectal or the rectosigmoid area (Chaudary & Truelove 1962; Latimer et al, 1981; Welgan et al, 1985). For these reasons we investigated the effect of a common physiological stressful event, i. e. sudden awakening, on proximal and distal contractile activity of the colon in man.

SUBJECTS and METHODS.

Fourteen stress-free healthy male volunteers, aged 25 to 35 yr, were entered in the study. Each volunteer gave informed consent after the aim of the investigation has been carefully explained. No subject complained of abdominal symptoms nor had undergone abdominal surgery. Manometric studies were done by means of a previously described equipment and technique (Narducci et al, 1987; Bassotti et al, 1987). After colonic cleansing with magnesium sulphate (30g per os 36 h before the procedure) and tap water enemas, a multilumen standard manometric probe (with 12 cm-spaced side openings) was inserted within the proximal colon with the aid of a colonoscope. The probe was then connected, after colonoscope withdrawal, to a low compliance infusion system and writing apparatus.

Recording points were selected in order to have registrations of contractile activity from proximal (data obtained from ascending and transeverse) and distal (data obtained from descending and sigmoid) colon. After three hours of basal adaptation, colonic motility was recorded until the subjects fell asleep. On average, this required four hours. Threfore, 30 mins of continuous sleeping were recorded; then, the subjects were suddenly awakened by one of the investigators by shaking them a shoulder, and the recording session continued for further 30 mins.

A motility index for both proximal and distal colonic portions was calculated, as previously described (Narducci et al, 1987; Bassotti et al, 1987). For each colonic portion, pre- and post-stress Motility Indices were compared by employing the Student's t-test for paired data. Values of p less than 0.05 were considered as significant. Results are expressed as means $\pm$ SEM.

RESULTS.

After comparison of pre- and post-stress Motility Indices, it was observed a striking influence of awakening on colonic contractile activity. In fact, in both the proximal (146 $\pm$ 102 vs 1498 $\pm$ 490, $p < 0.005$) and the distal (606 $\pm$ 422 vs 1737 $\pm$ 516, $p < 0.05$) portions of the viscus the stressful event elicited a significant increase in contractility. Interestingly one subject, after being suddenly awakened, manifested the appearance of high-amplitude propagated contractions, that represent the manometric equivalent of colonic mass movements (Narducci et al, 1987; Bassotti et al, 1988).

DISCUSSION.

The present investigation shows, for the first time, that the entire human colon is sensitive to a stressful event. It is our feeling that the stressor employed here, i.e. sudden awakening, simulated well a commonly occuring physiological event. In fact, this kind of stress is likely to occur sooner or later in everyone's life, so that it might be considered a good experimental (and, perhaps, reproducible) model even for comparison with groups of subjects complaining of functional colonic motor disorders. The results we obtained confirm previous observations about an increase in distal colon motility following a stressful event, and add data on proximal portions too, that appeared to behave like the distal ones. The fact that sudden awakening evoked high-amplitude propagated contractions in one subject is also, in our mind, interesting. This kind of activity is usually recorded following awakening in the morning and after meals, sometimes while occurring borborigmy, and is generally accompanied by defecatory stimuli (Bassotti & Gaburri, 1988). The present evidence suggests that this peculiar motor activity might be elicited by different stimuli also. In conclusion, this investigation shows that a) the entire human colon also, such as the esophagus (Rubin et al, 1962) and the upper gut (Stanghellini et al, 1983; Valori et al, 1986) is sensitive to stressful events and b) the viscus may be an important target organ after awakening.

REFERENCES.

Almy TP (1951): Experimental studies on irritable colon. Am.J.Med. 10:60–67

Almy T, Hinkle L, Berle B, Kern F (1949): Alterations in colonic function under stress. III. Experimental production of sigmoid spasm in patients with spastic constipation. Gastroenterology 12:437–439

Bassotti G, Gaburri M (1988): Manometric investigation of high-amplitude propagated contractile activity of the human colon. Am.J.Physiol. (in press)

Bassotti G, Imbimbo BP, Gaburri M, Daniotti S, Morelli A (1987): Transverse and sigmoid colon motility in healthy humans: effects of eating and of cimetropium bromide. Digestion 37:59–64

Bassotti G, Gaburri M, Imbimbo BP, Rossi L, Farroni F, Pelli MA, Morelli A (1988): Colonic mass movements in idiopathic chronic constipation. Gut 29:1173–1179

Chaudary N, Truelove S (1962): The irritable bowel syndrome. Q.J.Med. 31:307–322

Latimer P, Sarna S, Campbell D, Latimer M, Waterfall W, Daniel E (1981): Colonic motor and myoelectric activity: a comparative study of normal subjects, psychoneurotic patients, and patients with irritable bowel syndrome. Gastroenterology 80:893–901

Narducci F, Snape WJ, Battle WM, London RL, Cohen S (1985): Increased colonic motility during exposure to a stressful situation. Dig.Dis.Sci. 30:40–44

Narducci F, Bassotti G, Gaburri M, Morelli A (1987): Twenty four hour manometric recording of colonic motor activity in healthy man. Gut 28:17–25

Rubin J, Nagler R, Spiro HM, Pilot LM (1962): Measuring the effect of emotions on esophageal motility. Psychosom.Med. 24:170–176

Schuster M (1983): The measurement of colon motility. In Psychophysiology of the gastrointestinal tract, ed. R.Hölzl, W.Whitehead, pp.239–250. New York:Plenum

Stanghellini V, Malagelada JR, Zinsmeister AR, Go VLW, Kao PC (1983): Stress-induced gastroduodenal motor disturbances in man: possible humoral mechanisms. Gastroenterology 85:83–91

Valori RM, Kumar D, Wingate DL (1986): Effects of different types of stress and of 'prokinetic' drugs on the control of the fasting motor complex in humans. Gastroenterology 90:1890–1900

Welgan P, Meshkinpour H, Hoehler F (1985): The effect of stress on colon motor and electrical activity in irritable bowel syndrome. Psychosom. Med. 47: 139–149

Welgan P, Meshkinpour H, Beeler M (1988): Effect of anger on colon motor and myoelectric activity in irritable bowel syndrome. Gastroenterology 94: 1150–1156

Whitehead W, Engel B, Schuster M (1980): Irritable bowel syndrome: physiological and psychological differences between diarrhea-predominant and constipation-predominant patients. Dig.Dis.Sci. 25:404–413

N-methyl-D-aspartate receptors and stress : gastric ulcers, hippocampal long-term potentiation, and coping

Peter G. Henke

Neuroscience Laboratory, St. Francis Xavier University, Antigonish, Nova Scotia, Canada. B2G 1CO.

Hippocampal lesions are known to aggravate restraint-induced gastric erosions and increase "learned helplessness" in rats. Similar pathological effects in the stomach are produced by damaging input pathways from the entorhinal cortex to the dentate gyrus of the hippocampal formation. Stimulation of fibers in this pathway produces long-term potentiation (LTP), an increased efficacy of transmission, which seems to be mediated by N-methyl-D-aspartate (NMDA) receptors (Elmes, et al., 1975; Henke, 1982; Morris et al., 1986). The present studies investigated the effects of intra-ventricular (i.c.v.) injections of the selective NMDA receptor antagonist, aminophosphonovaleric acid (AP 5), on stress ulcers, LTP, and learned helplessness in male Wistar rats.

Table 1 shows that injections of AP 5 into the lateral ventricles aggravated the cold-restraint (3 hr at 4°C) induced stomach pathology in a dose-dependent manner.

Table 1

Mean cumulative ulcer length (mm)

Treatment (ug)	n	Ulcer Length
Saline	6	1.9
AP 5 (15)	6	2.3
AP 5 (30)	6	3.9*
AP 5 (60)	6	8.7*

*$p < 0.05$ (Mann-Whitney U-test, two-tailed).

Table 2 summarizes the effects of i.c.v. injections of AP 5 (30 ug) on the evoked population spikes recorded from the dorsal granule cell layer of the dentate gyrus of the hippocampal formation. Blockade of NMDA receptors by AP 5 prevented LTP, i.e., the evoked amplitudes did not increase, relative to baseline, during the 30 min recording period. However, LTP was produced in the vehicle-controls when a high-frequency burst (100 us, 7 V, 400 Hz, 250 ms) was applied near the angular bundle fibers. AP 5 did not affect the amplitude measures during the 30 min low-frequency (100 us, 7 V, 0.05 Hz) baseline stimulation period.

Table 2

Relative mean potentials

Treatment (ug)	n	Percent Change
Saline	5	+32
AP 5 (30)	5	- 3

In the next study, the so-called learned helplessness phenomenon was investigated after i.c.v. AP 5 (30 ug) injections. This effect is assumed to occur when the experience of uncontrollable aversive conditions interferes with subsequent coping behaviour (Seligman, 1975). Table 3 shows the escape performances in response to scrambled electric shocks (1.2 mA) in a runway apparatus. The goal box of the apparatus was not electrified,

Table 3

Mean escape speeds (1/s)

Treatment	n	Speed
Saline + uncontrollable shocks	6	.85*
AP 5 + uncontrollable shocks	6	.41**
Saline + no prior shocks	6	1.31
AP 5 + no prior shocks	6	1.28

*$p < 0.05$, relative to Saline + no prior shocks
** $p < 0.05$, relative to Saline + uncontrollable shocks

and running speeds were measured over a 90 x 20 x 15 cm section of the runway. Twenty-four hours prior to runway testing, some animals had received a 5-min session of inescapable shocks (1.2 mA) in a different apparatus. Controls were also placed in this apparatus, but were not shocked. Injections into the lateral ventricles were given 30 min prior to this session. The results showed that AP 5 aggravated the learned helplessness effect, i.e., it interfered with escape responses following inescapable shocks to an even greater extent than normally seen under such circumstances. However, AP 5 did not interfere with escape performances when no such helplessness-inducing experience had occurred.

Based on the present data, it is concluded that the blockade of NMDA receptors, probably located on dentate granule cells in the hippocampal formation, interfered with somatic resistance and behavioural coping in uncontrollable stress situations.

This research was funded by the Natural Sciences and Engineering Research Council of Canada.

REFERENCES

Elmes, D. G., Jarrard, L. E., and Swart, P. D. (1975): Helplessness in hippocampectomized rats: Response perseversation? Physiol. Psychol. 3: 51-55.

Henke, P. G. (1982): The telencephalic limbic system and experimental gastric pathology: A review. Neurosci. Biobehav. Rev. 6: 381-390.

Morris, R. G. M., Anderson, E., Lynch, G. S. and Baudry, M. (1986): Selective impairment of learning and blockade of long-term potentiation by an N-methyl-D-asparate receptor antagonist, AP 5. Nature 319: 774-776.

Seligman, M. E. P. (1975): Helplessness. San Francisco: W. H. Freeman.

Is MMC sick in intestinal disease ?

Sushil K. Sarna

Departments of Surgery and Physiology, Medical College of Wisconsin and Zablocki VA Medical Center, Milwaukee, WI 53295 USA

A migrating motor complex is a cyclic group of contractions that generally originates in the proximal small intestine and migrates caudad. In healthy humans and other non-ruminants, it occurs only in the fasting state. Its mean cycle length in humans is about 150 min. Each group of contractions lasts about 6 to 8 min and migrates caudad at a velocity of 2 to 8 cm/min. This cyclic occurrence of complexes is disrupted within a few minutes after the ingestion of a meal; cycling resumes when digestion is complete and the small intestine is nearly empty. The putative function of the migrating motor complex is to keep the small intestine clean of residual food and debris. It does so by the persistence of contractions in the complex which may dislodge the small debris from the villous surface. Once dislodged, the debris are propelled to the forefront of the complex by individual contractions. As the complex migrates caudad to the terminal ileum, the debris are emptied into the colon. Concurrent secretions of the stomach, pancreas and biliary tract aid in the cleaning process and digestion of the residues.

Since its original discovery in the dog (1) and subsequent confirmation of its presence in humans (2), several attempts have been made to determine if changes in MMC's can be related to small intestinal motility disorders in disease states. The following three questions have been asked for this purpose.

A. Do the characteristics of MMC's change in diseased states and, if so, what is their potential significance?

The MMC cycle length of MMC's is one of the most studied parameters in disease. In humans, this cycle length is studied most often in the duodenum or the proximal jejunum for the sake of convenience. It is tacitly assumed that all MMC's that start in the duodenum migrate to the terminal ileum. This is invariably the case in dogs but, in humans, MMC's recorded by intraluminal devices such as manometric catheters are not as regular in cycling or consistent in migration all the way to the terminal ileum (3). In our experience, sometimes MMC's are not present in normal human subjects for 4 to 6 h after intubation. Finally, when the subjects are relaxed and go to sleep, MMC's appear. Sometimes they recur with a very short period (20 min) and sometimes they migrate short distances (20-40 cm) and drop out. All of these observations indicate that the cycle length and distance of migration of MMC's in normal humans is very variable. Furthermore, if the function of the MMC's is simply to clean the small intestine after digestion is complete, it is not necessary that even a statistically significant change in cycle length would have a major effect on their cleaning function. In short, a significantly prolonged cycle length does not mean that the small intestine will be less clean. Only a few MMC's may be required after a meal to do the necessary cleaning and the rest may be redundant.

Although persisting contractions at their maximal frequency may be necessary to dislodge the debris from the inter-villous space, it is really not known what minimum duration of phase III activity is required to accomplish this job reasonably well. MM C duration in humans may vary from 3 to 10 min. Variations of phase III duration within the above range may not be of importance in determining the cleaning function.

Migration velocity also seems to be of less importance in cleaning function. It is really the individual contractions in phase III activity that propel the debris to the forefront of the MMC. How fast the MMC moves down may have little functional significance. The migration velocity of MMC's varies by a factor of 2 to 3 in normal humans and dogs.

The point of origin and distance of migration of MMC's may be an important factor in the cleaning function of the MMC's. Apparently, cleaning will be done only over the length of the small intestine that the MMC migrates. Kellow and Phillips (3) have very carefully defined variations of MMC characteristics in normal human subjects. Unfortunately, because of convenience of recording from the duodenum only, most investigators did not record from the entire small intestine in disease states. In IBS patients, the spatial distribution of MMC's and their point of origination is not different from normals (4).

B. Are MMC's absent in intestinal disease?

Complete absence of MMC's would certainly stop cleaning of the small bowel in between meals. In the long run, this may result in rotting of the residual food and bacterial overgrowth as suggested by Vantrappen et al. (2). However, complete absence of MMC's has not been reported unequivocally in any intestinal disease (See Ref. 5 for details). In some cases, MMC's were absent in a subgroup of patients with the same diseases studied at the same center. It is, however, not clear why MMC's were absent in some patients and not in others with the same disease.

Complete absence of MMC's may mean a major abnormality of the enteric nervous system because the enteric nerves are responsible for the spontaneous initiation and migration of MMC's (6, 7). Although at this time there is no clue to the relationship between the enteric nerves that initiate and propagate the MMC's and the nerves that cause postprandial contractions, there is likely to be some nerves common for these two functions, e.g., the postsynaptic motor excitatory and inhibitory nerves (5). The complete absence of MMC's is, therefore, a drastic situation and would likely be associated with a major motility disorder. But complete absence of MMC's has not been convincingly reported yet in any disease.

C. Do MMC's migrate orad?

An obvious implication of orad migration of MMC's is that the debris and residual food would be emptied into the stomach. This may, however, not be correct. It is sometimes forgotten that propulsion is not due to the MMC but due to the individual contractions in an MMC. If we assume for a moment that MMC's do migrate orad in disease, the debris would still be propelled distally as long as the spatial and temporal organization of Electrical Control Activity does not change. If MMC's do migrate orad, the debris will be left behind the trailing edge of the orad migrating MMC's.

However, the orad migration of MMC's has never been established. At least two groups of investigators suggested orad migration (8, 9), but such observations were made at only two recording sites. At least three recording sites are necessary to establish orad migration. Each small segment of the small intestine is capable of initiating an MMC on its own (6, 7). It is possible that an MMC may start prematurely in a distal segment and be followed shortly by an independent MMC in a slightly proximal segment. The MMC in the proximal segment may not propagate caudad due to the absolutely refractory state of the distal segment, but this is not orad migration. Orad migration must be established over a sufficiently long segment of the small intestine (at least 50-100 cm) by recording at multiple sites. Also, in defining orad migration, the end of phase III activity may be a more appropriate marker than the beginning because the latter is more ambiguous.

Two of the disturbances of MMC phenomenon that may have a significance on the intestinal motor function are 1) no disruption after a meal, and 2) premature recurrence after a meal. In either case, the MMC's in the fed state would have a major impact on transit time of the meal and may lead to a motility disorder. These disturbances have been reported in at least two abnormal states, during the period of fractionated abdominal irradiation (10) and after vagotomy in patients presenting diarrhea (11)

In summary, the MMC's in humans are highly variable in their cycle length, duration and migration velocity. It is not certain that even a significant statistical variation in these parameters would compromise the intestinal motor function of cleaning. The complete absence of MMC's in a disease state affecting intestinal motility has not been established. The orad migration of MMC's has also not been established and its occurrence is unlikely. Finally, although the recording of MMC's from one or two sites in the proximal small intestine may be convenient and sufficient for some purposes, it may not be enough for the complete characterization of MMC's in disease.

References

1. Szurszewski, J.H. A migrating electric complex of the canine small intestine. Am. J. Physiol 217:1757-1763, 1969.
2. Vantrappen. G. et al. The interdigestive motor complex of normal subjects and patients with bacterial overgrowth of the small intestine. J. Cl. Invest. 59:1158-1166, 1977.
3. Kellow, J.E., Borody, T.J., Phillips, S.F., et al. Human interdigestive motility: variations in patterns from esophagus to colon. Gastroenterology 91:386-395, 1986.
4. Kellow, J.E. and Phillips, S.F. Altered small bowel motility in irritable bowel syndrome is correlated with symptoms. Gastroenterology 92:1885-1893, 1987
5. Sarna, S.K. and Otterson, M.F. Small intestinal physiology and pathophysiology. In: Gastroenterology Clinics in North America. Bethesda:Am Physiological Soc., 1989. In press.
6. Sarna, S.K. Cyclic Motor Activity; Migrating Motor Complex: 1985. Gastroenterology, 89:894-913, 1985
7. Sarna, S.K., Condon, R.E. and Cowles, V. The enteric mechanisms of initiation of migrating myoelectric complexes (MMC's) in dogs. Gastroenterology 84:814-822, 1983.
8. Nowak, T.V., Anuras, S. and Brown, B.T. Small intestinal motility in myotonic dystrophy patients. Gastroenterology 86:808-813, 1984.
9. Malagelada, J-R and Stanghellini, V. Manometric evaluation of functional upper gut symptoms. Gastroenterology 88:1223-1231, 1985.
10. Otterson, M.F., Sarna, S.K. and Moulder, J.E. Effects of fractionated doses of ionizing radiation on small intestinal motor activity. Gastroenterology 95:1249-1257, 1988.
11. Thompson, D.G., Ritchie, H.D. and Wingate, D.L. Patterns of small intestinal motility in duodenal ulcer patients before and after vagotomy. Gut 23:517-523, 1982.

CONCLUDING REMARKS

J. Malagelada

Concluding remarks

In surveying the Symposium and what we heard during the last three days I like to tell you about what I learned myself. First of all, I learned about the importance of CRF. There was nearly general agreement that CRF is important since injection of CRF into the ventricular system appears to ellicit virtually the full spectrum of acute stress responses. There was convincing evidence as well that blocking CRF by specific antagonism will abolish most of these responses to stress. However, we also learned something about CRF perhaps not being the beginning of the chain of events elicited by stressing animals. CRF release may be itself regulated by norepinephrine release. These concepts may change in the years ahead, but for the time being they sounded convincing to me.

When we got into the area of animal models of stress things got a little bit more muddled because there wasn't as clear an agreement among the different speakers as to what these models show. What I learned on this subject was that different methods and species may be associated with different responses. However, I also learned that different types of inducing stress, and perhaps also the magnitude of stress, may be associated with different responses and, in particular, with different mediators. I recall, as an example, that cold stress in rats appears to start inicially a prearranged TRH mediated response which, if the cold stress goes on longer or it is more intense, slides into a typical CRF response. It is obvious that we have to be careful not only how we induce stress in animal models, but also to standarize the degree of stress we induce. There was at least one speaker that refered to the effects of chronic stress or, I would say more accurately, of sub-acute stress. This appears to be a very interesting avenue to pursue in the future. Most other speakers dealt with acute stress but we have to increasingly start worrying about both the lingering effects of acute stress and the effects of chronic stress.

In the section about behavioural aspects of stress there was one thought that stuck to my mind and that was that we should establish some paralels betwen the skin (the surface of the organism that interacts with environmental agents of stress) and the digestive system (the surface reacting to ingested agents of stress). The digestive system may react to ingested agents stress differently than to environmental stress. Yet, most of the animal models currently in use are, in fact, somatic or environmental models of stress. In this section there were also quite interesting comments about stressful life events and what stuck to my mind, in particular, is the importance of stressful life events as acute punctuating events that, in turn, originate several body responses. For instance, it was tantalising to learn that the imune system can be affected by such stressful life events and even more intriguing was to me one of the latest presentations in this regard, that suggested that the impact on the GI tract of stressful life events may not necessary always go through a psicological (depressive or anxiety type of reaction) but may somehow affect directly the GI tract. Such direct effect seems at least plausible given our current understanding of semi-autonomous gut control mechanisms.

There were a number of presentations on human studies and, in this regard, let me say first that I am not as enthusiastic about human stress research as I was a number of years ago. Such studies involve almost always acute stress and there is also an inherent element of subjectivity. But it is not to say that we cannot properly perform nature studies as long as we have the proper controls and, yes, a proper Protocol reviewed by Commitee. Anyway, as far as the human studies are concerned, what have we learned?. First, that we can perturb the normal GI function both during fasting and after a meal so we are able to change through acute stress the normal patterns of motility and secretion. Second, that different tests produce different responses and, in that regard, the results of human studies resemble some of the results obtained from animal studies. I think that we have also learned in the human studies that some GI functions are more perturbable than others. For instance, I was struck by the oesophageal experiments which suggest that the oesophagus is particularly resistant to acute stress; more so than the stomach and the small bowel. We do not know whether the mechanisms that mediate the alteration of human GI function in response to acute stress are the same ones that were identified in animal experiments and I think that this will be a major research task for the future; that is, to determine whether there is a paralelism between human and animal models. The bottom line, however, is that we still do not know whether the observations that have been made in man with these acute somatic and viceral stresses bear any relationship to chronic stress, functional disease etc. It will probably take a long time before we can develop, in the human laboratory, comparable modelsto a real-life situation.

In the pharmachology section there were a number of interesting aspects of the field brought up. One of them was on substances that seemed to have differential effects on the stress response whether they were administered intra-ventricularly, intravenously or orally. The oral route, I suppose, could theoretically act on afferent fibers that go to the brain and hence modify the stress responses in different ways that agents given parenterally. The clinical section mostly reminded me of the difficulties that performing these kinds of studies entail, as well as the difficulties in interpreting the results obtained. It may be important to continue to do descriptive studies and perhaps also experimental stress studies in patients but again, without wanting to sound overly pessimistic, I think it's going to be a long time before we learn how to link the information obtained with real clinical situations. As long as we don't understand the pathological mechanisms involved in patients with functional-type disorders of the gut, it will be an arduous task to learn how stress plays a pathogenetic role in their ailments. Thank you very much.

Reproduction photomecanique
IMPRIMERIE LOUIS-JEAN
BP 87 — 05002 GAP
Tél. : 92.51.35.23
Dépôt légal : 612 — Septembre 1989
Imprimé en France